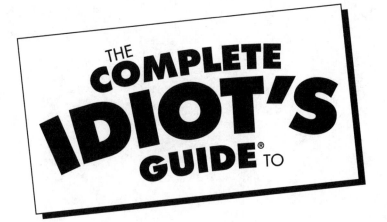

THE
COMPLETE IDIOT'S GUIDE® TO

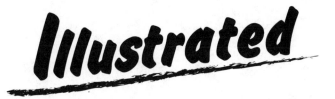
Functional Training

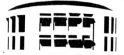
Illustrated

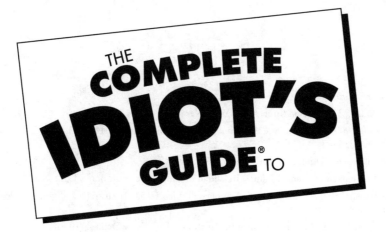

THE COMPLETE IDIOT'S GUIDE® TO

Functional Training

Illustrated

by Justin Price, M.A., and Frances Sharpe

ALPHA

A member of Penguin Group (USA) Inc.

ALPHA BOOKS

Published by the Penguin Group

Penguin Group (USA) Inc., 375 Hudson Street, New York, New York 10014, USA

Penguin Group (Canada), 90 Eglinton Avenue East, Suite 700, Toronto, Ontario M4P 2Y3, Canada (a division of Pearson Penguin Canada Inc.)

Penguin Books Ltd., 80 Strand, London WC2R 0RL, England

Penguin Ireland, 25 St. Stephen's Green, Dublin 2, Ireland (a division of Penguin Books Ltd.)

Penguin Group (Australia), 250 Camberwell Road, Camberwell, Victoria 3124, Australia (a division of Pearson Australia Group Pty. Ltd.)

Penguin Books India Pvt. Ltd., 11 Community Centre, Panchsheel Park, New Delhi—110 017, India

Penguin Group (NZ), 67 Apollo Drive, Rosedale, North Shore, Auckland 1311, New Zealand (a division of Pearson New Zealand Ltd.)

Penguin Books (South Africa) (Pty.) Ltd., 24 Sturdee Avenue, Rosebank, Johannesburg 2196, South Africa

Penguin Books Ltd., Registered Offices: 80 Strand, London WC2R 0RL, England

International Standard Book Number: 978-1-59257-925-9
Library of Congress Catalog Card Number: 2009928406

11   10   09   8   7   6   5   4   3   2   1

Interpretation of the printing code: The rightmost number of the first series of numbers is the year of the book's printing; the rightmost number of the second series of numbers is the number of the book's printing. For example, a printing code of 09-1 shows that the first printing occurred in 2009.

Printed in the United States of America

Note: This publication contains the opinions and ideas of its authors. It is intended to provide helpful and informative material on the subject matter covered. It is sold with the understanding that the authors and publisher are not engaged in rendering professional services in the book. If the reader requires personal assistance or advice, a competent professional should be consulted.

The authors and publisher specifically disclaim any responsibility for any liability, loss, or risk, personal or otherwise, which is incurred as a consequence, directly or indirectly, of the use and application of any of the contents of this book.

Most Alpha books are available at special quantity discounts for bulk purchases for sales promotions, premiums, fund-raising, or educational use. Special books, or book excerpts, can also be created to fit specific needs.

For details, write: Special Markets, Alpha Books, 375 Hudson Street, New York, NY 10014.

Publisher: *Marie Butler-Knight*
Editorial Director: *Mike Sanders*
Senior Managing Editor: *Billy Fields*
Senior Development Editor: *Christy Wagner*
Senior Production Editor: *Megan Douglass*
Copy Editor: *Emily Garner*

Cartoonist: *Steve Barr*
Cover Designer: *Kurt Owens*
Book Designer: *Trina Wurst*
Indexer: *Heather McNeill*
Layout: *Ayanna Lacey*
Proofreader: *Megan Wade*

Contents at a Glance

Appendixes

Contents

Introduction

If you look up the word *functional* in the dictionary, you'll find definitions like "practical" and "useful." That's exactly how I'd describe functional training. It's a new approach to fitness that offers practical, real-life benefits. Here's how it works: functional exercises mimic the way you move in real life so you can move better in your everyday activities, alleviate aches and pains, and perform better when participating in your favorite sports and hobbies.

Unlike most training programs that offer a cookie-cutter approach to exercise, functional training offers a completely customizable program so you can get exactly what you want out of it. Whether you're new to fitness or you've been playing sports your entire life, you can adapt the exercises in this book to help you achieve your fitness goals.

How This Book Is Organized

This book is divided into five parts that introduce you to the basics of functional training and lead you from beginner to advanced exercises.

Part 1, "Functional Training 1-2-3," introduces you to the ABCs of functional training, including what makes it different from every other fitness program and how it can benefit you regardless of your current fitness level. It also gives you a peek at the inner workings of your amazing body, offers an overview of a host of training tools you can use, and provides you with everything you need to know to start a functional training program.

Part 2, "Preparing for Your Workout," takes you through some simple steps to loosen up your muscles before your functional training session. It also shows you the best way to warm up your body so you can get the most out of your workout.

Part 3, "Beginner Functional Exercises," is the starting point for your functional training. For each beginner exercise, you'll find step-by-step instructions along with photos, tips, and precautions. Each chapter presents exercises using a different type of training tool. The exercises in these chapters give you the foundation necessary to perform the more complex exercises to come in later parts.

Part 4, "Intermediate Functional Exercises," introduces you to more challenging exercises that improve your strength, balance, and coordination. Here, you'll find chapters dedicated to each type of training aid as well as exercises that don't require any equipment at all. Detailed instructions and photos make it easy to follow along.

Part 5, "Advanced Functional Exercises," builds on everything you learned in the beginner and intermediate Parts 3 and 4 and takes your functional training to the next level. With chapters dedicated to each individual training tool, Part 5 is where you'll find the most demanding functional exercises. These powerful moves also provide the biggest payoff in your everyday life, in recreational activities, and in sports.

In the back of the book you'll find a couple appendixes to supplement what you've learned in the preceding chapters. Included are a glossary and sample workout plans to carry you further along your functional training path.

Extras

Throughout this book, you'll notice a number of sidebar boxes that include quick and helpful need-to-know information. These boxes include …

Definition _____

Read these boxes for definitions of terms you need to know.

Malfunction _____

Check these boxes for special cautions intended to help keep you injury-free.

Fit Fact _____

In these boxes, you'll find intriguing tidbits of information as well as tips to make the most of functional training.

Acknowledgments

From Justin: I would first like to thank Frances Sharpe for her amazing efforts in helping write this book. Without her wonderful skill of simplifying complex information, this book would not have been possible. Frances also went out of her way on many occasions to make trips to San Diego to ensure the photo shoots were a success.

I would also like to thank all my peers in the fitness industry who have helped me gain a better understanding of function and the wonderful capabilities of the human form.

Many of the exercises for this book were created over the past 3 to 5 years each morning before work when I took my dog Tui to the park to do my own functional workout. Tui's patience while I crawled, climbed, squatted, lunged, skipped, hopped, pulled, pushed, and reached have undoubtedly earned her a few extra treats.

Most of all, I would like to thank my wonderful wife and business partner, Mary Bratcher. She is my functional fitness idol. Mary has never had a structured exercise routine, but she is always active and participates in everything. As a result, during our past 18 years together, she has participated with me in some of the most extreme functional workouts imaginable. From scaling cliffs in New Zealand, to being dragged under a boat in a crocodile-infested river in Africa, to being stuck in the bush in the Dominican Republic, Mary is always ready and willing to try anything. It's her "ready for action" attitude that truly defines functional fitness, and I can only hope I'll continue to keep up with her as we grow old together.

From Frances: I would like to thank my coauthor, Justin, for his invaluable expertise on the exciting new field of functional training. To fitness models Chris and Jamie Renfro, I offer my appreciation for your tireless efforts and patience. A big thanks goes to Justin's wife, Mary, for all her assistance with the photo shoots.

I appreciate all the editorial direction from Mike Sanders, Christy Wagner, and the entire team at Alpha Books. As always, I am grateful to my agent, Bob Diforio.

I am indebted to all my fitness trainers and tennis instructors who help keep me functionally fit, especially Suzie Dimpfl, Diane Ekker, Stephanie Grimes, Sondi Kroeger Foley, Karen Voight, and Scott Wilson. My biggest thanks go to the most functionally fit person I know, my husband, Wil. I dedicates this book to the memory of my favorite outdoor workout buddy, my Chesapeake Bay Retriever, Itsa.

Trademarks

In This Part

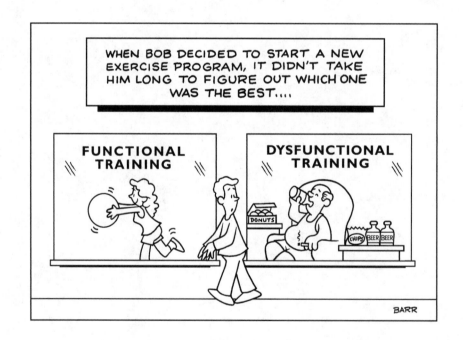

Functional Training 1-2-3

What if I told you that you could pump up your fitness and improve the way your body moves without ever picking up another barbell or doing another crunch? Don't believe me? It's true! Functional training is a new kind of workout that promises huge payoffs in your everyday life. Yes, like other workout programs, it will increase your strength, improve your balance, and stretch your flexibility. What makes functional training unique is that instead of training your body to perform movements you'll probably only ever use in a gym, it focuses on helping you do the things you already do in the real world.

Part 1 covers the many ways functional training is different from other fitness programs and how it can benefit you regardless of your current fitness level. In this part, you also discover how functional training works your entire body, from your fingertips to your toes.

In This Chapter

- ◆ Training so you can move better
- ◆ Exercises that mimic real-life movements
- ◆ Ways functional training differs from other types of exercise
- ◆ Who can benefit from functional training?
- ◆ Achieving ultimate functional fitness

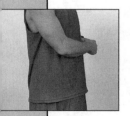 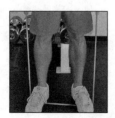 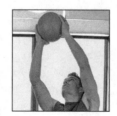 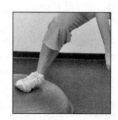 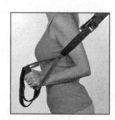 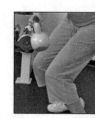

Chapter 1

What Is Functional Training?

Love to play golf? How would you like to swing your clubs with greater ease? Have a 2-year-old at home? Wouldn't you love to chase your toddler around the house without tweaking a muscle? Approaching your golden years? How great would it be if you could bend down to tie your shoes without feeling that twinge in your back? All these things are possible with functional training, a breakthrough type of workout that aims to help you do the things you love to do—only better!

Getting Your Body to Move Better

Helping you move better in your daily life, in recreational activities, and in sports—that's what functional training is all about. Forget about hitting the gym, lifting barbells, or doing endless crunches. You don't need any of these things to achieve functional fitness.

Instead, functional training relies on movements and exercises that mimic what you do in real life. Doesn't that make more sense than practicing a bunch of movements you would never do outside the gym?

Focusing on How the Body Functions

The human body is an amazing machine that's designed for all kinds of movement—walking, running, climbing, twisting, reaching, bending—the list goes on and on. You probably think you use your legs to walk and your arms to reach. You do, but those aren't the only body parts involved. What you may not realize is that to perform any of these movements, you have to get your whole body working together. That's because your body functions as an integrated system rather than a bunch of individual parts.

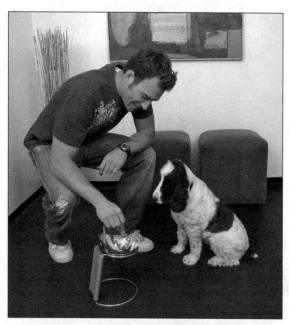

Everyday activities such as feeding your dog involve bending and squatting.

Here's how it works: let's take something as simple as feeding your dog. To give Fido (or Tui, my dog pictured in the photo here) a treat, you have to use your legs and butt to squat down to her level, you have to round your back to bend down, and you have to reach out your arm. Actually, you integrate a lot more of your body than just that—your feet, your hands, and your torso play a part, too. That's a lot of movement to coordinate for one little biscuit, don't you think?

If you still aren't convinced that your body operates as a whole, try this experiment: go open the refrigerator door. Don't bother setting down this book. Just take it with you in one hand and use your other hand to open the fridge. As you pull on the handle, notice how your feet plant a bit more firmly on the ground to provide stability, and notice the muscles in the side of your torso getting in on the act. Now close the door and try to open it using

nothing but your arm. You probably can't do it, can you? When you use only your arm, you probably end up pulling your body closer to the fridge rather than opening the door.

This little experiment should give you a better idea of how your body functions as an integrated unit. It's this concept that forms the basis for functional training, which focuses on training the body as a whole rather than as separate parts.

Eliminating Aches and Pains

If you're like a lot of people, you might feel a few aches and pains as you move throughout your day. It might seem that whenever you move you feel soreness, so you start to avoid activities that require you to move. Eventually, you're spending your entire day doing nothing but sitting at your desk, lounging on the couch, and lying on the bed. You've tried to alleviate your pain by restricting your movement, but in reality, you've made the situation worse due to inactivity.

 Malfunction _____

Life doesn't happen sitting down. If you don't move your body in your daily life, your body will become dysfunctional.

In the previous section, I talked about how the human body is designed for movement and how it functions as a whole. When you become inactive or you try to avoid moving specific body parts, you create dysfunction.

With functional training, you can begin to move again so you can regain the function you've lost. Back aches, neck pain, and knee troubles will all start to diminish so you can start moving freely again.

Making Everyday Chores and Activities Easier

For some people, housework, gardening, and routine household maintenance can be a real pain in the back, the knees, the hips, or the neck. I've trained a lot of people who, before they came to see me, had to head straight to the medicine cabinet for pain relievers every time they vacuumed, cleaned the windows, or did the weeding. It doesn't have to be this way.

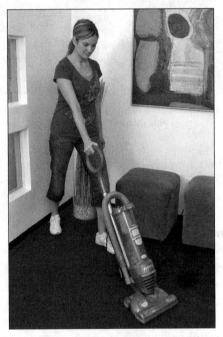

Vacuuming involves pulling, pushing, twisting, and walking.

With functional training, you retrain your body how to bend, twist, and reach the way you do when performing everyday chores. As your functional fitness progresses, activities that used to pose a problem for you won't seem so difficult anymore.

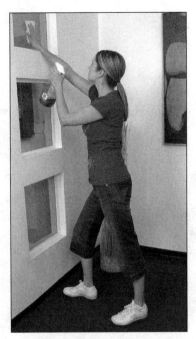

You have to reach up high to clean high windows.

Winning at Sports and Hobbies

Functional training can do a whole lot more for you than simply ease aches and pains. It can give you a competitive edge in sports and recreational activities. When you practice exercises that reflect the way your body moves on the court or on the field, you perform better. And when your body moves fluidly without any limitations or restrictions, you can get to the ball faster, swing a racquet or a golf club more freely, or hike up a steep trail with more ease.

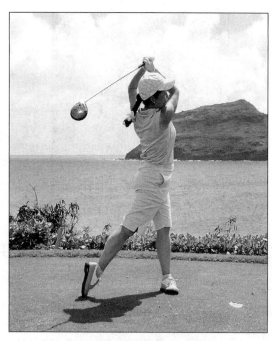

Functional training helps you swing
a golf club more fluidly.

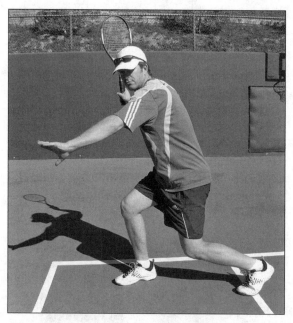

**Tennis is one of the most functional sports because it
gets you moving in all directions.**

Fit Fact

Any sport or activity that gets you moving is good, but some provide more functional exercises than others. The activities listed here involve quick starts and stops and changes in direction and get every part of your body moving every which way. And now—drum roll please—here are my picks for the top five functional sports and activities: tennis, soccer, dancing, rock climbing, and beach volleyball.

Achieving Perpetual Readiness

In addition to helping you perform everyday chores and play sports better, functional training helps you achieve something I like to call "perpetual readiness." That's when you're prepared to face any physical challenge life throws at you or you want to throw at life.

There's no better example of functional fitness and perpetual readiness than James Bond. In a single day, the secret agent might be forced to sprint from treacherous villains, shimmy up an elevator shaft, leap from one rooftop to another, slide behind the wheel of an Aston Martin and drive at breakneck speeds around hairpin turns, balance on a high-wire cable, dive off a cliff, and swim to shore. After shaking off the bad guys, he'd slip into a tuxedo and sweep a beautiful woman off her feet—literally.

In your life, you may not need to jump from a rooftop or crawl up an elevator shaft, but wouldn't you love to be ready for the kind of routine challenges we all face from time to time? What if you just moved and have to unpack boxes all day long? What if you get a flat tire and have to change it yourself? What if you want to play softball at the annual company picnic?

Functional training is intended to help you learn to move your body more freely so you can handle not only your everyday activities but also these unexpected physical challenges. That's perpetual readiness, and this book is going to help you get there!

A New Way to Exercise

Functional training is unlike any other fitness program. Most exercise routines target specific body parts or focus on a certain aspect of fitness, such as strength training. By contrast, functional training focuses on your body as a whole rather than a bunch of individual parts, and it aims to enhance all aspects of your fitness—strength, balance, flexibility, speed, and coordination.

What really makes functional training stand out from the crowd, though, is the way it applies to real-life activities. To hammer home this point, every exercise included in this book includes a handy list of everyday activities and sports it helps you do.

Rethinking Traditional Weight Training

Most weight lifting workouts involve sitting at a piece of equipment while you lift a barbell over and over again. In real life, how often do you sit down and lift something heavy like that? Probably never!

For years, fitness experts have advocated isolating muscles to build strength. Think about a typical biceps curl where you sit on a bench, hold a barbell in your hand, and raise it up to your shoulder. Isolating muscles, however, can create real problems in real-life situations.

 Malfunction _____

Exercise programs that encourage you to isolate specific muscles can actually make your body dysfunctional.

Let me explain why. Let's take the lat pull-down, a common weight training exercise, for example. In this upper back exercise, you sit on a bench at a machine, reach up to grab a horizontal bar with a wide grip, and pull the bar down to your chest. The idea is to work the back muscles you would use if you had to pull yourself up for some reason, say if you were climbing a tree or rock climbing.

But think about it. You wouldn't climb a tree or rock climb without using your legs. You would use your legs to help you scurry up faster, wouldn't you?

Doing isolated lat pull-downs can actually make your body more dysfunctional. Imagine a company with 100 employees who never talk to each other and have no idea what the company's overall goals are or what any of the employees in other departments do. Now, imagine that this is what's happening inside your body. Your lats might be strong individually, but they don't know how to communicate with the other muscles in your body. That means when you try to climb that tree or rock climb, your lats and lower body won't know how to coordinate to make you move faster and more efficiently.

Because of this, your lats may try to do most of the work while you climb, which can lead to overuse injuries. Or you might strain your leg muscles because they aren't used to working in tandem with your upper body. It seems a bit silly to think that your lower and upper body wouldn't know how to work together, but if you always train them separately, you're teaching them to work separately. That's why functional training focuses on whole-body integration rather than individual parts. It works your body the way you use it in real life.

Going Beyond Core Conditioning

Your core is basically the trunk of your body—all the muscles and connective tissues from your hips to your rib cage and around to your spine and back. Your core is involved in every movement you make, whether you're bending down, reaching up, or twisting. This area's primary job is to coordinate motion between your upper and lower body. Because this area is so important to human movement, a lot of fitness professionals are currently emphasizing core conditioning, which involves exercises that isolate this vital area of the body.

Uh-oh. There's that word *isolate* again. Remember what I said about isolating body parts? The same holds true here. How often in life do you do dynamic activities that only involve your trunk but don't require you to use your arms or legs? Almost never!

That doesn't mean that conditioning your core isn't an important part of functional training. It is. With functional training, however, you'll be doing exercises that involve both your upper and lower body as a way to get your core involved rather than isolating it.

Not Like Yoga or Pilates

Some aspects of yoga fit with the basic concept of functional training. For example, many yoga poses involve bending, twisting, or balancing—all good functional activities. That's great, but yoga typically requires you to hold these poses for long periods of time, and that can set you up for an injury.

Holding long, static stretches can actually lead to ligament problems. As you'll learn in Chapter 2 on anatomy, ligaments are connective tissues that connect bone to bone and help protect your joints. Those long yoga stretches tend to relax the ligaments so they begin to lose their ability to hold the joints in place. That can spell trouble for your joints.

Not a Single Crunch in the Bunch

How would you like it if I told you that you never have to do another crunch again? If you're like most of my clients, you'd probably jump for joy. This staple of most traditional

fitness programs isn't doing your body any good. In fact, doing crunches while lying on the ground actually creates dysfunction in your body. That's the opposite of functional fitness.

Your abs, which wrap all the way around your torso, are extraordinary multitaskers. In fact, they have more jobs than any other muscle in your entire body. Their primary task is to act like a sort of cross-your-heart bra within your torso to coordinate the movements of your arms and legs. If you're walking, running, bending down, rotating, leaning to the side, reaching up, or dancing, your abs are working.

 Fit Fact _____

Functional training works your abs in a whole new way—a way that helps you move more easily in real life.

When you do crunches lying on the ground, however, the floor prevents you from using the ab muscles to help your spine arch backward like when you reach upward or to rotate like when you throw a ball. Because of this, crunches only train the abs in one way, which can eventually lead to lower back pain.

Functional training aims to target all your ab muscles in the way they were intended to work in real life. That's why crunches have no place in a functional training workout.

Form Follows Function

Most fitness programs make a lot of unbelievable promises. *Flat abs in just 3 minutes a day! Lose 15 pounds in 2 weeks! Bikini-ready by summer!* Notice something about all these claims? They all focus on the way you *look*.

Functional training takes a different approach and focuses on helping you move with greater ease in real life. That may not sound as enticing as losing belly fat in a few minutes a day, but when you move your body the way it was intended, you will tone your muscles and lose body fat.

Fit Fact

If you're hoping to reshape your figure, functional training can help. It may not be the primary goal, but it's a great added benefit.

Is It for You?

The best thing about functional fitness is that anybody and everybody can benefit from it. I've seen it change the lives of people from all walks of life, all fitness levels, and all ages—from their 20s to their 90s. In this section, I show you just how it can help you.

Beginners and Hard-Core Couch Potatoes

Functional training offers an ideal introduction to fitness for beginners and sedentary folks. I meet a lot of inactive people who are afraid to try certain activities because they lack confidence in their abilities.

Typically, after even just a few short weeks of training with the beginner exercises in this book, you can start to get a better feel for the way your body moves and begin to gain some confidence.

Active Exercisers

If you're already an active exerciser, good for you! You can take your fitness to the next level by incorporating functional training into your current workouts and activities. Let's say you jog 6 days a week, but that's the only exercise you get. It's great that you're active, but doing the same thing over and over places stress on only a select group of muscles. Over time, this can lead to injuries.

With functional training in the mix, you can achieve a more balanced workout in which your entire body is sharing the load. Instead of only using the muscles involved in your favorite activity, you'll work all your muscles, which decreases your risk of injury and helps make your whole body stronger and more functional.

Weekend Warriors

Are you one of those people who works non-stop during the week but then participates in intense, heart-pounding sporting activities on the weekend? If so, I've got some bad news for you. Doing no physical activity all week and then stressing your body at maximum levels is a recipe for injury.

By incorporating some functional training into your week, you can help prevent injuries commonly experienced by weekend warriors.

Elite Athletes

Functional training is an ideal workout for elite athletes. If you're competing at the highest level of your sport, you probably won't benefit much from most traditional workout methods because they don't prepare you for your particular sport.

With functional training, however, you can practice using your whole body the way you use it in your sport.

Manual Laborers

People who perform manual labor tend to repeat the same motions over and over. If you're a bricklayer, for example, you probably bend over all day and use the same arm each time you move the bricks into position. Painters typically use the same arm to move the roller up and down walls. This type of repetitive use can cause serious imbalances in your body, with one side becoming much weaker than the other.

Adding functional exercises helps you strengthen that weaker side to create a body that's more balanced. It also helps unlock your body from familiar positions to get you moving in other directions to prevent aches and pains.

Seniors

If you're at the age where physical activities you used to do with ease—bending down to tie your shoe, playing with your grandchildren, putting on your clothing, or playing golf—are becoming more difficult for you, functional training can help. Functional exercises can help you perform daily activities with greater ease, which can make you feel younger!

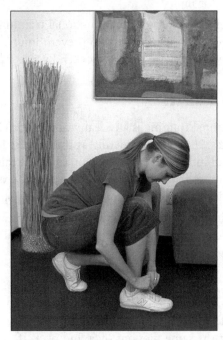

Functional exercises mimic real-life activities, such as bending over to tie your shoes, and make them easier to perform.

People Recovering from Injury

Functional training can help you recover from injury more quickly and more completely. Let's say you sprain your right ankle. Most people would try to protect the injured ankle by limping on their left leg. Unfortunately, this sort of compensation pattern sets you up for possible knee problems down the road and can limit your ability to regain full range of motion with that ankle.

With a functional training approach, you would rest your ankle for a few days until the inflammation goes down and then start moving it gently in all directions. This reintroduces you to using your ankle the way you did before it was injured. In this way, you're more likely to recover fully from the injury without any lasting limitations.

People Dealing with Chronic Pain

One of the most gratifying aspects of my work is helping people who live with chronic pain start to unlock their bodies and begin to move freely again. I've worked with many clients who couldn't stand for more than 2 minutes at a time without feeling searing back pain. After practicing functional training for some time, they leave with the ability to go dancing or play golf—things they never imagined they would ever be able to do again.

The Three Stages of Functional Training

The ultimate goal of this new style of training is to be highly functional in unpredictable situations when you have to move in every which way on a second's notice. Playing with your child, racing in from the rain while carrying groceries, reacting when your dog darts off after a cat, or playing sports are all examples that call for a high level of functional fitness. Unfortunately, I can't wave a magic wand to help you reach that goal. You'll need to progress gradually through stages to get there.

Acing the Lab Environment

In the first stage, you'll be learning to move functionally in something I call "the lab environment." That's a safe haven, such as your home or an exercise studio.

In this controlled environment, you can practice functional training exercises that get your body moving in all directions. With time, these movement patterns will start to become ingrained in your body's memory and you'll begin to feel more confident.

Awakening Body Awareness During Routine Activities

The second stage of functional fitness involves taking what you've learned in your lab environment and applying it to your everyday activities.

Thanks to all that practice, you'll develop better body awareness and, as you go through your day, you'll know how to move your body more efficiently. When you walk upstairs, for example, you'll have the body awareness to use your legs and butt to propel you upward. When you're in the driver's seat and have to reach into the backseat of the car, you'll know how to rotate your torso properly.

Peak Athletic Performance and Kinesthetic Change

When you reach the ultimate stage of your functional training, you'll have undergone something called *kinesthetic* change. That's when your movements become completely natural and fluid.

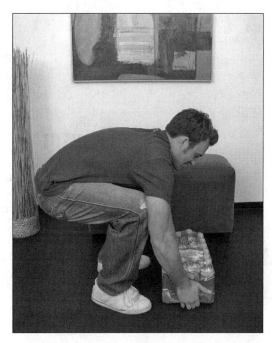

Learning to use the muscles in your legs and butt helps you lift heavy objects.

At this stage, you can reach peak athletic performance and react quickly to unpredictable physical challenges.

When you're able to handle unpredictability with ease, you'll know you've achieved true functional fitness and perpetual readiness. Now, let's help you get there.

The Least You Need to Know

◆ Functional fitness gives you the gift of perpetual readiness.

◆ Life doesn't happen sitting down, and neither does functional training.

◆ Functional training focuses on your body as a whole, not any isolated individual parts.

◆ Functional training tones your muscles and encourages weight loss.

◆ Functional training is for everyone— young, old, active, inactive.

Definition

Kinesthetic changes are those related to the sensation of movement in the muscles or the body as a whole.

In This Chapter

- ◆ Seeing your body as a whole
- ◆ Movement takes more than muscles
- ◆ Getting to know your connective tissues
- ◆ Using teamwork to move your body

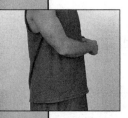
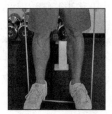
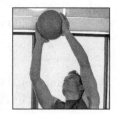
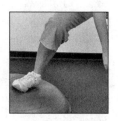
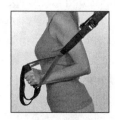
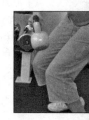

Functional Training and Your Anatomy

Did you know that the human body is made up of more than 600 muscles, 200 bones, hundreds of ligaments and tendons, and about 45 miles of nerves? That's a lot of body parts. Scientists have come up with hard-to-pronounce names for each and every one of these parts. Don't worry—even though I want to introduce you to the inner workings of your amazing body in this chapter, I won't be giving you a pop quiz on anatomy.

In fact, I'll let you in on a little secret: as far as functional training is concerned, there are no separate body parts. All those muscles, bones, ligaments, tendons, and nerves are interconnected. Each and every time you move, all those parts have to coordinate and work together. That's why functional training doesn't focus on specific muscles, but rather on getting all your parts to work in harmony so you can move with the greatest of ease.

Bone Up on Your Bones

When you're going to build a new house, you start by pouring a solid concrete foundation. The human body has a similar sturdy foundation: bones. Human bones are far tougher than concrete, though. In fact, they're one of the strongest materials on the planet.

Your bones make up your skeleton, which provides the framework to support your body and give it shape. That's not all your bones do. They also protect your vital organs and enable you to move. Actually, it's the joints between the bones at your knees, hips, shoulders, elbows, wrists, fingers, and toes that permit movement.

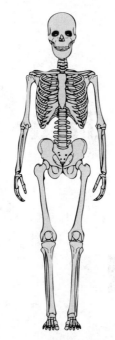

Your bones provide the framework
for your body.

Also designed to help you move is one of
the most mobile parts of your skeleton, your
spine. Made up of 24 bones called vertebrae
plus 2 more called the sacrum and coccyx, your
spine runs from your neck to your lower back.
In between each vertebra is a cushioned disc
that provides movement. Thanks to these guys,
you can bend and twist your back and neck in
an almost limitless number of directions.

Ligaments: The Ties That Bind

Your bones would be lying in a heap on the
floor if it weren't for your ligaments. These
tough, fibrous tissues cross your joints to connect bones to other bones. Basically, your ligaments are designed to protect your joints from
experiencing too much stress or from moving
too far in the wrong direction.

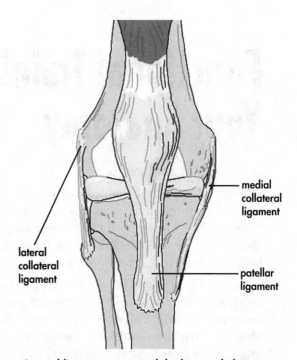

lateral collateral ligament

medial collateral ligament

patellar ligament

Several ligaments surround the knee to help protect
it from injury. The lateral collateral ligament (LCL)
and medial collateral ligament (MCL) attach bone to
bone, and the patellar ligament attaches the patella
to the fibula.

In everyday life, your ligaments usually do an adequate job of keeping your joints where they need to be. Certain high-impact situations, however, such as a hard tackle in football, a car accident, or a tumble down the stairs, can stretch the ligaments past their limits. This is especially common with the ligaments that protect the knees. In these types of situations, you may end up with a sprained knee, or worse, a tear in the ligament.

The goal of functional training is to teach you to use the other tissues around your joints, such as muscles, so you put less stress on your ligaments and joints. By learning to use your body correctly, you can reduce your risk of injuring important tissues.

Fit Fact _____

The knee's anterior cruciate ligament (ACL) is the most commonly injured ligament. By improving the strength of the muscles in your thighs, glutes, and calves with functional training, you can help prevent injuries to the ACL.

Tendons: Connecting with Your Connective Tissue

Tendons are thick, sinewy tissues that attach muscles to bones. You've probably heard of your Achilles tendon, the best-known of all these hard-working tissues, which connects the calf muscle to the heel. According to legend, the mythical hero Achilles died from an injury to this particular tendon.

I'm not sure if a person could actually die from an injury to a tendon, but I do know that tendons play an important role in your ability to move. Tendons work in tandem with muscles to cause your bones move, which is what makes you move.

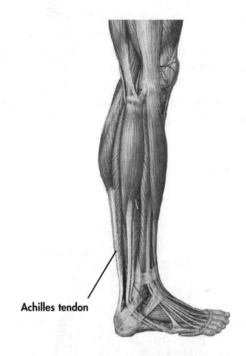

Achilles tendon

A tendon's primary job is to attach muscle to bone. The Achilles tendon attaches the calf muscle to the heel bone.

When your muscles aren't doing their share of the job, your tendons have to pick up the slack. With time, this can lead to something called tendonitis, an inflammation of the tendon. Thanks to functional training, you'll discover how to use your muscles so you can avoid overtaxing your tendons.

Meet Your Muscles

Remember how I told you that you have more than 600 muscles in your body? All those muscles have a single job to perform: they must contract to produce motion.

Some of your muscles work 24/7 without any effort on your part. Take your heart, for example. You don't need to do anything to make it beat. Can you imagine what it would be like if you had to constantly remind your heart to beat? You wouldn't have any time left over to do anything else with your day.

Other muscles take direction from you. It's as if you're the CEO of a company with 600 employees, and you get to boss them around all day long. For example, if you want to take a stroll, you tell your muscles, "Hey guys, let's go for a walk." This causes the muscles in your legs to contract, which activates the tendons that pull your bones and make you move forward.

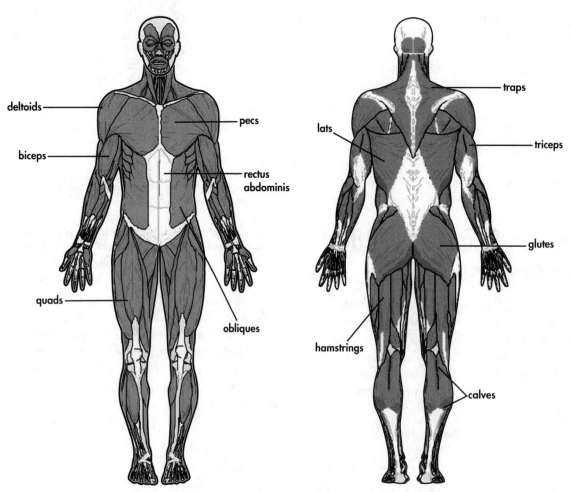

deltoids

pecs

biceps

rectus abdominis

quads

obliques

traps

lats

triceps

glutes

hamstrings

calves

The 600-plus muscles in your body produce movement.

At the same time, a host of other muscles get in on the act. Your abdominals help rotate your torso, and your arms swing into action to keep you balanced. With just one simple step forward, you engage muscles from your fingers all the way down to your toes. Pretty neat, huh?

By now, you understand that contracting your muscles produces motion. But that's not all your muscles do. I don't want to start sounding like a science teacher, but have you ever heard the phrase "for every action, there's a reaction"? This concept applies to your muscles. As one muscle contracts, another muscle has to relax. For example, let's say you want to lift a gallon of milk out of the refrigerator. To lift it, you have to contract your biceps muscle—that's the one on the front of your upper arm. At the same time, your triceps muscle located on the back of your upper arm has to lengthen.

This lengthening action plays a key role in protecting you from injury by slowing down and controlling your movements. Let's go back to that gallon of milk. If your triceps didn't keep the movement under control, you would probably lift the milk jug so fast that you'd smack yourself in the face with it. Ouch!

Fit Fact _____

Whenever one of your muscles contracts, an opposing muscle relaxes. This contract-relax phenomenon is yet another example of how all your body parts are interconnected.

You've Got a Lot of Nerves

Your muscles, tendons, ligaments, and bones all play a part in moving your body, but there would be no movement if it weren't for your brain. This 3-pound supercomputer inside your skull is where all movement begins. Your brain gives orders to your spinal cord, which transmits those orders to your various body parts so you can lift a milk carton, swing a baseball bat, or run up a hill.

This complex system is called the central nervous system, and it regulates numerous body functions, including movement. In order to move properly, your brain and spinal cord need to be in tip-top shape. Your spine is what protects your spinal cord, so it's important to keep your spine in alignment. If your spine is out of whack, it can put pressure on the nerves that tell your arms, fingers, legs, feet, and toes what to do.

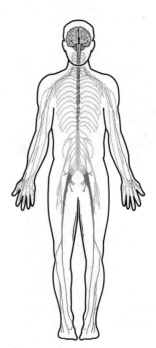

The central nervous system alerts your body when you want to move.

Fascia: Holding It All Together

Holding together all your muscles, ligaments, tendons, and other body parts is something called fascia (pronounced *fash-ee-uh*). Fascia is like a cool, three-dimensional web of tissue that wraps around and through your body parts. Fascia goes from your head to your toes and around every layer of tissue.

Here's a good example of how fascia works: imagine I'm wearing a Spiderman costume. Okay, you can stop laughing now. If you pulled hard on the toes of my outfit, it would stretch the fabric all the way to my head. Similarly, if I bent forward, it would stretch the material on my backside. That's what fascia does. It helps coordinate your movement.

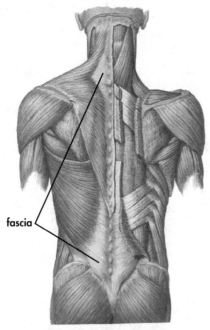

Fascia is like a 3D web that holds together all your body parts.

Working on the Kinetic Chain Gang

Have you ever noticed how major corporations always emphasize teamwork rather than individual accomplishment? Your body is no different. Your muscles, ligaments, tendons, and other tissues work in teams to help you move with greater power, speed, and grace. These teams are referred to as *kinetic* chains.

Definition

Kinetic refers to anything that produces or is related to motion.

Your body has three main kinetic chains:

◆ The anterior chain includes all the muscles and connective tissues on the front side of your body from your foot to your jaw.

◆ Starting under your foot and running up your backside to your scalp is the posterior chain.

◆ Lateral chains go from the side of your neck all the way down to the side of your foot and under the toes.

In addition to the big three, your body also houses a number of other teams called spiral chains or oblique chains. These chains wrap around your body and help your torso twist and untwist as you move.

As you move throughout the day, you often have more than one kinetic chain working at the same time. It's like the CEO is bringing in teams from two or more departments to work together on a project. In this case, the project might be getting down on the ground to play with your kids, running uphill, or playing basketball.

Fit Fact

Functional training doesn't focus on individual muscles the way many other exercise programs do. Instead, it targets kinetic chains to help you move better.

Here's an example: let's say you're walking with your right foot forward and your left arm swinging forward at the same time. The team or chain of muscles and connective tissues that are working include your posterior oblique chain from the back of your right foot up to your right butt, crosses over to the left side of your back, and up into your left shoulder and arm. Think of how thrilled corporate bosses would be to see this kind of teamwork from their employees. Lucky you, you've got teams of employees eager to pitch in.

Always keep this concept of teamwork in mind in your functional training. Forget about trying to isolate a certain muscle or spot on your body. The human body just doesn't work that way. Instead, think of your body as a big corporation with hundreds of employees and dozens of departments just waiting to team up to get you moving.

Getting Grounded

One of the most fascinating things about the human body is how it interacts with the ground. I don't want to sound like a physicist here, but when the human body applies force to an object—say you hit a punching bag—it causes the object to move. It's like being at the gym, where you sit on a machine and press your legs against a weight to make the weight move. In this example, your leg muscles create the force to lift the weight, but the weight doesn't press back. That's what exercise scientists call open chain movement.

Now, let's say you apply force by stepping on an object that doesn't move freely, like the ground. Physics dictates that if you apply force and the ground doesn't move, your body has to. Your body absorbs the shock of your foot hitting the ground, which causes every muscle in your feet, legs, and hips to respond. This is referred to as closed chain movement.

With closed chain movement, your body gets twice the benefit for every movement. In addition to the effort it requires to take that step forward, your muscles have to react to the force of your foot hitting the ground. Functional training focuses on closed chain movement, which means you get the maximum benefits possible from all the exercises in this book.

The Least You Need to Know

- Your body is a series of integrated systems rather than a collection of individual parts.
- Movement starts in the brain, and muscles, ligaments, tendons, fascia, and nerves are all involved when you move.
- Your ligaments help protect your knees, elbows, and other joints from injury.
- Your muscles, ligaments, and tendons use teamwork to help you move more effectively.

In This Part

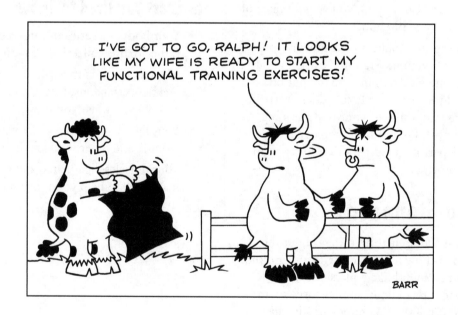

Part 2

Preparing for Your Workout

If you were going to drive across the country, you wouldn't just jump in the car and go, would you? No. You'd first get your car a tune-up to be sure it was in tip-top condition. If you didn't, and your wheels were out of alignment or the oil was low, you could end up stranded by the side of the road.

The same concept holds true for starting your functional training workout. Before you dive in, you need to be sure your body is ready to go. In Part 2, you learn everything you need to know to start your functional training program so you can begin to move better and feel better. Also in this part, you learn the best ways to loosen up your muscles and warm up your body before your workout. With the proper preparation, you'll be able to perform the movements safely so you can reach your final destination: functional fitness.

In This Chapter

- ◆ Testing your body alignment
- ◆ Starting at the beginning
- ◆ Creating a program just for you
- ◆ Mixing it up
- ◆ Making functional training part of your day

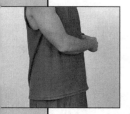 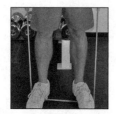 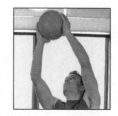 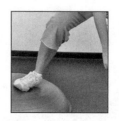 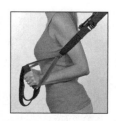 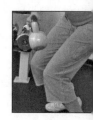

Getting Started

By now, you're probably very excited about all the great things functional training can do for you, and you should be! Even though you're ready to start incorporating functional exercises into your life, you may be wondering where to begin. You've come to the right place. In the following pages, you learn everything you need to know to get started with functional training.

Remember, functional training is supposed to improve *your* movement to help *you* do the things *you* want to do. What you want to do may not be the same as what your neighbor, co-worker, sister, or father wants to do. Because of this, there's no cookie-cutter approach that works for everyone.

With this in mind, I help you learn how to choose the exercises that will provide the most benefit for you. You also discover how to mix up your training program so you never get bored, and you find out how to pump up the intensity of your workouts as your functional fitness progresses. Ready? Let's get started!

Assess Yourself for Functional Success

Whenever I train a new client, I always do some quick tests to check their body alignment and basic movement. This is just as important for people who have never exercised a day in their lives as for athletes who have played professional sports. Over the years, I've found that even high-level athletes can have imbalances in their alignments. They're just really good at compensating for them!

Having good body alignment is the same concept as having a solid foundation when you're building a house. If your foundation is crooked or weak in one spot, the whole house is going to fall down. Body alignment issues probably won't actually make you fall down, but over time, they can cause aches and pains. Also, when you try to perform some of the more complex and demanding functional exercises in this book, those alignment imbalances might actually lead to injuries.

Having basic structural problems doesn't mean you can't begin functional training. It just means you need to be aware of these issues and choose exercises that help you correct them.

> **Fit Fact** _____
>
> Before starting any exercise program, you should have a check-up with your doctor to be sure you're healthy enough for exercise.

Here, I show you how you can give yourself a few quick tests to check your own alignment and movement. Luckily, you don't need to study for these tests!

Check Your Body Alignment

The same way your car needs to be in alignment so it drives in a straight line, your body needs to be aligned properly to move correctly. What exactly is good body alignment? When standing, your lower back should be slightly arched and your upper back should be slightly rounded. Sounds easy, right?

Unfortunately, most people don't come close to this picture-perfect posture. Years of hunching over desks have rounded our upper backs too much so we compensate by adding a more pronounced arch to our lower backs. To make matters worse, when the upper back rounds forward, the head goes with it. Then we have to arch our necks upward so our eyes can remain even with the horizon. Not a pretty picture, is it?

With this posture, it's no wonder so many people complain about neck and back pain.

> **Fit Fact** _____
>
> The most common body alignment problems I see are too much arch in the lower back and too much rounding of the upper back. I blame desk jobs and a sedentary lifestyle for these problems.

To check the alignment of your lower back, shoulders, and head, try the following tests. Ideally, you should do these with a partner, but you can also try them in front of a mirror if nobody else is around.

For your lower back assessment, stand with your heels, back, and head against a wall. Just stand naturally rather than trying to press your back to the wall. Take your left hand and slide it between your lower back and the wall with your palm on the wall. With proper alignment, you won't be able to slide your hand past about the third knuckle where your fingers meet your palm. If you can slide your entire hand behind your lower back, you've got too much arch.

As a rule, an exaggerated arch means your lower back is probably working too hard. If this is the case, you may experience back pain whenever you have to stand for long periods of time. The pain isn't due to any weakness in the lower back. On the contrary, it's because your lower back is doing all the work.

Let's move on to your shoulders now. Stand in front of a full-length mirror and turn so your left side is facing the mirror. Turn your head to the left so you can see yourself and place your left index finger in the spot where your collarbone meets and makes a V. Place your right index finger behind your neck on the vertebra that protrudes the most at the base of your neck. With perfect posture, your fingers will be parallel. In most people, however, the right finger is much higher than the left. This indicates that your upper back has rounded so much that your rib cage has drooped.

Go back to the wall now and stand with your back to it. Tilt your pelvis under without bending your knees. Lift your rib cage without arching your back, and pull your head back to the wall. This helps align both your lower and upper back. Now ask your assessment buddy if your line of sight is parallel to the floor or if you're looking upward. If it's parallel, your alignment is good. Most people, however, have to arch their neck and tilt their head upward. If this is the case for you, you're placing too much stress on your neck throughout the day.

Don't feel bad if these tests show that your posture needs a tune-up. You aren't alone. In my business, most of the people I train have alignment issues. Think of your initial assessment as a baseline test. As your functional training progresses, come back and do the tests again to see how much your posture has improved. And use this information to help you choose functional exercises that help correct any alignment problems. (More on selecting exercises later in this chapter.)

Test Your Body in Motion

Another test I perform assesses how well you transfer weight from side to side—basically whether or not you can walk in a straight line. Stand in front of a full-length mirror and try to position yourself in front of a corner of a wall or door running down your center so you can see it in the mirror. This helps you see how much your body shifts to the side as you move. Place a chair in front of you, and lift your right foot on it. Notice how far your head and body move to the left.

Now try the same thing with your left foot on the chair and see how much you shift to the right. It's normal to see slight movement

to each side, but if you go much farther to one side than the other, you've got some imbalances. This can eventually lead to hip and back pain.

 Fit Fact _____

> One way to tell if you don't walk in a straight line is if you constantly run into your spouse or significant other while walking together.

If your test reveals imbalances, it doesn't mean you aren't ready for functional exercise. Just pick exercises that can help you overcome imbalances so you can get back on the straight and narrow.

Where Do You Begin?

Over the years, I've worked with a lot of elite athletes who think they can just jump right into an advanced functional workout. Wrong! I recommend that everybody, regardless of your fitness level, start at the beginning.

Why would I make a professional athlete bother with beginner exercises? As you learned in the previous sections on body alignment, even high-level athletes can have problems with their body mechanics. It's important to go back to the basics and fix those faulty movement patterns before tackling more advanced exercises. Remember, the goal of functional training is to help you move better. The only way to achieve that is to be sure you're starting with a good foundation.

Beginners: Start at Square One

The beginner exercises in Part 3 help you get a feel for the way your body moves. If you're like most people, you'll quickly discover that you have differences from one side of your body to the other. One side may be stronger, more flexible, or more balanced. Use this feedback, and focus your workout on your weaknesses so you can begin to balance out your body.

If you're truly a beginner, keep practicing the beginner moves until you feel comfortable and confident with them. If you're a regular exerciser or athlete, use the beginner moves to reveal any fundamental problems with your movement and start correcting them. In many cases, you won't need to spend much time with these basic moves and you'll progress quickly to the higher levels.

Intermediate: On Your Way to Better Movement

With the intermediate exercises in Part 4, you increase the challenge. These more dynamic exercises involve a bigger range of motion, use more parts of the body at the same time, and introduce speed to your workout. Can you see why it's important to have your basic movement patterns ingrained before trying these moves?

When you're feeling good about the beginner moves, start adding a few intermediate exercises to your routine. Then gradually shift to more intermediate moves. If any beginner exercises still give you trouble, keep them in your repertoire.

🚫 **Malfunction** _____

Don't ever rush ahead to the next level of exercises. If you aren't prepared for the more demanding moves, you put yourself at risk for injury.

Advanced: For Expert Movers Only

The advanced exercises involve flowing very rapidly through some pretty complex movements—jump up, bend down, twist, shuffle, pivot. Because you're moving quickly,

you don't have time to think about each individual movement. They all have to come to you naturally. That's why you need to have all the basic movement patterns etched in your memory.

When you feel ready to tackle these moves, progress slowly. Add no more than one or two advanced exercises at a time as you transition from the intermediate level. With time, you can focus most of your workout on the advanced moves. This doesn't mean you should completely eliminate the beginner and intermediate exercises from your routine. Even when you're starting to feel like a functional dynamo, it's okay to keep some simpler moves in the mix. In fact, I recommend it.

Graduating to the Next Level

Reaching the advanced-level exercises is a tremendous accomplishment, but it isn't the ultimate goal of functional training. You'll know you've achieved the highest level of functional fitness when you're enjoying life, moving without any limitations, and engaging in physical activities you never dreamed possible.

Take my client Joan, for example. She came to see me at age 55 because she couldn't feel her hands or feet and was suffering from pain in her neck, back, knees, and feet. The pain was so severe that she had eliminated virtually all physical activity from her daily life. After 9 months of functional training, she felt great. The feeling had returned to her extremities, and the pain had disappeared. Now, when she hikes, she can do 18 to 20 miles in a day and can also play golf. Her whole life turned around thanks to functional training. Yours can, too.

Go for the Goal

To get the most out of functional training, think about your overall fitness goals. Whether you're simply hoping to be able to lift up your grandkids without wrenching your back, or you'd like to be more competitive in your basketball league, write down the things you'd like to do better.

When writing down your goals, be sure they're SMART goals. *SMART* stands for Specific, Measurable, Achievable, Realistic, and Time-oriented. By setting specific and realistic goals you can measure the success of over time, you're more likely to be successful with functional training.

Fit Fact _____

I've found that people who write down their fitness goals are more likely to achieve them.

Include both short-term and long-term goals. Short-term goals allow you to experience a series of successes along the way, which helps keep you motivated to stay with the program. Long-term goals give you something to continually strive for.

Remember that your goals aren't set in stone. Review them from time to time and alter them as your fitness level improves. Take Joan, for example. Her initial goals were simply to alleviate her pain and recover feeling in her hands and feet. Now, her goals include lowering her golf score and hiking more challenging trails.

Choosing the Best Exercises for You

Forget about taking a one-size-fits-all approach to functional training. With this new type of fitness program, you get to create a workout that's tailor-made just for you. To choose the best exercises for you, consider any issues with your body alignment or basic movement, your current activities, and your goals.

Let's go back to those assessment tests you did earlier. If you discovered that you have too much arch in your lower back, you need to strengthen your upper back. Doing so will take some of the pressure off your aching lower back. When choosing exercises, be sure to include moves that target your upper back muscles. Choose some exercises that involve extending your arms overhead and some that make you bend forward from your lower back. When you do exercises that involve raising your arms overhead while standing, tilt your pelvis under to prevent arching your lower back too much. In exercises where you bend forward, focus on rounding your lower back rather than just your upper back.

Malfunction _____

Don't avoid doing exercises that point out your weaknesses. To improve your functional fitness, those are the exercises you need to focus on.

Remember the body in motion test from earlier? If you shifted really far to the left when lifting your right leg, you need to strengthen your left butt and outer thigh as well as the muscles that bring your right leg forward in a straight line from your hip. (These muscles are called hip flexors.) Exercises that include lunges and single-leg squats in all three planes of motion (more on these in the next section) are ideal for strengthening these areas. In this particular case, when performing lunges or single-leg squats, pay particular attention to how your body shifts toward your left side when your weight is on your left leg. Try to use your glutes and foot muscles to help stop your body from shifting too far to the left. This helps you achieve a more balanced body.

The Holy Trinity: Sagittal, Frontal, and Transverse

The human body moves in three planes of motion: forward and back, side to side, and rotating. In scientific terms, these movements are called sagittal, frontal, and transverse. All the exercises in this book get you moving in one or more planes of motion.

To be functionally fit, you need to be able to move well in all three planes of motion. That's why you need to include a good mix of sagittal, frontal, and transverse exercises for your functional training routine.

Most of us spend the majority of our days in the sagittal plane—going forward and back. If you like to jog or ride a bike, you're basically moving in only one direction. If this sounds like you, you're missing out on a lot of great side-to-side and rotational movements. For those of you who spend a lot of time in the sagittal plane, be sure that at least two-thirds of the functional exercises you choose involve frontal (side-to-side) and transverse (rotating) movements.

Fit Fact _____

In most traditional weight lifting routines and gym classes, the most overlooked plane of motion is the transverse, or rotational, plane. Be sure you include some twisting exercises every time you work out.

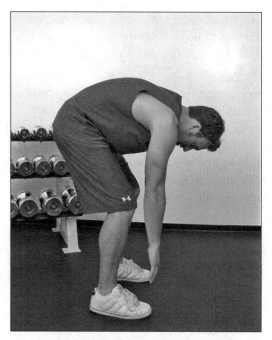

Bending forward in the sagittal plane.

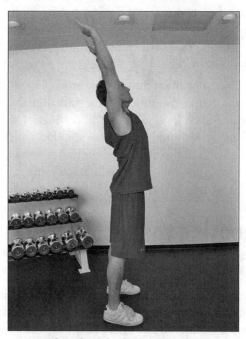

Arching back in the sagittal plane.

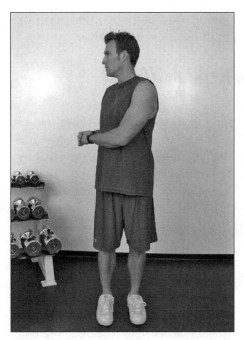

Rotating to the right in the transverse plane.

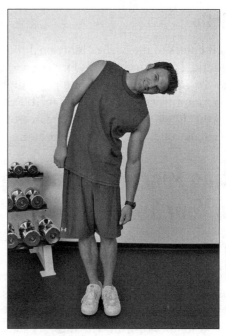

Bending to the left side in the frontal plane.

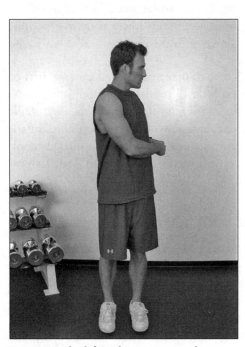

Rotating to the left in the transverse plane.

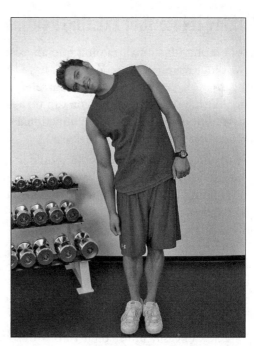

Bending to the right side in the frontal plane.

Mix It Up

When it comes to the perfect functional training routine, I have three words for you: *variety, variety, variety!* Ideally, you should never do the same workout twice. With more than 100 exercises in this book, you can mix and match to create an almost endless array of routines.

Fitting Functional Training into Your Busy Day

Are you excited about the idea of moving better but wondering just how you'll find the time to fit functional training into your busy life? I've got good news for you: functional training is something you can do anytime, anywhere. And because it mimics real-life activities, it's something you can do as you go about your normal day.

Working It into Your Existing Routine

Incorporating functional training into an existing workout routine is easy. You don't have to throw away all the exercises you're currently doing. With just a few tweaks, you can turn those traditional moves into fully functional exercises that help you in the real world.

For example, if you typically do shoulder presses use a medicine ball or kettlebells and do them standing up. As you press up, step to the right and squat. Then step in the other direction on the next press up. You've now taken an exercise that isolated only one area of the body in one plane of motion and expanded it to incorporate your entire body in two planes of motion. Same amount of time, but triple or even quadruple the benefit!

Joggers can easily infuse their runs with some functional training. Instead of running straight ahead in one plane of motion, add bursts of side steps, shuffles, or crossover steps.

How Much? How Often?

Functional training doesn't mean spending an hour at the gym and then forgetting about it until your next workout. It's your entire life! You should be thinking about incorporating functional training into every aspect of your day. I'm not saying you have to exercise 24/7, but you do have to get off that couch and move.

Here are some simple ways to rev up your functional fitness:

◆ Always vacuum using your right hand? Use your left instead.
◆ Use your legs and butt to propel you upstairs rather than leaning forward and gripping the railing.
◆ Every time you sit down in a chair, avoid using the armrests and instead use the muscles in your lower body to ease you slowly into the chair.

It's best to make functional training part of your everyday life. Ideally, in addition to using functional training throughout the day, you'll also be able to devote 30 to 45 minutes or so a few times a week to the exercises in this book. With a dedicated approach, you'll see faster results.

How Many Sets?

In fitness speak, sets are the number of times you perform a series of repetitions of a particular exercise. The number of sets you should perform depends on your fitness level. As a beginner, you should limit yourself to one set of each exercise with a 1- to 3-minute rest period between each exercise. This helps introduce you to a lot of new movements without overloading your muscles or risking injury by doing too much too fast.

When you shift into the intermediate exercises, try doing 2 sets of each exercise with a brief, 1- or 2-minute rest between each exercise and each set. At the advanced level, aim for 2 or 3 sets per exercise and eliminate the rest periods between sets so you're going straight from one exercise to the next.

Functional Cardio

I have designed the exercises in this book so that if you perform them quickly without much rest in between, you can really get your heart pumping for a great cardiovascular workout. In fact, with some of the more advanced moves, your *heart rate* should zoom toward maximum, leaving you breathless. This is a good thing.

Definition _____

Your **heart rate** is the number of times your heart beats per minute. It can be used as a measure of your workout intensity.

Many people, however, are afraid to let their heart rate go very high because they've read articles or been told by a trainer that they need to stay in their "training zone." A training zone is often described as 50 to 85 percent of your maximum heart rate. For example, if you're a 50-year-old man whose maximum heart rate is 180, this would mean training with your heart rate between 90 and 153 beats per minute. (The American Heart Association defines your maximum heart rate at about 220 minus your age.) Unfortunately, this notion of training zones doesn't make sense for functional training. For true functional fitness, it's better to have your heart rate spike near your maximum for short bursts and then rest.

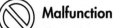

Malfunction _____

If you have a heart condition or any health issues, you should check with your physician before engaging in any cardio activities.

If you really want to improve your cardio conditioning, flow rapidly from one functional exercise to the next and choose exercises that get you moving from low to high. To really pump up the intensity, skip or do high knees for 1 minute in between each exercise. If at any time your heart is beating so fast that you feel like you need to stop, listen to your body and stop for a rest. It's that simple.

The Least You Need to Know

◆ Most body alignment problems can be improved with functional training.

◆ Everybody should start with the beginner exercises. *Everybody.*

◆ There's no cookie-cutter approach to functional training. Make it as personal as you want.

◆ Vary the pieces of equipment you use and the exercises you do to keep your workout fresh.

◆ Functional training can be incorporated into your daily life very easily.

In This Chapter

- ◆ Your body = your best piece of equipment
- ◆ Toys to help your body move better
- ◆ Deciding where to work out
- ◆ Tips for working out with a trainer
- ◆ The best shoes for functional training

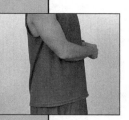
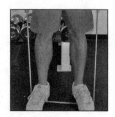
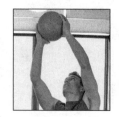
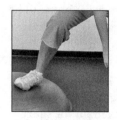
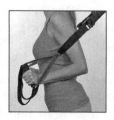
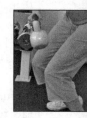

Chapter **4**

Tools of the Trade

One of the best things about functional training is that your own body is your number-one tool. That means you don't have to invest in a gym membership or buy a lot of fancy equipment to benefit from functional training. In fact, you can do functional training anytime, anywhere, using no equipment at all.

A host of aids are available to take your functional training to the next level, though, and in this chapter, you discover the many tools that can jump-start your progress.

Toys! Toys! Toys!

Although functional training doesn't require any equipment other than your own body, it can be more challenging and more fun if you use a variety of tools. In this book, I cover five different pieces of equipment—in addition to your body—you can use to improve your functional fitness. (I discuss these in more detail later in the chapter, but if you're curious, the five tools are resistance bands, medicine balls, the TRX, the BOSU, and kettlebells.)

What makes these tools so special? In essence, they force you to use your body the same way you do in real-life situations, which is the fundamental philosophy behind functional training. For example, this equipment can do the following:

◆ Work every part of your body from your neck to your feet.
◆ Require you to use your balance, strength, flexibility, mobility, agility, and concentration.
◆ Force you to coordinate all the working parts of your body at the same time.

The Best Piece of Equipment: Your Body

Your body is by far your best piece of equipment for functional training. Because the main goal of functional training is to improve the way your body moves, it makes sense that your body is the key component of every exercise.

Here's how your body creates its own resistance: each part of your body has weight, including your arms, your legs, your torso, and your head. When you move any of those body parts, your muscles have to kick in to work against that weight to generate the movement.

Let's say you're standing with your arms at your sides, and I ask you to lift your arms straight out to the front to shoulder height. The muscles in your shoulders and back must work to raise the weight of your arms. That's a pretty easy movement for most people, but now try a push-up. While lying face down on the floor with the palms of your hands on the ground at about shoulder height, push yourself up while keeping your body straight. Not so easy anymore, is it? That's body weight resistance.

Irresistible Resistance Bands

If you think fitness equipment means heavy barbells and complicated machinery, think again. Resistance bands are about as light and simple as it gets. These long, stretchy hollow tubes look like elongated rubber bands, and they weigh only a few ounces at most. In fact, they're so small and light, you can fold them, stick them in your purse or briefcase, and take them with you anywhere. How can something so simple and portable possibly be an exercise tool?

The way they work is easy. You simply anchor one part of the tube to something solid—a door frame, a tree limb, or even a part of your body—to create resistance. Then you push, pull, kick, twist, or reach against that resistance to work your body. Resistance bands are ideal for functional training because they make you

incorporate more muscles and coordination than traditional weight training. Plus, they reduce the amount of stress on your joints compared to traditional weight training, and they encourage you to use your full range of motion.

There's a lot to love about resistance bands. They cost less than $10 each. They come in a variety of styles designed to target various parts of the body. They're available in a number of lengths and thicknesses that vary the resistance.

Malfunction _____

If resistance bands aren't securely anchored, they can snap back and hit you. Ouch!

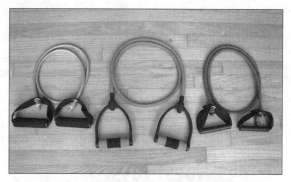

Resistance bands come in many sizes. Thinner bands provide less resistance than thicker bands.

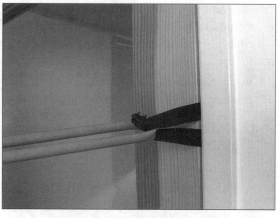

A resistance band door anchor is one of many ways to secure resistance bands safely.

Master the Medicine Ball

The medicine ball is a weighted ball made of rubber or leather, comes in a variety of sizes and weights, and may or may not bounce. People from all walks of life and all fitness levels can use this tool to improve their conditioning.

Fit Fact

The medicine ball, which dates back more than 3,000 years to Persia, is considered the oldest piece of fitness equipment still in use today.

To catch a medicine ball, your muscles have to stabilize your pelvis, hips, spine, and rib cage. That's good for any kind of strength training program, but what makes the medicine ball a good functional training tool is its round shape. Unlike barbells that are designed to make it easier for you to lift them, the medicine ball more closely mimics everyday objects that don't have a handle you pick up all the time—think of how you'd pick up a tire to change a flat or pick up a large box.

Fit Fact

Which piece of equipment do my clients like best? Hands down, it's the medicine ball. Everybody thinks it's fun to play with a ball, and many of my clients say it makes them feel like a kid again.

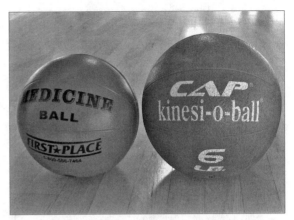

Medicine balls are available in a variety of sizes and weights.

Rx for the TRX

The TRX is a suspension training device that uses your body weight to create resistance. This relatively simple tool consists of straps with handles that you anchor to a secure object, such as a door, a tree, or a fence post. You either place your hands in the handles or put your feet in the straps to perform any number of exercises for a whole-body workout.

The minute your feet or hands are in the TRX straps, your entire body has to start working to stabilize. This gets you moving in three planes of motion, which is one of the basics of functional training.

The real beauty of the TRX? It allows you to adjust the level of difficulty of any exercise to fit your abilities. Depending on the height of the anchor point and how you position your hands and feet, it can make a move easier or more challenging. That means people of any fitness level can benefit from the TRX, and as your fitness improves, you can incrementally pump up the intensity. And if you're feeling sluggish one day, you can tone down the challenge and make it easier.

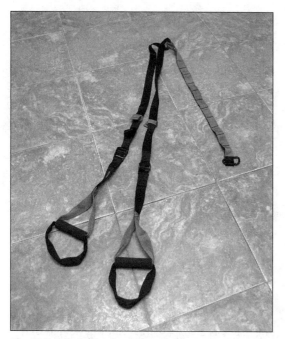

The TRX is lightweight and portable so you can take it with you wherever you go.

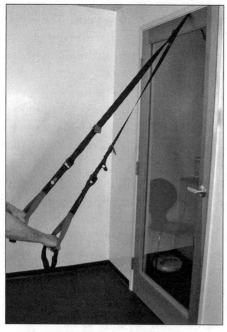

The TRX can be anchored to a door, a tree, or other objects.

Bravo for the BOSU

A BOSU is a piece of fitness equipment that looks like a *stability ball* that has been cut in half and attached to a firm platform. In fact, that's basically how the BOSU, which stands for "both sides utilized," was created. Priced at about $100, this squishy device creates a dynamic surface that helps your body integrate all its parts to improve your balance. That's something that comes in handy in your everyday life, whether you're playing sports, engaging in recreational activities, or doing daily chores.

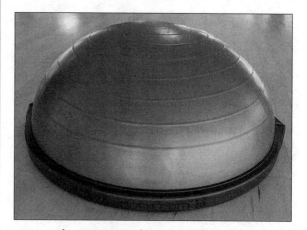

The BOSU provides a dynamic surface that improves balance.

 Definition

The **stability ball**—also called a Swiss ball or exercise ball—is a large, inflatable plastic ball commonly used for strength training and conditioning. It isn't considered a tool for functional training, however, because it doesn't mirror real-life situations. Think about it: in real life, how often do you find yourself sitting or leaning against a ball?

Go Crazy with the Kettlebell

The kettlebell, a weight that looks like a cannonball with a flat bottom and a handle, is one of the key pieces in the functional training toolbox.

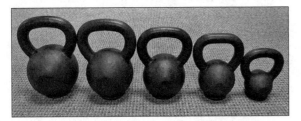

Kettlebells are sold individually or as a set.

The kettlebell teaches you something traditional weight training doesn't. Typical weight workouts emphasize lifting the weights, whereas the kettlebell focuses on both lifting and lowering the weights. Thanks to the kettlebell's unique shape and handle, it can also be used to mimic lifting motions you use on a daily basis.

Getting Loose with the Foam Roller

A long, cylindrical foam tube, the foam roller isn't used for any of your functional training exercises, but it's a great tool to help you get ready for your workout. You just get down on the floor and position the foam roller under an area of your body, such as your thighs or back, and roll your body back and forth on it to create a massaging effect. The pressure from the roller provides something called *myofascial* release. This means it loosens up tight muscles as well as the connective tissues that bind all the muscles together, so they'll be able to handle the tasks involved in your workout.

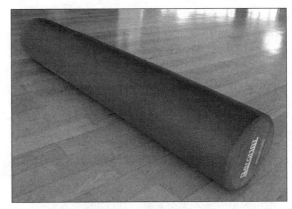

The foam roller helps prepare your muscles for a functional training workout.

Definition

The **myofascial** tissues targeted by the foam roller include the muscles (*myo*) and the connective tissues (*fascia*) that connect your muscles to each other.

Hit the Gym or Train at Home?

One of the things my clients like best about functional training is that they can do it anywhere—in a gym, at home, in a park, or even in a hotel room. Although you don't have to join a gym to do a functional training workout, there are a lot of good reasons why you may want to include a health club in your routine.

For example, if you're new to exercising, you may want to start at a fitness center where you can solicit advice when you need it. Plus, gyms should have most of the equipment covered in this book, so you can test it all out to see which tools you like best and might want to purchase for home use.

Even if you enjoy going to the health club, don't let yourself get into the mind-set that you can only do your functional training at the gym.

⊘ **Malfunction** _____

Avoid what I call the "gym mentality." That's when you think you can only perform an exercise at the gym with a particular piece of equipment, and if that equipment isn't available, you don't do the exercise. With functional training, you learn ways to exercise your body without any equipment.

I teach my clients to think about functional training in any setting, and they do. My clients are always telling me about the crazy places they've done their workouts—on a boat, in the back of a plane, or even in a hotel bathroom.

Work with a Trainer or DIY?

A personal trainer can be a great asset if you're just starting a functional training program. A professional trainer can assess your fitness level and can help you learn how to use the proper form while exercising so you can attain your goals and prevent injuries. After three or four sessions with a personal trainer, you should have enough knowledge to go it alone. You may want to schedule a monthly or bi-monthly follow-up with the trainer for a tune-up and to add new exercises as your fitness level progresses.

Although starting a program with a personal trainer is a good idea, learning to do it yourself is key to long-term success.

If you'd like to jump-start your functional training program with a personal trainer, look for one who is certified by the National Strength and Conditioning Association (NSCA; www.nsca-lift.org), American College of Sports Medicine (ACSM; www.acsm.org), American Council on Exercise (ACE; www.acefitness. org), or National Academy of Sports Medicine (NASM; www.nasm.org).

⊘ **Malfunction** _____

When it comes to functional training, one size definitely doesn't fit all, so avoid personal trainers who offer cookie-cutter fitness programs. Be sure any trainer you're considering creates a program that's custom tailored for you based on your individual fitness level and goals.

Be sure you ask any potential trainers if they specialize in functional training.

Fashion Police: What Not to Wear

The shoes you wear while performing functional training exercises can either help or hinder your movement. Unfortunately, most people work out wearing running shoes, which aren't ideal for functional training. In fact, they're terrible.

Running shoes are designed with more padding in the heel to tilt and propel your body in a forward motion, which is great for running. With functional training, though, you're moving your body in all different directions, so you don't want a shoe that's tilting your body in a single direction. In fact, it can throw off your body alignment, prevent you from moving your body properly, and potentially lead to injury. Ideally, you should wear cross trainers or tennis shoes for functional training. These shoes allow more freedom of movement for going side-to-side, backward, and forward, as well as for twisting and turning.

If you're used to wearing running shoes, don't switch to cross trainers or tennis shoes overnight. The padded heel in running shoes can lead to a shortened Achilles tendon. Abruptly changing to shoes with a lower heel could aggravate your Achilles tendon. To prevent this, make changes in your footwear gradually.

The Least You Need to Know

◆ Your number-one functional training tool is your own body.

◆ A few pieces of training equipment—namely, resistance bands, medicine balls, the TRX, the BOSU, and kettlebells—can help take you to the next fitness level.

◆ You can do functional training anywhere—at home, at the gym, in a hotel, or outdoors.

◆ If you're new to exercise, consider hiring a personal trainer to help you get started.

◆ Don't wear running shoes for functional training. Opt for cross trainers or tennis shoes to avoid injury.

In This Chapter

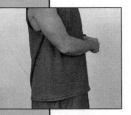
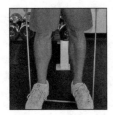
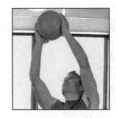
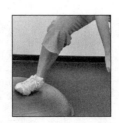
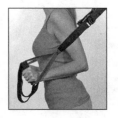
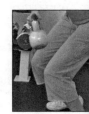

Chapter 5

The Dynamic Duo: Foam Roller and Warm-Up

If you're in a hurry to achieve functional fitness, you may be tempted to skip over this warm-up chapter and dive right into the exercises. Don't! Preparing for your workout is essential for functional training. I think it's so important I make everybody I train—from total beginners to elite athletes—start with the moves in this chapter.

Preparing for your workout only takes about 15 minutes and helps you get the most out of your functional training. If you don't take the time to wake up your body, you'll struggle more during your workout and, even worse, risk injury. With a good warm-up, you help keep your body safe and improve your performance.

Fun with the Foam Roller

In Chapter 4, you got a quick introduction to the foam roller, my favorite preworkout tool. In this chapter, I show you how to use this long, colorful foam cylinder to condition your muscles so they're ready for action.

To use the foam roller, just get down on the ground and position the part of your body you want to target on top of the foam roller. Then shift your body back and forth on the foam roller to create a massaging effect. This helps hydrate your muscles and connective tissues to make them more pliable and mobile so you'll be better able to perform the exercises in the upcoming chapters.

The following exercises show you how to use the foam roller before your functional training workout.

Fit Fact

When using the foam roller, if you shift onto a spot that's extremely sore, stay static, or motionless, on it for a few moments and then roll back and forth to help release the tension.

Good for the Glutes

You'll feel the effects of this rolling massage throughout your butt and hip.

What It Targets

Butt muscles

Hip rotators

Movement

1. Sit on the foam roller with your hands resting on the ground behind you and your legs out in front of you with your knees bent.

2. Place your right ankle on your left knee so your right knee faces out to the side.

3. Shift your weight into your right hand and right butt cheek, and bring your left arm around your right knee and pull it toward your torso as if you were hugging your knee to you. Don't let your back slouch or round as you pull in your knee.

4. Move around on the foam roller until you find any sore sports and then roll back and forth for 1 or 2 minutes or until you feel the discomfort subside. Be aware that the soreness should diminish but may not go away completely. Be sure you don't hold your breath when you hit those sore spots. Breathing helps minimize the pain.

5. Relax and repeat on the other side.

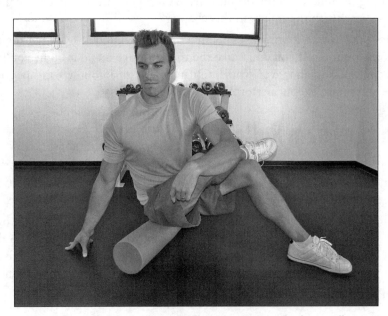

Work one side of your hips and butt at a time on the foam roller.

Say Hi to Your Thighs

With this exercise, you'll be massaging your iliotibial (IT) band, a thick connective tissue that runs all the way down your outer thighs from your hip to just below your knee. When your IT band is in good condition, it helps you avoid hip, back, and knee pain.

What It Targets

IT band

Movement

1. Lie on your side on the foam roller, with the upper area of your right thigh on the foam roller.
2. Place your right forearm and your left hand on the ground to help you balance.
3. Stack your hips on top of each other so your left leg is on top of your right leg.
4. Roll down your thigh to just below your knee. If you find any sore spots, keep the pressure on that area until you feel the pain subside. Usually, 1 or 2 minutes of rolling is enough to ease the discomfort.
5. Roll over to the other side and repeat on your left thigh.

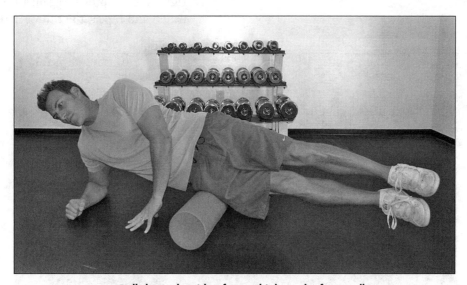

Roll down the side of your thigh on the foam roller.

Prep Your Quads

This rolling action specifically targets the quad muscle on the outside edge of the front of your thighs. By conditioning this area, you help protect your knees and lower back.

What It Targets

Quadriceps, with an emphasis on the rectus femorus

Movement

1. Lie face down on the foam roller, with the front of your left thigh on the foam roller. Shift your weight slightly to the left so the top outer edge of your left thigh is in contact with the foam roller.

2. Let your right knee bend in front of your left leg.

3. Place your left forearm and your right hand on the ground to help you balance.

4. Roll down to your knee, staying along the outer edge of your thigh. Go back and forth over any sore places until you feel some relief. Then shift your weight to the front of your thigh and continue rolling.

5. Shift your body to the other side so your right thigh is pressed against the foam roller, and repeat the rolling action.

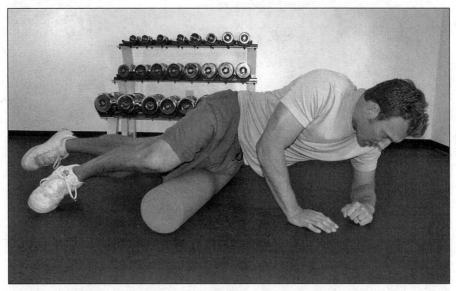

Target your quadriceps by rolling down the front of your thigh.

Get Your Back Into It

When you sit at a computer all day, your shoulders and spine tend to hunch forward. The rolling massage featured here helps you unlock your body from that rounded position.

What It Targets

> Spine
>
> Rhomboids
>
> Trapezius
>
> Erector spinae
>
> External rotator cuff muscles

Movement

1. Lie with your upper back on the foam roller.
2. Support your head with your hands, and open your elbows out to the side.
3. Bend your knees, and keep your feet flat on the floor.
4. Roll down to the bottom of your rib cage and then up to the top of your shoulder blades. The goal here is to gently arch the top of your back without arching your lower back or letting your head fall backward.
5. Gently roll over any sensitive areas for 1 or 2 minutes.

🚫 **Malfunction**

Holding static stretches for a long time can relax your ligaments, which reduces their ability to contract back into place. It's like taking a rubber band and stretching it out until all the elasticity is gone and it no longer snaps back. When your ligaments become loose, they can no longer do their job, which is to protect your joints from injury when you're moving. That's why there's no place for static stretching when warming up for functional training.

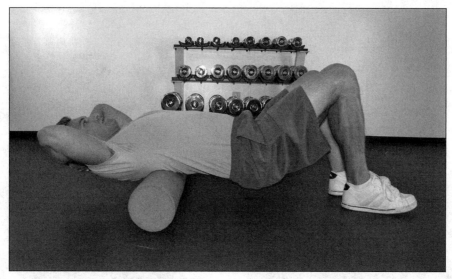

Be very gentle when rolling your back on the foam roller.

Do a Dynamic Warm-Up

I always recommend warming up before a functional training workout.

A good warm-up should last about 5 to 10 minutes. When you add that to your foam roller routine, your total preparation time should be about 15 minutes. I think this preparation is so important that even if you only have a short time to work out, you should still devote 15 minutes to your warm-up rather than jumping straight to the exercises. If you skimp on the warm-up, you'll have a tougher time doing your workout.

Leg Swings Back and Forth

This move wakes up your entire body and primes you for your body's most basic movement patterns—going forward and backward and swinging your opposite arm and opposite leg in the same direction.

What It Targets

Hamstrings

Hip flexors

Trunk

Shoulder girdle

Feet

Movement

1. Stand on your left leg, and keeping your right leg straight, swing it forward the way you might kick a ball. Simultaneously, swing your right arm back and your left arm forward.

2. Without pausing, swing your right leg back as you bring your right arm forward and your left arm back.

3. Keep your torso fairly erect as you continue swinging your right leg and both arms forward and back 10 to 15 times.

4. Repeat on the other side, swinging your left leg back and forth like a pendulum.

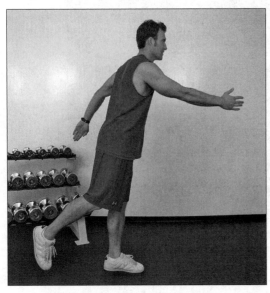

Leg swing to the back.

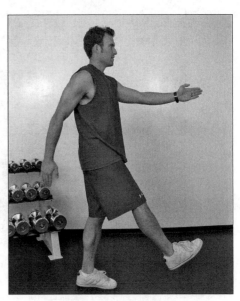

Leg swing to the front.

Leg Swings Side to Side

These leg swings activate the sides of your body so you'll be ready for side-to-side movements. They also gently rotate your upper body from one side to the other to wake up your abs and torso.

What It Targets

Inner and outer thighs

Obliques

Feet and ankles

Deep hip rotators

Shoulder girdle

Movement

1. While standing on your left leg, swing your right leg in front and to the left of your left leg as if you were kicking a soccer ball to the side. You'll feel the muscles in the side of your left leg kick in.

2. At the same time, swing both of your arms to the right to activate the muscles in the right side of your torso.

3. In a fluid motion, shift your right leg out to your right side while you move your arms in the opposite direction to the left. As you swing your arms and leg side to side, try to keep your body upright rather than leaning to one side or the other.

4. Swing from one side to the other 10 to 15 times and then switch to your other leg.

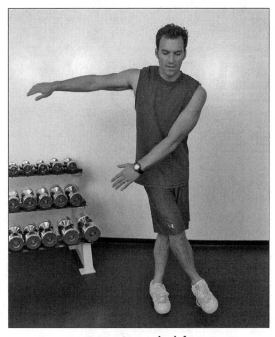

Leg swing to the left.

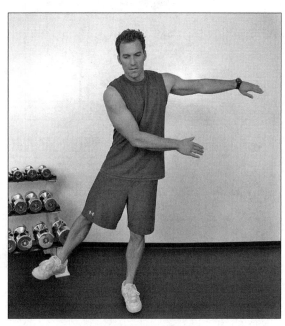

Leg swing to the right.

High Knees with Rotations

Here, your upper and lower body twist in opposite directions the way they do when you walk or run. This loosens up your hips and trunk, which reduces the amount of stress you feel in your hips and back.

What It Targets

Abdominals (rectus abdominus and obliques)

Hip flexors

Glutes

Shoulders

Latissimus dorsi

Movement

1. Stand with both feet facing forward about hip-width apart. Raise your left knee in front of you and across to the right.

2. In the same motion, swing both arms across to the left and behind you, similar to the way can-can dancers perform knee lifts.

3. Place your left foot back on the floor, and raise your right knee while you swing your arms to the right.

4. Keep alternating sides without pausing, and do 10 to 15 knee lifts on each side.

Left high knee lift with trunk twist to the left.

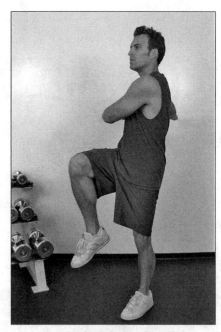
Right high knee lift with trunk twist to the right.

Toe Touch to Overhead Reach

This move uses rotation to prepare the muscles in your trunk for exercises that involve twisting. At the same time, you are moving up and down to increase your heart rate and opening your arms out wide to stretch the muscles in your chest and shoulders.

What It Targets

Obliques

Shoulders

Chest

Glutes

Hamstrings

Hip flexors

Inner thighs

Latissimus dorsi

Movement

1. Stand with your feet about 3 feet apart, and stretch your arms out wide to your sides a bit higher than shoulder height, as if you were going to make a snow angel while lying in the snow.

2. Keeping your arms straight, reach down and touch your right toes with your left hand while your right arm swings up behind you.

3. Return to your snow angel position, and reach your right hand down to touch your left foot, letting your left arm reach behind you.

4. Keep going from side to side for a total of 20 to 30 toe touches, returning to the snow angel position after each toe touch.

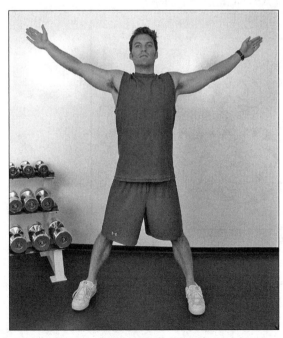

Return to the snow angel position after each toe touch.

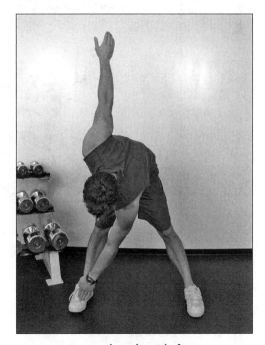

Toe touch to the right foot.

In This Part

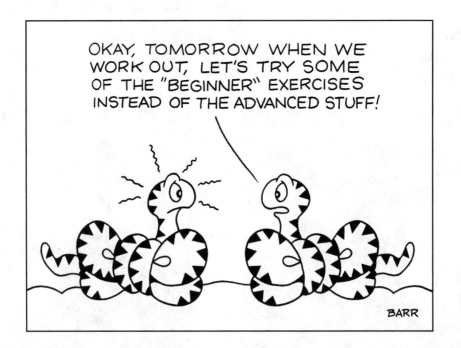

Part 3

Beginner Functional Exercises

Just like a baby needs to crawl before it walks, and a child needs to ride a tricycle before trying a two-wheeler, you need to ease into functional training. Even if you're a fitness enthusiast who works out on a regular basis, it's a good idea to start with this part rather than jumping ahead to the more advanced exercises in Parts 4 and 5. These beginner moves are designed to give you the foundation you need to perform the more complex moves in later chapters.

To help you get in the swing of functional training, each exercise includes easy-to-follow, step-by-step instructions along with photos of real people performing the moves. You'll also find tips and precautions to help you perform the exercises for maximum benefit or to modify moves if they're too difficult or too easy for you.

In This Chapter

- ◆ Using your body weight as resistance
- ◆ Working against gravity
- ◆ Improving your posture
- ◆ Using balance and coordination
- ◆ Moving in more than one direction at the same time

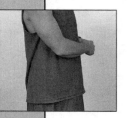 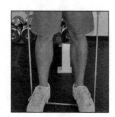 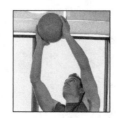 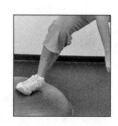 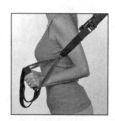 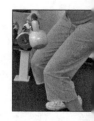

Chapter 6

Beginner Body Weight Exercises

The number of hamburgers and doughnuts you've chowed down throughout your lifetime isn't the only thing that creates body weight. In fact, the main culprit that gives your body weight is that universal element Sir Isaac Newton described more than 300 years ago: gravity. This nifty force of nature pushes your body down to the ground every second of every day of your life. Whether you're lying down, standing up, or jumping as high as you can, your body has to work against gravity at all times. Because of this, your body weight is an ideal tool for functional training. The fact that it's completely free and it goes with you everywhere makes it even better!

The beginner movements in this chapter rely on nothing more than your body weight for resistance. At first glance, they may look effortless because they don't require you to heft any equipment. They can be surprisingly challenging, though, especially if you're recovering from an injury or you're new to a fitness program. As your functional fitness improves, these movements will get easier for you. When you feel they're too easy, you can move on to the intermediate and advanced body weight movements or the exercises that involve resistance bands, medicine balls, the TRX, the BOSU, or kettlebells.

Pelvic Tilt

The pelvic tilt is one of the most basic exercises in functional training. This seemingly simple exercise strengthens the muscles that support the hips and lower back, specifically the abdominals, glutes, and hamstrings. In addition, it's designed to increase mobility of the lower back and can improve posture. This move also helps prepare you for the more complex, whole-body movements later in this book.

Although the pelvic tilt seems easy, it can be challenging if you're new to a fitness program or if you suffer from low back pain, which may indicate weakness of the muscles that support the lower part of the spine and hips. Back pain is second only to headaches as the most common neurological ailment in the United States, so you're not alone if your back's supporting muscles are weak.

Real-Life Activities It Helps You Do

Mastering the pelvic tilt can help you with a variety of daily activities, such as turning over in bed or bending over to brush your teeth, tie your shoes, or pick up the dog bowl.

Starting Point

1. Lie on your back on an exercise mat or a carpeted surface, and bend your knees, keeping your feet flat on the floor. Keep your arms down at your sides with your palms facing down, and look up at the ceiling.

Movement

2. Gently tilt your pelvis up so your lower back flattens against the floor, but don't lift your hips off the ground. Hold this position for 2 or 3 seconds.

3. Slowly relax, letting your pelvis return to the starting position. You should feel your lower back raise away from the floor slightly.

4. Rest for 2 or 3 seconds, and do another repetition. Work up to 12 to 15 repetitions.

Tips and Precautions

Although this exercise is intended to strengthen the muscles that support the lower spine and hips, it's not an exercise for the lower back per se. You shouldn't feel any tension in your lower back while performing the pelvic tilt. If your upper back and shoulders have become rounded as you've aged, it can place stress on your neck when you lie flat. To avoid this, place a small pillow under your head while performing this exercise.

Variations

Keep lifting your pelvis until your hips come off the ground and your knees, hips, and shoulders are in a straight line. This is called a bridge.

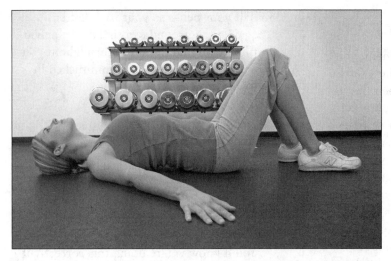

Starting/ending position.

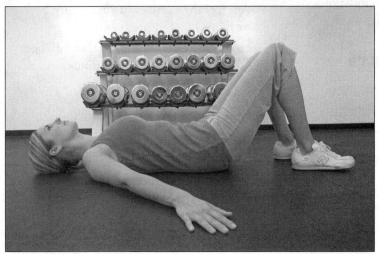

Midpoint position.

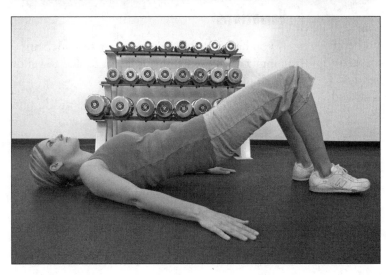

Variation: bridge position with hips off the floor.

Lying Wave Good-Bye

After you try this upper body movement, you'll never want to say good-bye to it. This exercise targets the shoulder area to strengthen the stabilizers of the shoulder blade and rotator cuff. For those of you who sit at a computer all day long, it's likely that your shoulders have started to roll forward, which can cause all kinds of problems with your body mechanics as you age. The lying wave good-bye can help you reverse the dreaded forward shoulder roll. It also prepares you for any movement that requires you to move your arm back and forth while it's above your shoulder, and it lays the foundation for more complex upper body movements.

Real-Life Activities It Helps You Do

Whether you're brushing your hair, putting on a jacket, using a hairdryer, or throwing a ball, you can benefit from this beginner shoulder movement.

Starting Point

1. Lie on your back on an exercise mat or a carpeted surface, and bend your knees, keeping your feet flat on the floor.
2. Raise your arms out to the sides to shoulder height so the backs of your arms are touching the ground, and bend your elbows to raise your forearms to a 90-degree angle, as if a burglar had just told you "Hands up!" Your palms should be facing the ceiling.

3. Tilt your pelvis so your back flattens against the ground (this is called a pelvic tilt and you'll do it often throughout your training), and keep your chin tucked in toward your neck.

Movement

4. Pull your shoulders back so they maintain contact with the ground, and pull them down away from your neck. At the same time, push your forearms back so the backs of your hands push into the ground. You'll know you're doing this correctly if you feel the muscles in your upper back working.
5. Hold for 30 seconds, and relax for about 15 seconds. Repeat 2 or 3 times.

Tips and Precautions

The movement in this exercise is very subtle and from the looks of the photo, it may not appear to be an exercise at all. Learning to keep your shoulders down and back, however, is one of the best things you can do to improve your functional movement.

Variations

If you have trouble keeping your shoulders in contact with the ground, place a folded towel or small pillow under your elbows.

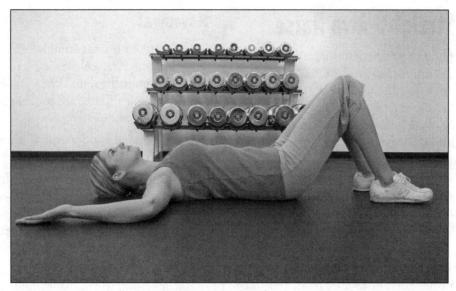

Starting/ending position.

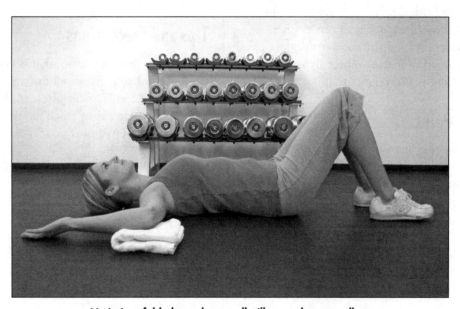

Variation: folded towel or small pillow under your elbows.

Lying Straight-Arm Raise

It's always good to aim high in life, and that's what this exercise encourages you to do. Essentially an upper body exercise, the lying straight-arm raise is designed to help you reach over your head while maintaining the correct posture. Although it primarily targets the muscles in your upper back and shoulders, it also involves your glutes and abdominals because you need to do a pelvic tilt while performing the exercise.

With so many muscles involved, this move can be harder than it looks. Many of my clients initially struggle to keep their backs flat against the ground while their arms are raised. Usually, it doesn't take long before they're comfortable with this important move.

Real-Life Activities It Helps You Do

This movement improves your ability to do everyday things like placing an object on a high shelf or adjusting the shower nozzle. For athletic types, it prepares you for dynamic overhead activities like serving in tennis.

Starting Point

1. Lie on your back on an exercise mat or a carpeted surface, and bend your knees, keeping your feet flat on the floor.

2. Hold your arms out to your sides and straighten them while looking up at the ceiling.

Movement

3. Swing both arms straight over your head as if you were celebrating a touchdown at a football game. When you finish, be sure your thumbs are touching the ground behind you.

4. In the same motion, tilt your pelvis so your back flattens against the ground.

5. While keeping your arms straight and in contact with the ground, pull your shoulders back so they touch the floor and pull them down away from your neck. Keep your chin tucked in toward your neck.

6. Hold for 30 seconds, release your arms back down to your sides, and relax your pelvis so your back raises up slightly off the ground.

7. Rest for 30 seconds, and try it again 2 or 3 times.

Tips and Precautions

If you have shoulder issues that prevent you from getting your hands all the way to the ground in the movement phase of this exercise, place a folded towel or small pillow under your hands when they're over your head.

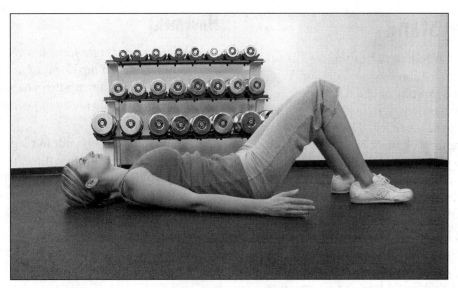

Starting/ending position.

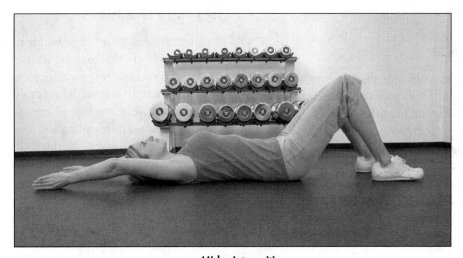

Midpoint position.

One-Leg Stand

This exercise introduces a healthy dose of balance and coordination to your workout. With this move, the muscles of one leg have to hold up your entire body weight instead of sharing the load with the other leg. This means your muscles have to work twice as hard to coordinate to keep your foot, ankle, knee, hip, spine, shoulders, and head aligned. Expect to feel a bit wobbly when you lift your foot off the ground. You'll also immediately notice the muscles in the standing leg fire to keep you balanced.

Don't be surprised if you can't keep your leg lifted for long at first. With practice, you'll be able to stand on a single leg for a longer time period with less shaking.

Real-Life Activities It Helps You Do

This move helps you perform any activity that requires you to transfer weight from one foot to the other, such as walking or running.

Starting Point

1. Stand with your legs slightly bent and hip-width apart. Lift your torso tall with your head in alignment with your spine and your eyes facing forward.

2. Lift your right foot off the ground until your shin is parallel to the ground. Your right knee should be slightly in front of your left leg, and your right foot should be behind your left leg.

Movement

3. Hike up your right hip a few inches. This brings your left hip down to mimic the way your hips move when you walk. This also activates the glutes in your standing leg.

4. While standing on your left leg, push the big toe of your left foot into the floor to help you balance, but don't let your left ankle roll inward. This integrates the foot and glute and helps stabilize your standing leg.

5. Hold this position for up to 15 seconds, and lower your right foot back down to the ground.

6. Rest for 5 to 10 seconds, and repeat the balance position by lifting your other leg. Your goal should be to perform 2 or 3 repetitions on each side.

Tips and Precautions

If you can't keep your leg lifted for more than a few seconds, do this exercise near a table or countertop you can rest your fingertips on it lightly. Be sure to use the fingers of the hand opposite your standing leg. Using the fingers on the same side as the standing leg will cause you to lean, which defeats the purpose of the exercise. Eventually, you'll get the hang of it and won't need the balance aid anymore.

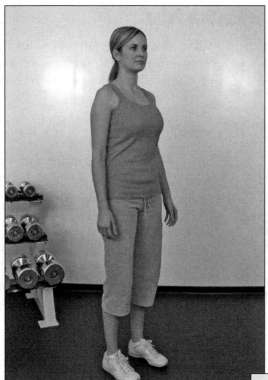

Starting/ending position.

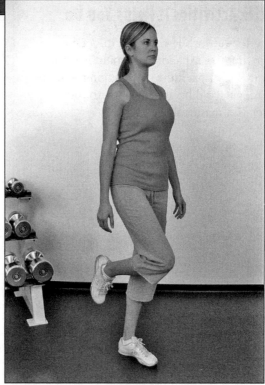

First position.

Partial Lunge with Crossover Reach

Ready to do the twist? This exercise adds rotation to your functional training repertoire. Life often calls for you to twist and rotate your body, but this seemingly basic movement actually requires serious coordination among numerous muscles.

This exercise trains and strengthens all those muscles, but that's not all. When added to the partial lunge, which targets nearly every muscle in the lower body, this becomes a whole-body exercise. Because it works so many muscles at once, this is a highly effective and efficient exercise to include in your workout, especially if you're short on time. With this multimuscle movement, you'll learn how to transfer weight properly through the hips, spine, and shoulders.

Real-Life Activities It Helps You Do

Stepping forward while reaching to open a door, moving toward a kitchen counter while stretching to grasp a knife, and jogging—these are all things you'll be able to do with more ease after you master this exercise.

Starting Point

1. Stand with your feet slightly wider than hip-width apart with your arms down at your sides. Be sure your torso is erect.

Movement

2. Step forward about 12 inches with your left leg, keeping both legs slightly bent.

3. At the same time, reach your right arm out as if you were reaching down to shake a small child's hand. Reach your arm straight across your left knee and rotate your torso to the left, keeping your shoulders level. As you reach your arm across your body, pull your left hip back so your hips are squared.

4. Return to the starting position, and repeat 10 to 12 times. Then switch sides so your right leg and left arm are doing the work for another 10 to 12 repetitions.

Tips and Precautions

For some people, the lunge portion of this exercise can cause knee pain. If you feel a twinge when you take a step forward, try taking a smaller step. Also, don't lean forward, which can put added stress on your knee joint.

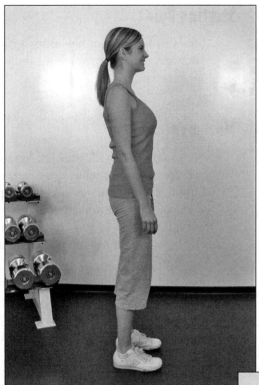

Starting/ending position.

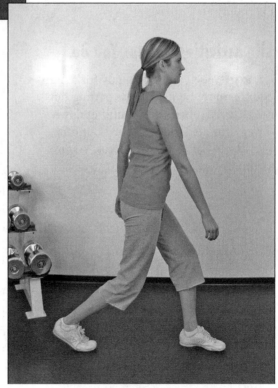

Midpoint position.

Partial Side Squat with Lateral Reach

You'll get a lot of bang for your buck with this beginner movement that combines upper body rotation with a side-to-side motion. Like the partial lunge, the partial side squat hits all the major muscles in your lower body, including the glutes, hamstrings, inner thighs, quadriceps, and calves. Add that to the rotational element, which targets the muscles in your upper body, including the obliques, lats, shoulders, and arms, and you've got another all-in-one exercise.

Even though this is a beginner movement, it can be tricky to perform because it combines upper and lower body movements, so pay attention to your form. Practicing this kind of exercise lays the foundation for the more complex intermediate and advanced movements later in the book.

Real-Life Activities It Helps You Do

This combo exercise comes in handy for a number of routine movements, such as getting out of your seat at the movies and shuffling down the row to get to the aisle or getting out of a car. If you like to dance or play tennis, you'll benefit from this exercise, too.

Starting Point

1. Stand with your feet hip-width apart with your arms down at your sides and your torso erect.

Movement

2. Step to the side with your left leg so your feet are about 24 inches apart, keeping both feet facing forward. As you step out with your left leg, squat back with your left hip as if you were going to sit in a chair. Your right leg can be either straight or slightly bent.

3. As you step and squat to the left, reach your right arm out across your body and rotate your torso to the left, keeping your shoulders level. Rotate only as far as is comfortable.

4. Push off of your left leg to return to the starting position as you bring your right arm back to your side.

5. Repeat 10 to 12 times. Then switch sides so your right leg and left arm are doing the work for another set of 10 to 12.

Tips and Precautions

Whenever you're in a squat position with your hips pushed back, be sure your weight is mainly in the heel of your foot rather than in the ball or the toes. By sitting back into your hips, you engage the glutes, which helps support your knees. In this exercise, many people who have difficulty rotating their torsos try to compensate by lowering one shoulder and rounding their back. Doing so can stress the lower back, so pay attention to keeping your shoulders level as you rotate.

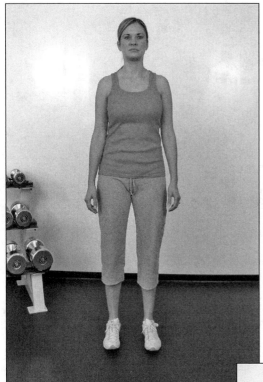

Starting/ending position.

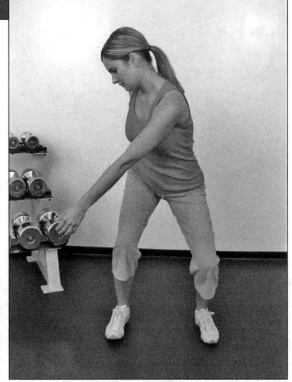

Midpoint position.

In This Chapter

- Working against resistance
- Learning to react to external forces
- Increasing coordination
- Targeting your upper body
- Creating power

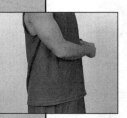
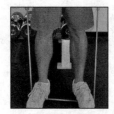
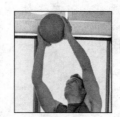
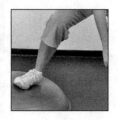
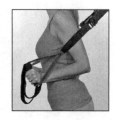
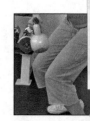

Chapter 7

Beginner Resistance Band Exercises

Join the resistance—the resistance band movement, that is! Similar to a long rubber band with handles on the ends, these handy tools have become some of the most popular exercise equipment around. That's no surprise when you consider that they weigh next to nothing and they're extremely portable. Oh, and did I mention that they can work just about every single part of your body—at the same time? Talk about getting a lot of bang for your buck!

The resistance band moves in this chapter begin teaching your body how to work against resistance in addition to gravity, which you learned how to control in Chapter 6. The exercises in this chapter get the entire chain of muscles, ligaments, nerves, and other tissues of your lower body, core, and upper body coordinating to work together. Now, that's functional training because anytime you move your body in real life, you have to get all those parts to work in unison.

Before you start exercising with resistance bands, you need to ensure that they're properly anchored. If there's a bed or couch around, wrap the band around one of the legs. If you're outside, you can loop it around a sturdy tree limb. You can also safely secure resistance bands using a neat device called a door anchor. This tool is a loop of heavy nylon fabric that you stick in the hinge side of an open door. Then you close the door to secure it in place. Just slide the band through the loop, and you're ready to go.

Band Shuffle

The band shuffle sounds kinda like a dance move, and it gets you shimmying from side to side. What it's really designed to do, though, is strengthen the muscles on the outer side of your hips to help you balance, stabilize, and create power as you move laterally.

This exercise is tougher than it looks because the resistance from the band tries to knock you off your balance. To fight that resistance and stay upright, you have to coordinate your muscles, nerves, and more. When you get the hang of it, you may just want to hit the dance floor!

Real-Life Activities It Helps You Do

If you want to walk in the ocean with the waves crashing against your legs, go ice-skating, or go dancing, this exercise is a must. It also helps you keep your balance and prevent falls on uneven surfaces, such as cobblestone streets or icy sidewalks.

Starting Point

1. Start with your feet facing forward about shoulder-width apart with the resistance band under both feet and your arms down at your sides with your hands in the handles. Pull up slightly on the band so there isn't any slack.

2. Keep your torso erect and your eyes facing forward rather than looking down at your feet.

Movement

3. With your feet facing forward, slide your left foot about 18 inches away from your right foot, as if you were making your way down a long bookshelf at the bookstore (perusing the titles of *Complete Idiot's Guides*, of course). Lift your left foot up only as much as necessary to shuffle it to the side rather than lifting it up high.

4. Slide your right foot over toward your left foot so they're back to approximately shoulder width. Keep shuffling to the left, working up to about 10 steps with your left foot, and switch and do 10 more to the right.

Tips and Precautions

Be aware of the amount of tension you have in the band. If it's too easy, pull the handles of the band up higher to increase the intensity. If you have trouble shuffling your feet far enough to the side, lower your hands so there's less tension on the band, or try a lighter band.

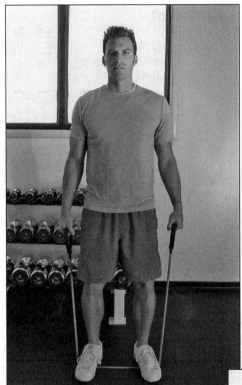

Starting/ending position.

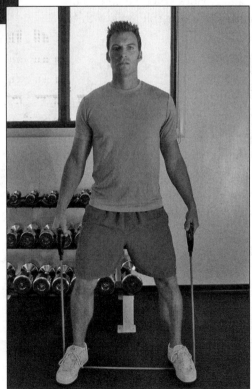

Midpoint position.

Side Walk with Band

This exercise takes the band shuffle to new heights. A more dynamic move, it integrates more muscles and makes it harder for you to stabilize against the resistance. And because you lift your leg higher as you side walk, your standing leg gets much more of a balance challenge.

Like the band shuffle, it isn't as easy as it looks. With practice, however, it'll become like second nature to you. In fact, you'll probably find that after some time, you'll want to add more tension to the band to increase the difficulty.

Real-Life Activities It Helps You Do

Putting on your pants while balancing on one leg, getting in or out of a car, shuffling down a hiking trail, or walking up a mountain sideways on skis are all activities you'll be able to do more easily thanks to the side walk with band.

Starting Point

1. Start with your feet facing forward about shoulder-width apart with the resistance band under both feet and your arms down at your sides with your hands in the handles. Pull up slightly on the band so there isn't any slack.

2. Keep your torso erect and your eyes facing forward rather than looking down at your feet.

Movement

3. Lift your right foot about 12 inches off the ground, and step to the right as if you were stepping over a big rock.

4. As soon as your right foot hits the ground, lift your left foot up about 12 inches and bring it toward your right foot until they're back to about shoulder-width apart. A good goal for this exercise is 10 steps to the right and then 10 more to the left.

Tips and Precautions

Don't look down at your feet as you step, or you'll throw your body out of alignment, which means your body won't be working functionally.

Variations

To add more of a balance challenge, close your eyes as you perform this exercise or step back at an angle with your leading leg each time to make yourself rotate in a circle.

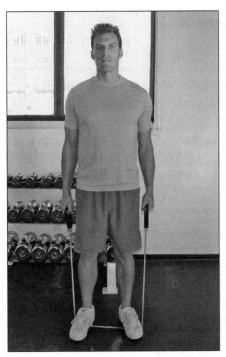

Starting/ending position.

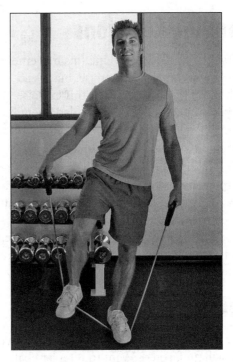

First position.

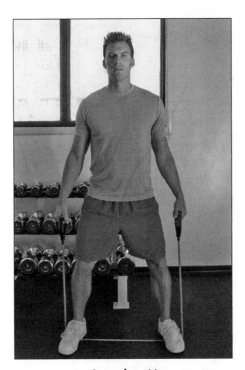

Second position.

Standing Rotations

At first glance, you may think this movement looks like a simple arm exercise, but it's so much more than that. In fact, this exercise gets you to practice one of the fundamentals of movement—rotating your hips and torso in opposite directions at the same time.

This basic maneuver stretches your midsection to create more mobility through your torso while improving flexibility in your hips. That adds up to an ability to create more power. How do mobility and flexibility help you create power? It's the same concept as a rubber band—the more you stretch it, the harder it will fly.

Real-Life Activities It Helps You Do

Want to take a bigger backswing in golf so your drive will go farther? Want to hit a baseball with more power? Want to be able to reach behind you to grab a pot off the stove? If so, start practicing this exercise.

Starting Point

1. Secure the resistance band at approximately chest height, and turn your body 90 degrees to the right of the anchor point.
2. Stand with your feet shoulder-width apart.
3. With your arms straight out in front of you at shoulder height, hold the handle with both hands, overlapping your fingers.

Movement

4. Keeping your torso erect and your shoulders level, rotate your torso—not your hips—and your arms to the right as you step back with your left leg about 12 inches.
5. As the heel of your back foot strikes the ground, tilt your pelvis under. You'll probably feel the tilt in your back leg only. You won't notice much of a change in your other leg.
6. Return to the starting position. Do 10 to 12 repetitions on one side before switching to the other side.

Tips and Precautions

If you feel any stress in your lower back as you rotate, take a smaller step back or don't take your leg behind you at all. Instead, keep both legs in the starting position about shoulder-width apart. You can also try bending your arms to bring them closer to your body.

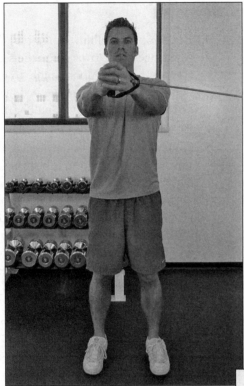

Starting/ending position.

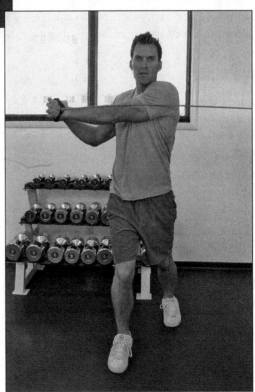

Midpoint position.

One-Leg Stand with Row

Remember the one-leg stand from Chapter 6? This exercise combines that lower body balance movement with upper body resistance work. The real beauty of this exercise is that it targets nearly every muscle from your working hand all the way down to your opposite foot. In exercise physiology speak, that chain of muscles is called the *posterior oblique system*, and it's one of the essential keys to better movement. Working the entire chain at the same time increases mobility, gives you more potential for strength, and creates stability in the lower back and hips. You simply can't get all those benefits by doing rows while sitting at a machine in the gym because when you're sitting, you break the chain.

Real-Life Activities It Helps You Do

Working the posterior oblique system helps you every time you take a step, reach out to open a door, or reach down to pick up a heavy object.

Starting Point

1. Secure the resistance band at approximately waist height, and face the anchor point with your eyes looking straight ahead.

2. Grasp the handle with your left hand with your palm facing to the right. Your arm should be pulled straight in front of you at about shoulder height. Let your other arm relax down at your side.

3. Lift your left leg and bend it so your shin is parallel to the ground. Your left knee should be slightly in front of your right leg, and your left foot should be behind your right leg.

Movement

4. Bend your left elbow as you pull the resistance band toward you the same way you would pull a door handle to open a door. Be sure your shoulders don't shrug or round forward as you pull back on the band.

5. Slowly straighten your arm back to the starting position without bending or rotating your torso. You'll know you have the proper amount of tension in the band when you can only complete 10 to 15 repetitions with your left arm. If you can do more, you don't have enough tension on the band, and if you can't get to 10, you need to reduce the amount of tension. Switch to do 10 to 15 additional repetitions using your right arm while balancing on your left leg.

Tips and Precautions

If the balance challenge is too much for you, tap the raised foot on the ground. You may only have to tap for a brief moment before raising it up again. As you progress, you'll be able to keep it in the air longer.

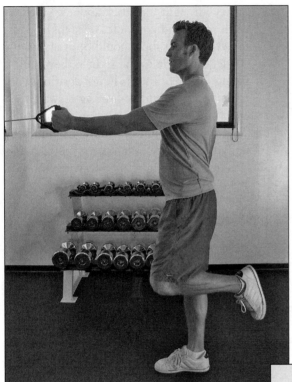

Starting/ending position.

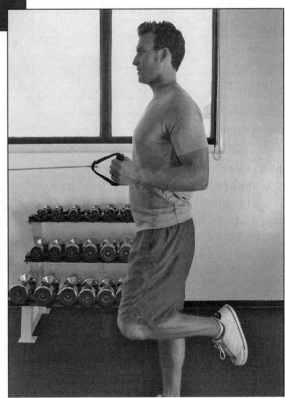

Midpoint position.

Lunge to One-Arm High Row

Like the one-leg stand with row you just did, this all-in-one exercise trains that chain of muscles that runs from your hand to your opposite foot. With the added lunge in this exercise, you get a nice prestretch throughout those muscles, which helps you create more power to perform the high row. This exercise also pumps up your flexibility and strength.

For this exercise, start with light resistance until you get the form down and then begin challenging yourself with higher intensity.

Real-Life Activities It Helps You Do

This useful exercise has hundreds of everyday applications, such as starting a lawn mower, pulling clothes out of a dryer, putting your luggage in the overhead compartment, and picking up a case of water from under a shopping cart and putting it in the car.

Starting Point

1. Secure the resistance band at foot height, for example, underneath a door or under something heavy, such as the leg of a couch or bed.

2. Face the anchor point and lean down to grasp the handle with your right hand with your palm facing the ground. Keeping your right arm straight, step back until there isn't any slack in the band. Your left arm can relax down at your side.

3. Step your right foot back about 24 inches while you bend your left knee, ankle, and hip. Your right foot should be at about a 45-degree angle to the right rather than facing forward. In this lunge position, your upper body should be leaning forward and your back should be slightly rounded. The tension from the band helps pull your body forward to stretch the chain of muscles from your right hand to your left heel.

Movement

4. Push off of your left heel to straighten your left leg and transfer your weight to your right leg. Lift and straighten so your torso is upright.

5. At the same time, pull the band the same way you would pull the cord on your lawn mower up to about ear height on your right side. Let the elbow of your right arm bend as you pull back on the band. Depending on your flexibility, your right elbow and hand may end up anywhere from in front of your shoulder to behind it.

6. Return to the starting position, and repeat the movement 8 to 12 times on this side before switching sides for 8 to 12 more.

Tips and Precautions

Lean your body only as far forward as is comfortable. If you feel any discomfort in this position, lift your upper body higher.

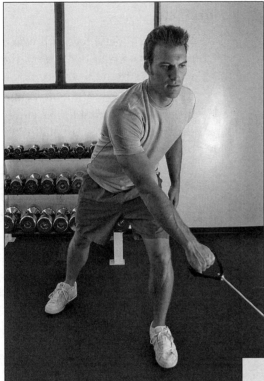

Starting/ending position.

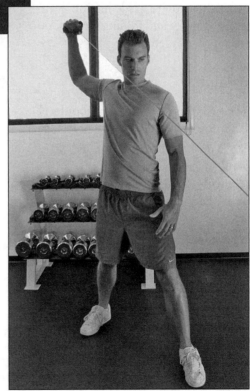

Midpoint position.

Standing Alternating High Pulls

Even though this exercise looks like it's all about arm strength, it isn't. It's designed to teach you how to use your back muscles and abs to create the power you need to lift your arms rather than relying solely on your arm muscles.

This basic functional movement pays off in a lot of ways in your everyday life by helping you lift more weight than you could otherwise and by preventing injuries when you lift heavy objects. That's a lot of good stuff from one simple exercise!

Real-Life Activities It Helps You Do

You'll reap the benefits of this exercise anytime you have to get down low and then come up high, such as when you're gardening or weeding, doing the laundry and folding clothes, or playing soccer or racquetball.

Starting Point

1. Secure two resistance bands at foot level under a door or under a heavy object, such as the leg of a couch or bed.
2. Face the anchor point, and grasp each handle with one hand so your arms are straight and your palms are facing the floor.
3. Step back until there's no slack in the band. With your feet shoulder-width apart, bend your knees slightly, keeping your torso erect. It's okay to round your spine slightly because that creates a pre-stretch for the movement.

Movement

4. Step back about 2 feet with your right foot as you rotate your body to the right about 45 degrees from the anchor point.
5. At the same time, straighten your spine, lifting your chest high, and pull back on the band as if you were pulling the chain to start a chainsaw. Lift your right arm as far back and as high as you can, keeping it as straight as you can. You can keep your eyes on the anchor point throughout the exercise, or you can look back at your hand as you raise it.
6. Return to the starting position, and repeat the movement on the other side. Keep alternating sides until you do a total of 20 repetitions.

Tips and Precautions

Remember, the goal here is to use your torso rotation to help lift your arm rather than trying to muscle the arm movement.

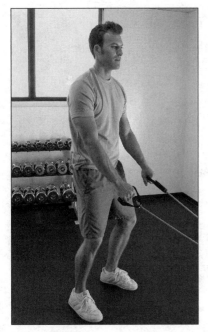

Starting/ending position.

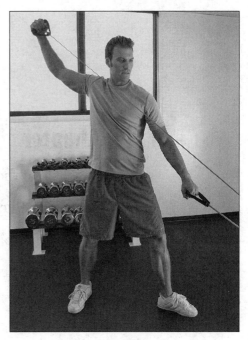

First position.

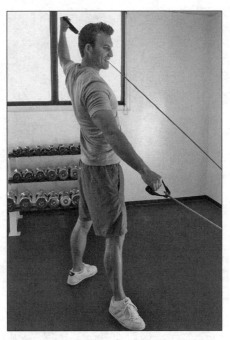

Second position.

In This Chapter

- ◆ Learning to love the medicine ball
- ◆ Handling the medicine ball
- ◆ Fancy—but functional—footwork
- ◆ Reaching the medicine ball away from your body

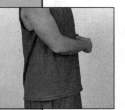 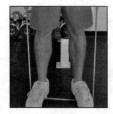 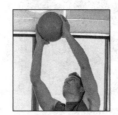 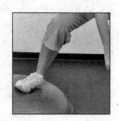 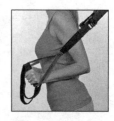 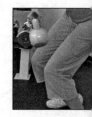

Chapter 8

Beginner Medicine Ball Exercises

There's a good reason why the medicine ball has been used as a fitness tool for thousands of years—it's fun! I'll bet you're going to have a ball with it. Here are some of the things my clients love best about the medicine ball: there's no *wrong* way to hold it; it won't break your foot if you drop it (can't say that about a dumbbell); thanks to its bright colors, it doesn't seem intimidating; and it comes in all different sizes and weights so it's easy to find one that matches your fitness level. Best of all: it reminds you of playing with a ball when you were a kid.

I think the medicine ball is such a great functional training tool because it's heavy. Just picking it up off the floor to begin your exercise activates your muscles. It isn't ergonomically designed to make exercises easier for you. You have to hold it in front of you the way you have to hold things in real life. Some medicine balls bounce, which adds unpredictability to any exercise. It can roll on the ground, too, which offers unique ways to train.

That's not all. It also adds momentum, which means that once you get the ball moving, you have to engage your muscles to bring it to a halt. The faster you move the ball, the harder it is to stop it. Plus, the medicine ball mimics gravity by becoming exponentially heavier as you reach it away from your body. That multiplies the intensity of the exercises. That's a lot to love about a single piece of equipment!

Bend Down, Reach Up

Just as its name suggests, this exercise is designed to help you become more comfortable bending down and reaching up, two of the most basic functional movement patterns. Thanks to the weighted medicine ball, this exercise also introduces you to the effect of momentum on your muscles.

With this exercise, you get your first taste of moving the ball and then trying to stop it. Start slowly at first so you can rein in the ball, and gradually pick up the pace as you go from bending down to a full stretch.

Real-Life Activities It Helps You Do

You probably need to bend down numerous times throughout the day to tie your shoes, get something out of a low drawer, or pick up something off the ground. Plus, in many sports, including baseball, football, and basketball, you need to bend down to pick up a ball and then reach up to throw it.

Starting Point

1. Stand with your feet hip-width apart.
2. Hold the medicine ball with both hands in front of you below belly button height with your arms slightly bent.

Movement

3. Bend down by bending at your hips and slightly bending your knees as you gently lower the ball to the ground—or as close as you can get—as if you were placing a heavy box on the ground. It's okay to round your back as you bend. Be sure to follow the ball with your eyes throughout the exercise.
4. In one swift movement, roll back up to standing as you swing the ball over your head with your arms almost straight, always keeping your eye on the prize, er, ball. Keep bending down and reaching up 12 to 15 times.

Tips and Precautions

Because this is your first exercise using the medicine ball, be sure to choose a size and weight that's appropriate for your fitness level. If you aren't sure what weight to use, it's better to start with a lighter ball. Only if you can easily surpass the recommended number of repetitions should you switch to a heavier ball. Also, when you reach down to pick up a medicine ball for the first time, be aware that it's heavy.

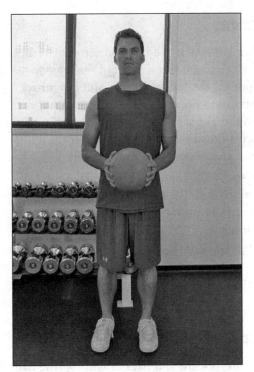

Starting/ending position.

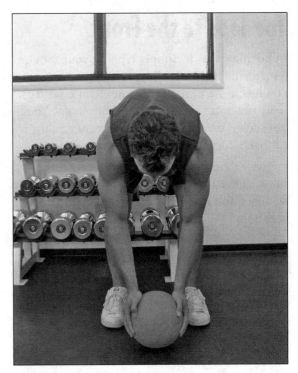

First position.

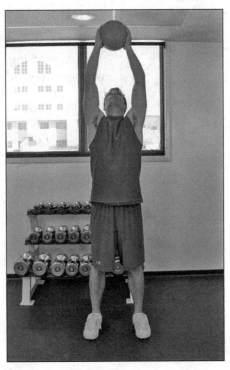

Second position.

Toe Taps to the Front

Who knew that by simply tapping your foot on a medicine ball and rolling it back and forth you could activate nearly every muscle in your legs, feet, and butt? Even better, it's fun to do. You'll get such a kick out of this movement you'll probably forget you're actually exercising.

Even though it may not feel like it, your muscles get a workout with this one—becoming stronger and increasing stabilization and coordination.

Real-Life Activities It Helps You Do

The footwork in this exercise makes you more comfortable when stepping onto a moving escalator, going up or down stairs, walking, playing soccer, or playing kickball.

Starting Point

1. With the medicine ball on the ground, stand on your left foot and tap your right foot on top of the ball. The middle of the ball should be level with your left toes and in front of your right hip. Keep your torso erect and your hands down at your sides.

Movement

2. Look down at the ball and use your right foot to make it roll forward. Take your foot off the ball as it rolls, and tap it back on top to bring the ball to a stop, the way you might stop your bowling ball if you set it down on the ground and it started to roll away from you. Pause briefly.

3. Using only your right foot, make the ball roll back to the starting position, and tap your foot on top to hold it there for a moment.

4. Roll the ball back and forth 10 to 12 times with your right foot, and switch legs for 10 to 12 on the left.

Tips and Precautions

Don't lean forward and back as you roll the ball back and forth.

Variations

As you get more comfortable with this movement, try closing your eyes or swinging your arms in opposition to your legs as you roll the ball.

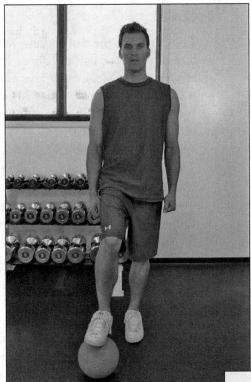

Starting/ending position.

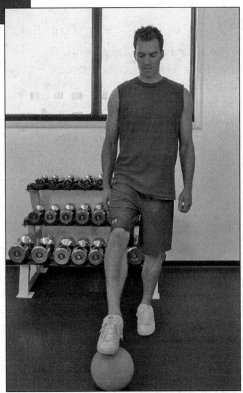

Midpoint position.

Toe Taps to the Side

Your feet, knees, and hips will thank you for this exercise. Because most of us wear shoes all day and walk around on carpeted surfaces, our feet begin to lose the ability to adapt to changing terrain and the arches may collapse. When this happens, it can cause pain in your feet and heels and eventually in your knees and hips. This exercise can help prevent this common problem by working the muscles in the foot as it taps and rolls the medicine ball from side to side.

As an added bonus, this exercise also targets the inner and outer thighs.

Real-Life Activities It Helps You Do

The fancy footwork in this exercise prepares you to walk sideways, dance, or dip your toes in a pool to test the water.

Starting Point

1. With the medicine ball on the ground, stand on your left foot and tap your right foot on top of the ball. The middle of the ball should be level with your left toes and in front of your right hip. Keep your torso erect and your hands down at your sides.

Movement

2. Look down at the ball and use your right foot to make the ball roll about 18 inches to your right side, exactly how you might use your foot to push something away from you. Take your foot off the ball as it rolls, and tap it back on top to bring it to a halt. Pause momentarily.

3. Using only your right foot, roll the ball back to the starting position, and tap your foot on top to hold it there briefly.

4. Roll the ball side to side 10 to 12 times on the right and then switch sides for 10 to 12 times on the left.

Tips and Precautions

Ideally, you should be able to perform this exercise without following the ball with your eyes. If that's too difficult for you, use your peripheral vision to follow the ball rather than turning your head.

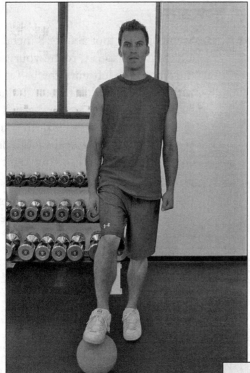

Starting/ending position.

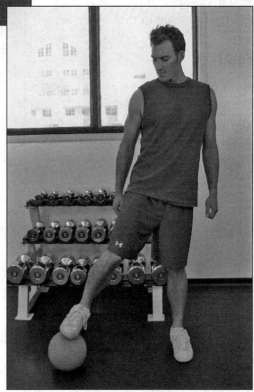

Midpoint position.

Rotations with Side Step

I explained earlier how your arm muscles have to work against gravity to hold something heavy without dropping it. Now you're going to learn how much heavier an object can get and how much harder your muscles have to work when you hold that object—in this case, the medicine ball—farther away from your body. Yes, this basic functional movement primarily gets you stepping from side to side and rotating to work your abs, glutes, and feet, but your arms will be working, too.

Real-Life Activities It Helps You Do

You probably use this movement on a routine basis without realizing it, such as when you take items from a shopping cart and place them on the conveyor belt, reach to pick up your luggage from the baggage carousel, or take heavy pots out of the sink to load them in the dishwasher.

Starting Point

1. Stand with your feet about hip-width apart and your torso erect.
2. Hold the medicine ball about 6 inches in front of your belly button with your arms slightly bent.

Movement

3. Step your left foot about 18 inches to the left. Simultaneously, rotate your torso and the ball to the left until the ball is in line with your left heel. The ball should be facing to your left side now, as if you were ready to hand off a sandbag to someone on your left. Your right heel should naturally come off the ground so your right foot can pivot as you rotate.
4. Rotate back to the front, and return your feet to the starting position. Immediately change directions by stepping and rotating to the right.
5. Keep alternating sides until you do a total of 20 to 30 repetitions.

Tips and Precautions

If your spine is stiff and you can't twist very far, you can hold the medicine ball with your fingertips so you don't have to rotate so far.

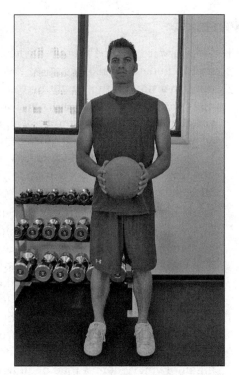

Starting/ending position.

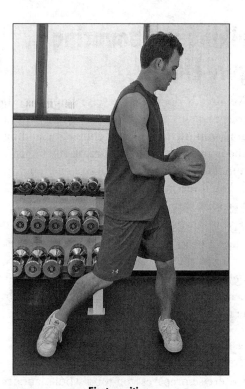

First position.

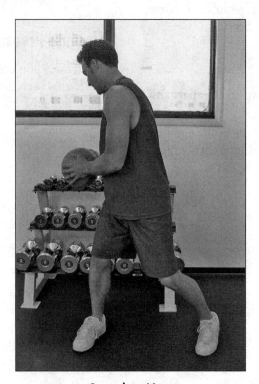

Second position.

Walking and Bouncing Figure Eights

You've already done this exercise a million times without realizing it because it mimics the same motions you use to walk. Of course, by adding the medicine ball to the picture, it takes this routine movement to a new, more challenging level. You'll feel your abs kick into gear as you try to coordinate the movements of your legs and spine.

A lot of people tend to overthink the movements when they first try this exercise, and they end up getting all discombobulated. Stop concentrating so hard, and the movement will come naturally.

Real-Life Activities It Helps You Do

This exercise prepares you for a whole laundry list of everyday and athletic movements, including walking, running, hiking, paddling a canoe, or even playing games on the Wii.

Starting Point

1. Stand with your feet hip-width apart and your torso erect.
2. Hold the medicine ball in front of you at belly button height with your arms slightly bent.

Movement

1. Step forward about 1 foot with your left foot to initiate a walking gait. At the same time, in a smooth motion, bring the ball up toward your right shoulder and swing your arms down as if you were swinging an axe and bounce the ball down to the left side of your left foot. Catch it as it bounces back up, and bring it up to your left shoulder.
2. Without stopping, step forward about 1 foot with your right foot as you complete your figure eight by swinging your arms down and bouncing the ball down to the outside your right foot. Catch it and bring it back up to your right shoulder. The shape your arms make as you flow through the motions should resemble a horizontal figure eight. Keep walking and bouncing until you've done a total of 30 figure eights.

Tips and Precautions

The closer you hold the ball to your body, the easier this exercise is. As you progress, start to hold the ball farther away and bounce the ball higher to add more stress to the muscles in your back and hips.

Variations

When you feel very comfortable with this exercise, try doing it walking backward.

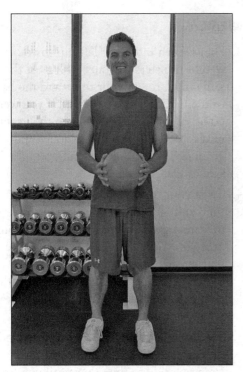

Starting/ending position.

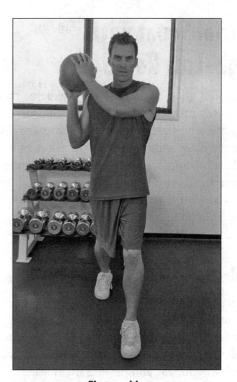

First position.

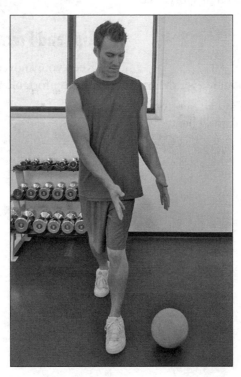

Second position.

Partial Squat with High-Low Rotation

Talk about good medicine—this medicine ball movement provides a healthy dose of challenge for your butt, thighs, calves, and abs. By strengthening these muscles, you gain a more solid foundation, which is a key component of all functional movement. With the added high-low twist, you're training your body to rotate while lifting a heavy object—something you probably do nearly every day of your life.

Real-Life Activities It Helps You Do

Many moves will be easier thanks to this exercise, including taking things out of the trunk of your car, clearing the dinner table and passing the dishes to another person, and washing the wheels of your car and passing the bucket of water to someone else. It also prepares you for the athletic movements involved in sports like basketball and baseball.

Starting Point

1. Stand with your feet shoulder-width apart.
2. Hold the medicine ball at belly button height with your arms slightly bent.

Movement

3. Squat down into your left hip so your weight transfers to your left leg. At the same time, rotate your torso and the ball to the left the way you would if you were going to put a heavy box onto the ground next to you, but don't let it touch the ground. The ball should end up to the left side of your left knee.

4. Twist your torso back to the forward position, and push off of your left leg to return to standing while you lift the ball up high over your right shoulder as if you were putting that heavy box away on a high shelf. Remember to follow the ball with your eyes—a good rule of thumb with all medicine ball exercises.

5. Now go the other way, rotating your body in the other direction. Keep changing from one side to the other until you finish 20 to 30 repetitions.

Tips and Precautions

Keep your movements small until you start feeling comfortable with this exercise.

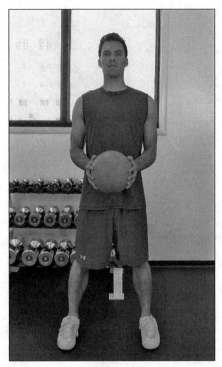

Starting/ending position.

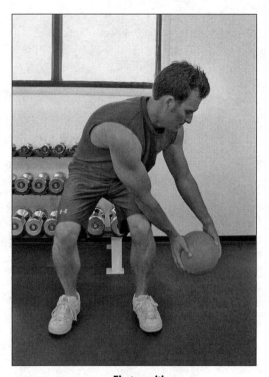

First position.

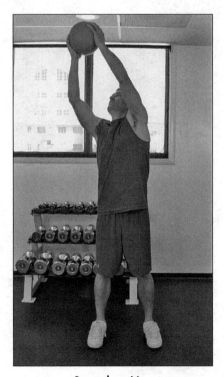

Second position.

In This Chapter

- ◆ Getting your spine moving

- ◆ Activating your core

- ◆ Positioning your body to make exercises harder or easier

- ◆ Increasing your range of motion with the TRX

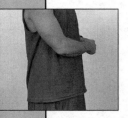
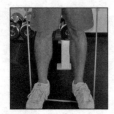
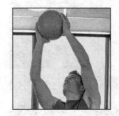
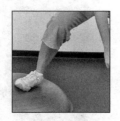
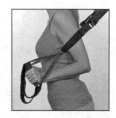
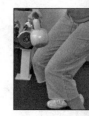

Chapter 9

Beginner TRX Exercises

Compared to the centuries-old medicine ball, the TRX is the new kid on the block. Originally developed by a Navy SEAL in the mid-1990s, the TRX hit gyms and sporting goods store shelves about a decade later. Consisting of long nylon straps, handles, and foot cradles, the TRX is about as low-tech as you can get, but it really delivers results. It hasn't taken long for this suspension-training system to be recognized as one of the best functional exercise tools for people of all fitness levels.

Among the many reasons why it's gaining popularity, the TRX requires nothing more than your own body weight for resistance. Thanks to its versatility, you can perform more than 200 functional exercises with the system. The fact that it weighs less than 2 pounds and can be folded up into a purse or briefcase makes it ideal for fitness on the go. Plus, it takes less than a minute to set up. A versatile, portable training tool that builds strength, stability, balance, and flexibility—what could be better?

For safety purposes, the TRX must be anchored securely to support your body weight. For indoor use, consider an affordable TRX door anchor that fits on almost any door, or try a permanent wall mount. Outdoors, you can anchor the TRX to a fence, pole, or tree.

Hip Flexor with Partial Lunge

Here's a great strength and flexibility exercise for desk jockeys who sit hunched over from 9 to 5. Similar to the lunges you performed in previous chapters, this move opens the anterior chain—the front side of your body—to increase flexibility in your hip flexors, abdominals, and shoulders. In earlier lunges where you took your arms overhead, you stopped raising your arms when it became uncomfortable. Here, with your hands secured in the handles, the TRX makes you take your arms a bit farther than comfortable so you really feel the stretch. Your body will thank you for this one!

Real-Life Activities It Helps You Do

Anytime you have to stand up for a long time—at work, at a concert, at church—you'll be able to maintain better posture, which can help keep you pain free. When your hips and spine are aligned properly, any kind of movement, including walking, running, and more athletic moves, are improved.

Starting Point

1. With your feet hip-width apart, face away from the anchor point. Grasp the handles, and raise your arms straight overhead with your palms facing away from the anchor point. Scoot away from the anchor point until there's no slack in the system.

Movement

2. Step forward with your left leg, and lunge down so your right knee comes close to the ground as if you were going to kneel down. Keep your torso erect, and tilt your pelvis under to increase the stretch in your right hip flexor. As you lunge, the system will pull your arms toward the anchor point, creating a deep stretch throughout your shoulders and abs.

3. Push off of your left heel to return to standing, and then lunge forward with your right leg. Continue alternating sides 16 to 20 times.

Tips and Precautions

The TRX system controls how far back your arms will go, you don't. If the stretch is too much for you, bend your elbows until you gain flexibility. Or if you're tight throughout your shoulders, work only one arm at a time while letting your other arm rest at your side. Work the opposite arm of the leg that steps forward.

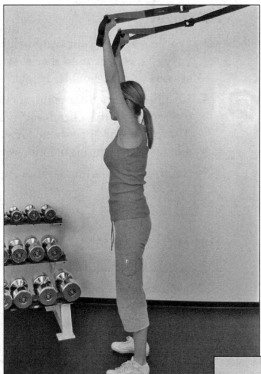

Starting/ending position.

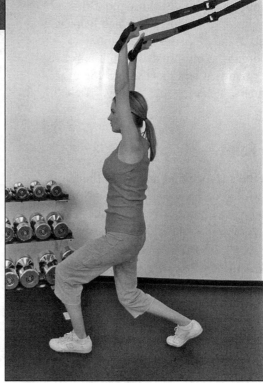

Midpoint position.

Isolated W

Remember the lying wave good-bye exercise from the beginner body weight moves in Chapter 6? That exercise showed you how to keep your shoulder blades down and back as you raise your arms overhead. In this version of that move, you work against gravity and your body weight to pump up the challenge.

In addition to focusing on your upper back, the isolated W targets your abs and shoulders. Want to know a simple trick that will make this exercise work the muscles of your hips and spine more? Keep your body straight like a plank rather than letting it collapse like a wet noodle. By maintaining a firm posture, you'll move through the exercise more efficiently.

Real-Life Activities It Helps You Do

Keeping your body straight throughout this exercise improves your posture, which helps you breathe better and increases blood supply to your vital organs. Not only that, you'll improve your performance at any sport where you use your shoulders, including kite surfing, baseball, and tennis.

Starting Point

1. Face the anchor point and grasp the handles with your arms straight out in front of you a little higher than shoulder height with your palms facing down. Be sure there's no slack in the system.

2. Walk your feet forward until they're slightly ahead of your hands about hip-width apart. Your body should be angled slightly back at this point as if you were leaning back against an angled wall.

Movement

3. Working against your body weight, pull your elbows back until they're straight out at your sides at shoulder height.

4. Keeping your body straight, rotate your forearms up into a "hands up" position. This pulls your upper body forward so you end up in a normal standing position.

5. Return to the starting position, and repeat 10 to 12 times.

Tips and Precautions

The isolated W is a perfect example of how the TRX can make an exercise easier or more difficult based on your body position. If you don't have enough strength to pull up your body weight, shift your feet farther away from the TRX in the starting position so you aren't leaning back as far. If the exercise seems too easy, you can add more body weight by starting with your feet closer to the anchor point so your body is leaning back more.

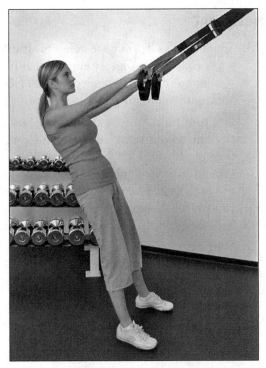

Starting/ending position.

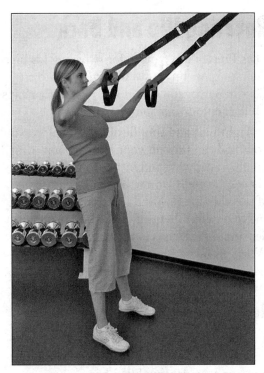

First position.

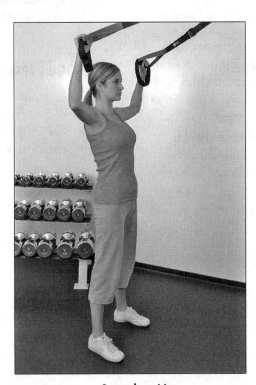

Second position.

Rotating Hip and Back

Elvis Presley was famous for swiveling his hips. I don't expect this move to turn you into an Elvis impersonator, but it will loosen your hips while rotating your spine.

Tight hips and an inflexible spine plague millions and can prevent your body from moving fluidly in daily life and in sporting activities. Having flexibility in the hips and spine is one of the keys to improved functional movement and gives you a better foundation for the more demanding exercises in upcoming chapters. When you start feeling the results of this exercise, you'll be saying, "Hip, hip, hooray!"

Real-Life Activities It Helps You Do

This exercise teaches you how to rotate your hips and torso, which helps with walking, running, or even dancing like Elvis.

Starting Point

1. Face the anchor point, and grasp the handles with your arms straight out in front of you a little higher than shoulder height with your palms facing each other. Be sure there's no slack in the system.

2. Walk your feet forward until they're slightly ahead of your hands about hip-width apart. Your body should be angled slightly back at this point as if you were leaning against an angled wall.

Movement

3. Squat back as if you were going to sit into a low chair. Squat deeply enough that if you let go of the handles, you would fall back onto your rear end.

4. Lift your right foot off the ground, and straighten your right leg in front of you; then place your right heel back on the ground with your foot flexed so it's pointing in the air, similar to the way you would step on the brakes in your car. Your right heel should be in line with your left toes.

5. Without moving your feet, rotate your right hip and torso to the right. Look under your right armpit. You'll feel a deep stretch on the right side of your body in this position.

6. Return to the starting position, and switch sides so you're straightening your left leg while rotating to the left. This completes 1 repetition. Keep alternating sides until you've done 8 to 10 reps.

Tips and Precautions

The placement of your feet determines the difficulty of this exercise. Starting with your feet farther forward will be more strenuous; placing them farther back will lighten the load.

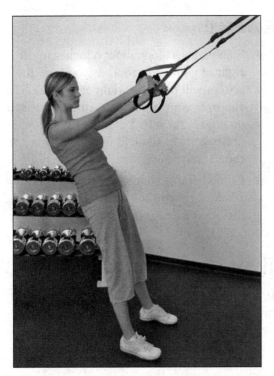

Starting/ending position.

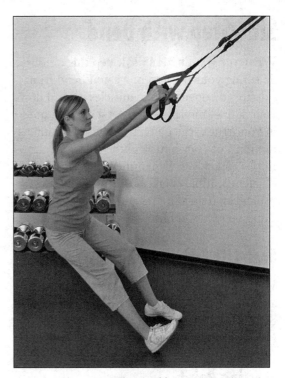

First position.

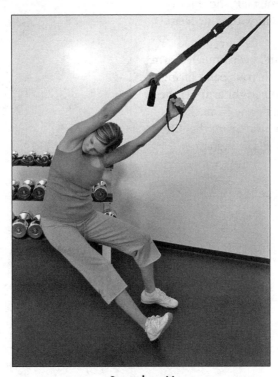

Second position.

Side Step with Bend

Whatever you do, don't sidestep this exercise! Teaching your body to move and bend from side to side opens all the muscles up and down your sides—the latissimus dorsi and obliques in your trunk, the gluteus medius and gluteus minimus of your butt, and the sides of your thighs and calves. When these muscles work efficiently, it helps take stress off your back, which can help alleviate and prevent back pain. Can you say "Ahhhhhh"?

Real-Life Activities It Helps You Do

When you reach over in bed to turn off your alarm clock, when you're reaching up to pull the curtains shut, or when you're dusting along a high shelf, you're using these side muscles.

Starting Point

1. Turn your body so your left shoulder is facing the anchor point with your feet hip-width apart.

2. Grasp the handles, and keep your left arm down at your side with your palm facing your thigh. Reach your right arm overhead with your palm facing away from the system. Scoot your feet away from the TRX until there's no slack in the system.

Movement

3. Step your left foot about 6 inches to the right of your right foot. As you step, the system will pull your right arm to the left and over your head, increasing the stretch on your right side. Let the TRX pull your upper body to the left, but don't rotate or round your spine.

4. Come back to your starting point, and do 10 to 12 repetitions before switching to the other side.

Tips and Precautions

If your back is really tight, take a smaller step to minimize the amount of bending. As you gain flexibility, take larger steps.

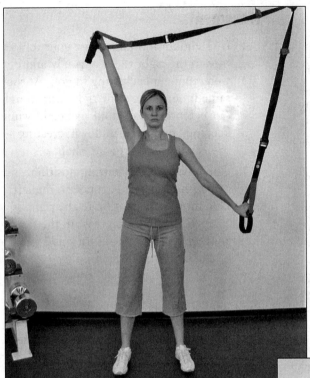

Starting/ending position.

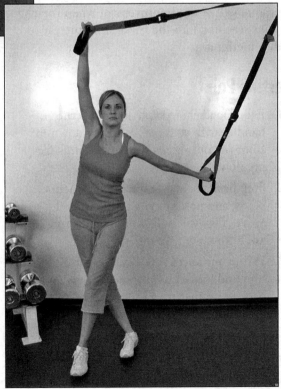

Midpoint position.

Trunk Rotations

To keep your car running smoothly, you head to your local mechanic for a lube job. What if you could do the same for your back? That's the basic concept behind this exercise. Just like your car needs oil, the discs in your back need fluids to maintain mobility. The best way to hydrate these discs is to get your spine moving with exercises like trunk rotations.

If your back is tight, ease into these spinal twists gently. Start with small movements, and gradually increase the twist as you get more comfortable.

Real-Life Activities It Helps You Do

If you're a golfer, baseball player, or tennis player, you'll love this move because greater trunk rotation can add power to your game. Everyone will notice improvement when rotating and reaching into the backseat of the car to grab something.

Starting Point

1. Face the anchor point, and grasp the handles with your arms straight down in front of your thighs with your palms facing down.

2. Step back about 3 feet from the anchor point, and position your feet hip-width apart. This will pull your arms up and away from your thighs.

3. With your knees soft, bend forward at the hips and look at the handles. Keep your back flat rather than rounding it. This position is similar to the way your body would look if you were diving off a diving board into a pool.

Movement

4. In a smooth motion, rotate your torso and hips to the right the way you would if you were taking a backswing in golf. At the same time, swing your right arm straight out behind you at shoulder height while keeping your left arm down, creating something similar to a T shape.

5. Come back to the starting position, and without pausing, rotate to the left. Counting each rotation to the right as 1 repetition and each twist to the left as another, keep swinging back and forth for a total of 20 to 30 repetitions.

Tips and Precautions

Remember that the TRX can pull you into a greater range of motion than you're used to, so move through this exercise slowly at first.

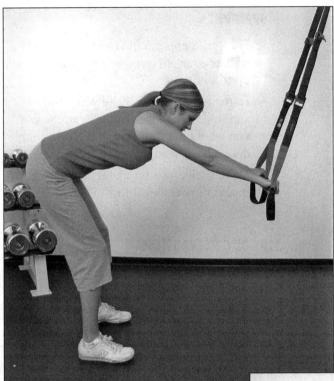

Starting/ending position.

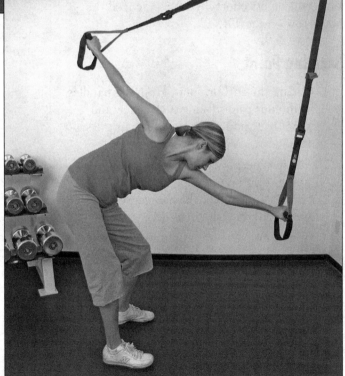

Midpoint position.

Squat Row

The squat row gets your whole body involved, strengthening your legs and butt while also targeting your upper body. As you've learned, anytime you work your upper and lower body at the same time, you have to engage your abs to coordinate the movement.

Even better, this full-body exercise also trains you to use good posture. When your body is aligned properly, you can work against gravity much easier, no matter what activity you're doing. Think of your body as a house of cards—if all the cards are stacked correctly, you can build it sky-high, but if a single card is in the wrong place, the whole thing will tumble down.

Real-Life Activities It Helps You Do

Standing for long periods of time, walking, climbing stairs, jumping, and lifting heavy objects take less effort if you've practiced the squat row on the TRX.

Starting Point

1. Facing the anchor point, grasp the handles with your palms facing each other, and scoot back until there's no slack in the system.

2. Squat as deeply as possible as if you were going to sit on the floor. You should feel that if you let go of the handles, you would fall on your backside.

Movement

3. Using the muscles in your legs and butt as well as your upper body, pull yourself back up to standing.

4. In the same motion, bend your elbows and pull the handles toward you the way you would pull on the handles of a double door. Avoid shrugging your shoulders.

5. Drop back down into your squat, and repeat the exercise 10 to 15 times.

Tips and Precautions

Here's another example of how the TRX can work with you as your fitness level progresses. When you're first starting your functional training program, you may not have adequate strength in your legs and butt to come up out of this deep squat, so you may need to rely more on your upper body to pull you up. As your fitness level improves, you'll find that you don't need to use your arms as much to return to standing.

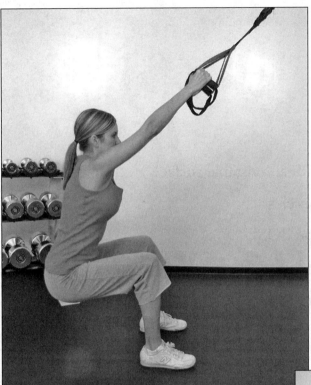

Starting/ending position.

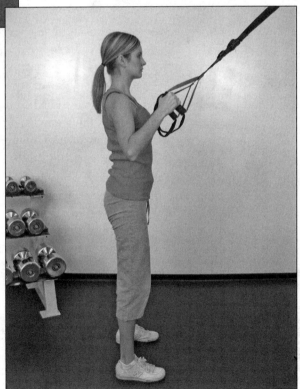

Midpoint position.

In This Chapter

- Getting acquainted with an unstable surface
- Engaging your feet muscles
- Stepping on and off the BOSU
- Standing on the BOSU
- Waking up your brain

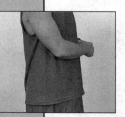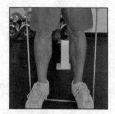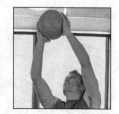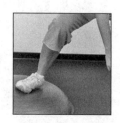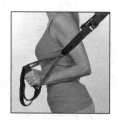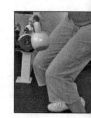

10

Beginner BOSU Exercises

The BOSU is going to rock your world—literally. This ingenious exercise tool provides an unstable surface that will have you shaking and wobbling as you try to keep yourself balanced. For many people, the BOSU is the most challenging of all the functional training tools because it takes away that nice, stable surface called the ground that we've all become accustomed to.

The exercises in this chapter are intended to introduce you to the one-of-a-kind feeling of the BOSU. When you first step onto it, you might feel like you're standing on a really firm mound of Jell-O. Because the sensation is so different from standing on terra firma, approach the BOSU with caution. The first time you give it a go, you might want to position it near a wall or countertop so you can reach out to support yourself if you feel like you're going to topple over. A good rule to remember when using the BOSU is if you feel like you're going to do a face plant and absolutely can't right yourself, just step off of it and get right back on to continue your exercise. No harm, no foul.

With practice, you'll become more comfortable on the BOSU, and you'll notice your balance improving dramatically. Thanks to these exercises, you'll begin to feel a lot more confident when facing uneven surfaces in the outside world, whether you're hiking on a trail, walking on cobblestones, or running in the sand on the beach.

Alternating Front Step with Partial Lunge

This exercise is designed to introduce you to the BOSU and the way it wiggles and jiggles when you step on it. To keep you safe as you're starting out, you'll keep one foot firmly on the ground at all times as you alternate placing one foot and then the other on the BOSU. As soon as your foot touches the BOSU, you'll feel it start to twitch like crazy. Those are your stabilizing muscles kicking in to keep you balanced.

This basic move lays the foundation for all the other BOSU exercises to come so be sure you master it before moving on.

Real-Life Activities It Helps You Do

By practicing this move, you'll find it easier to step onto an ice rink, step up into one of those bouncy castles to retrieve your child, hike on a rocky trail, or walk on cobblestone streets.

Starting Point

1. Stand about 18 to 24 inches behind the BOSU with your feet hip-width apart, your torso erect, and your arms down at your sides. Keep your eyes on the BOSU throughout the exercise.

Movement

2. Step your left foot onto the BOSU so the ball of your foot is slightly behind the top of the dome toward you. As if you were walking normally, swing your right arm forward at the same time.

3. Push off your left foot to return to standing on the ground, and step onto the BOSU with your right foot while swinging your left arm forward. Continue stepping left and right 20 times.

Tips and Precautions

Consider placing the BOSU near a wall or countertop at first in case you need help balancing. As you get more comfortable with this move, start farther behind the BOSU so you have to take a bigger step, swing your arms higher, and don't look at the BOSU.

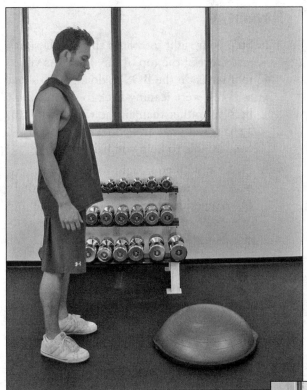

Starting/ending position.

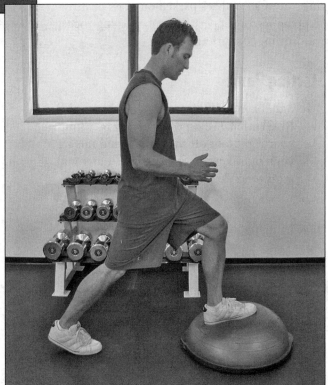

Midpoint position.

Side Step with Partial Squat

In the preceding exercise, you learned how to step onto the BOSU going forward and backward. Here, you'll be stepping to the side instead. Your side step will wake up all the muscles on the outer side of the leg that's stepping onto the BOSU while engaging the inner thigh muscles of the leg that remains on the ground.

Because you're standing to the side of the BOSU and aren't looking directly at it, this exercise also poses a bigger balance challenge than the forward steps. You'll probably find that this side move requires more concentration than moving straight ahead, so put on your thinking cap and get started!

Real-Life Activities It Helps You Do

Learning to step to the side onto an unstable surface gives you an advantage when you're getting out of a car that's parked on grass or dirt, stepping into a slippery bathtub, playing soccer, windsurfing, or surfing.

Starting Point

1. Stand about 2½ feet to the left side of the BOSU. Balance on your left leg by lifting your right foot off the ground and raising your right knee in front of you. Let your arms relax down at your sides.

Movement

2. Step your right foot onto the BOSU so it's just short of the top of the dome. As your foot lands on the BOSU, do a partial squat as if you were leaning back to sit on a high barstool rather than all the way down into a chair. Let your arms do whatever feels comfortable to help you balance.

3. Push off with your right foot to come back to your one-leg stand, and do a total of 12 repetitions before moving to the other side of the BOSU to repeat the exercise using your other leg.

Tips and Precautions

To increase the amount of work your feet have to do, try this exercise with bare feet. This tip applies to nearly every BOSU exercise.

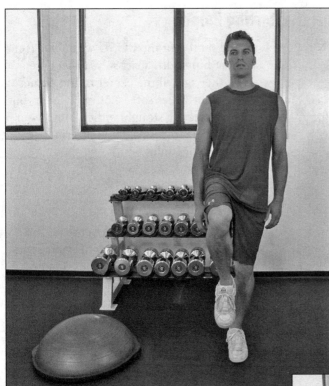

Starting/ending position.

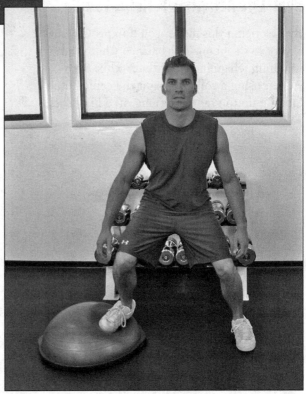

Midpoint position.

Stand with Reach-Up and Head Tilt

Now that you've mastered stepping on and off the BOSU, you're ready to try standing on it with both feet. Having both feet on the unstable surface intensifies the balance challenge and activates all the stabilizing muscles throughout both sides of your body.

What can really throw you for a loop, though, is the seemingly easy head tilt at the end of this exercise. Anytime you look up, it upsets your inner ear fluid, which is instrumental in your body's ability to maintain balance. By combining the unstable surface of the BOSU with the head tilt, this exercise makes your muscles and nervous system work overtime to keep you upright.

Real-Life Activities It Helps You Do

By practicing this move, you'll improve your ability to maintain your balance while bird watching, changing a lightbulb while on a ladder, using a roller to paint the ceiling, and looking up to grab something off a high shelf.

Starting Point

1. Stand on top of the BOSU with your feet almost hip-width apart so your feet are on either side of the center of the dome. Keep your knees soft—not really bent, but not completely straight either. With your eyes looking forward, let your arms relax down at your sides.

Movement

2. Swing both arms straight overhead, and when you feel comfortable, tilt your head back and look up at your hands. Come back to the start position and repeat 10 to 12 times.

Tips and Precautions

Be sure you feel relatively stable on the BOSU at each stage of this exercise before proceeding to the next move. If you don't feel confident, eliminate the head tilt or the arm reach and gradually work up to those moves.

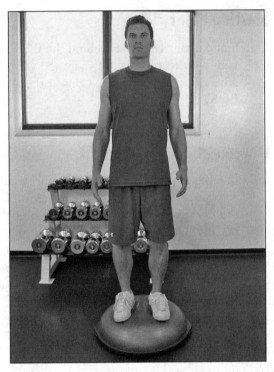

Starting/ending position.

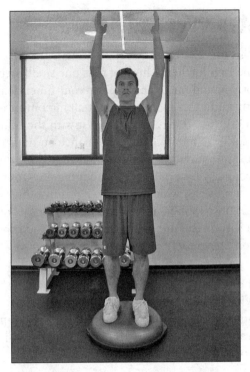

First position.

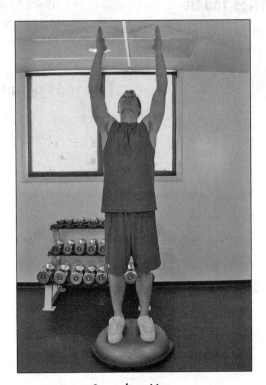

Second position.

Step Over and Back

This exercise takes the alternating front step one step further. Think of it as one small step for you and one giant leap for your functional fitness. In this move, you're stepping onto the BOSU and then walking over it with the other leg so one foot will have to balance on the unstable surface while the other foot is off the ground. This really starts strengthening your foot muscles, which can have a positive effect on the muscles in your legs and hips. Think about it: if your feet are stronger, your legs and hips won't have to work as hard when you move.

If you're like most people, you'll find that one side is much easier to do than the other. With practice and attention to proper technique, these imbalances should begin to disappear, which will greatly improve your overall movement and balance.

Real-Life Activities It Helps You Do

Thanks to this exercise, you'll feel more comfortable rock hopping, hiking on uneven surfaces, stepping over a picnic blanket onto the grass on the other side, or walking over a speed bump in the road.

Starting Point

1. Stand about 18 inches behind the BOSU with your feet hip-width apart and your arms down at your sides. Look at the BOSU.

Movement

2. In a regular walking motion, step forward with your right foot onto the center of the BOSU, and bring your left leg over the BOSU onto the ground in front of it as you bend your knees slightly. Let your arms swing naturally as you walk. Lift your left leg back over the BOSU to where you started. As your left foot hits the ground, step back to the starting position with your right foot. That equals 1 repetition.

3. Repeat the exercise by stepping onto the BOSU with your left foot and stepping over it with your right. Keep alternating sides until you've completed a total of 20 to 24 repetitions.

Tips and Precautions

Imagine there's a gymnast's balance beam under the BOSU and you have to keep the foot that's stepping over the BOSU in line to stay on the beam.

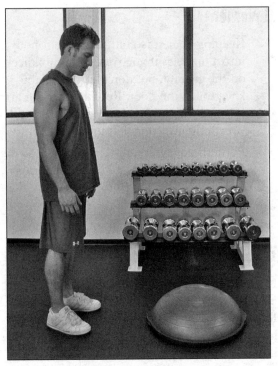

Starting/ending position.

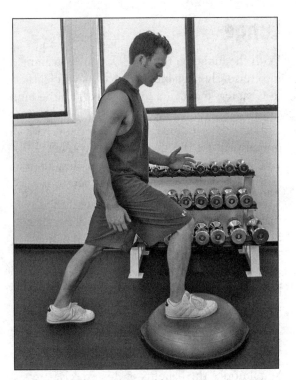

First position.

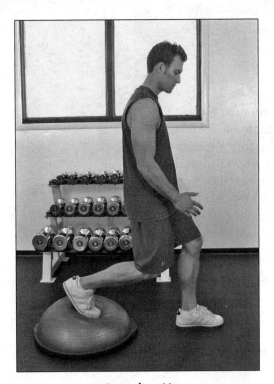

Second position.

Lunge

With the lunge on the BOSU, you're heading into seriously unstable territory. As you learned in Chapters 6 and 7, a lunge targets all the big muscles in your calves, hamstrings, quads, inner and outer thighs, hips, and glutes. Now, with one of your feet on the BOSU as you lunge, you'll be asking all the smaller muscles, known as the stabilizers, to get in on the act, too.

At first, this will seem a lot more difficult than the simple forward steps you did earlier, but as you progress, it will feel much easier. With all those small stabilizing muscles contributing, it's like you now have 100 employees helping you maintain your balance rather than just 5.

Real-Life Activities It Helps You Do

You'll notice the benefits of this exercise anytime you ski, ice skate, shovel snow, pick up leaves in the garden, or bend down to clean up after your dog.

Starting Point

1. Stand about 2 feet behind the BOSU, and step forward with your left foot as if you were walking normally and let it land on top of the dome with your left knee bent. Keep your right foot on the ground behind the BOSU, with your torso erect and your eyes facing forward, and let your arms hang down at your sides.

Movement

2. Keeping your torso tall, lower your body into a lunge as if you were going to kneel on the ground, but don't let your right knee touch the floor. Reach your right arm forward without leaning forward and feel your weight in your left foot.

3. Push off your left foot to come back to the starting position. Do 10 to 12 repetitions, and change legs for 10 to 12 more on the other side.

Tips and Precautions

If you start to lose your balance as you lunge, push down with the big toe of the foot on the BOSU. You'll be surprised how much this can help. You can turn this into an alternating lunge if you like by bringing both feet onto the floor after you lunge and then lunging forward with the other foot on the BOSU.

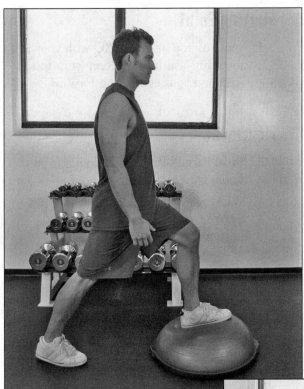

Starting/ending position.

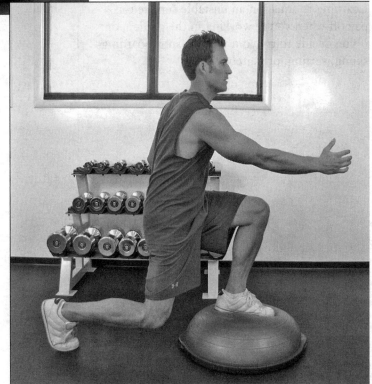

Midpoint position.

Partial Squat

By now, you're already familiar with the partial squat, which targets all the major muscles in the lower body. You're about to discover how much more challenging this move can be when it's performed on the BOSU. Because squatting changes your center of gravity, you're going to have to fight really hard to stay steady. In the beginning, your arms will probably flail around to keep you from falling off as if you were trying to surf or snowboard for the first time. With practice, however, you should be able to keep your body relatively still in the partial squat position.

Your goal should be to feel comfortable in this position before moving on to the intermediate BOSU exercises.

Real-Life Activities It Helps You Do

Learning to squat on an unstable surface can pay off when you're working in the garden, or if you decide to try your hand at snowboarding, skiing, surfing, or skateboarding.

Starting Point

1. Stand on top of the BOSU with your feet about hip-width apart. Keep your torso erect and your eyes facing forward.

Movement

2. Squat back as if you were trying to sit on a high barstool, and reach your arms out in front of you to help you balance.
3. Return to standing and repeat 10 to 12 times.

Tips and Precautions

Don't be surprised if you start to shake while squatting—that's just your nervous system freaking out from the new sensation of the unstable surface. With practice, the shaking should diminish.

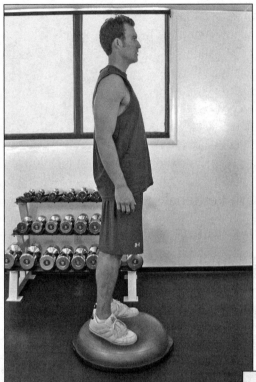

Starting/ending position.

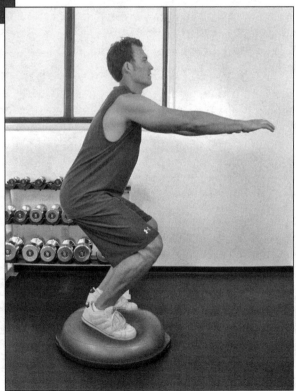

Midpoint position.

In This Chapter

- Building strength with kettlebells
- Improving coordination with kettlebells
- Increasing range of motion with kettlebells
- Getting more flexible with kettlebells

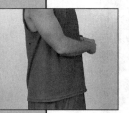 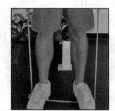 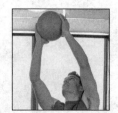 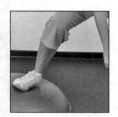 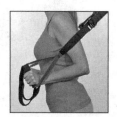 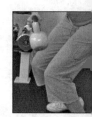

Chapter 11

Beginner Kettlebell Exercises

More than 300 years ago, when kettlebells were first designed, they weren't intended for functional training. Originally, Russian lifters used them to perform a limited series of traditional lifting exercises in strongman competitions. In this chapter, I've taken some of those time-honored kettlebell movements and put a new spin on them to create truly functional exercises that help you move better. When you use the kettlebells in this new way, they become one of the best tools available to improve your functional fitness.

More than any other tool in this book, kettlebells help you build strength, which makes it easier to perform all kinds of everyday tasks. But that's not all. Strengthening tendons and ligaments provides better joint stability to help you avoid common injuries like ankle and knee sprains. Another plus: swinging the cannonball-like weights increases your range of motion as you work out, which adds up to better flexibility.

Exercising with kettlebells also forces you to improve your timing and coordination. If you don't time your movements just right, you'll end up whacking yourself. Ouch! Because of this, the exercises in this chapter involve smaller movements to help you get a feel for the kettlebells. Be sure you master these basic moves before attempting the more dynamic exercises in later chapters.

Two-Arm Carry

With this exercise, you're taking everything you've learned so far about walking better and adding weight to the equation. With the two-arm carry, you'll be walking while carrying the kettlebells, the same way you would tote shopping bags or luggage. When you perfect this move, you might want to ditch the car, walk to the grocery store, and carry your groceries back home.

Real-Life Activities It Helps You Do

Two-arm carry helps make activities like carrying shopping bags, luggage, a bike, or a surfboard at your side easier. You'll also notice improvement when using a wheelbarrow or bowling.

Starting Point

1. With your feet hip-width apart, place the kettlebells on the ground just to the outsides of your feet.

2. Bend down at your hips and knees, and round your spine to grasp the kettlebells. Use the muscles in your legs and butt to help you stand up. Don't flatten your back and use it like a crane to come up to standing.

3. Hold the kettlebells down at your side.

Movement

4. Keeping your torso erect and your eyes facing forward, step forward with your right foot and then your left foot in a typical walking motion. As you walk, let your arms hang down by your sides rather than swinging them back and forth. If you can take about 50 to 75 steps, you're using the proper weight. Adjust the weight of the kettlebells higher or lower until you can take that many steps. In a small area, you can walk to one end of the room, turn around, and continue walking.

Tips and Precautions

The first time you pick up the kettlebells, be aware that they are heavy. A lot of my clients have trouble holding their arms down at their sides with the increased weight, and they hunch forward. Wrong! Walking tall with your spine erect and your shoulders back and down causes less stress on your body.

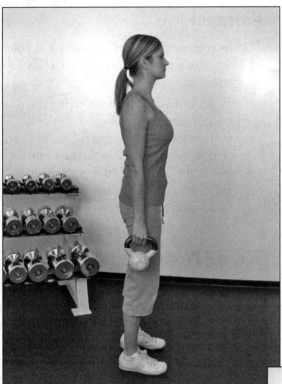

Starting/ending position.

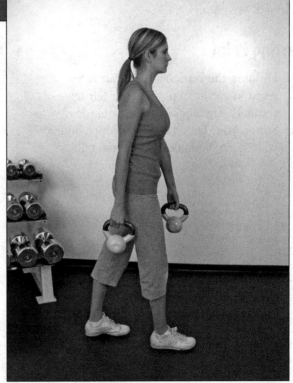

Midpoint position.

Split Step with Two-Arm Swings

You'll definitely get into the swing of the kettle-bells with this move. Swinging your arms back and forth while holding the kettlebells primarily targets your obliques but also engages the muscles in your lower body to keep you stabilized. Just how hard your abs have to work depends on how far you swing the kettlebells. The farther you swing them, the more you'll feel it in your midsection. (At first, keep the swinging to a minimum until you get a feel for them.)

Real-Life Activities It Helps You Do

As you might expect, swinging a golf club, a baseball bat, or a tennis racquet will feel more fluid after you practice this move. You'll also notice improvement when walking, running, or opening a car door.

Starting Point

1. Holding the kettlebells by your sides, stand in a split step with your left leg about 1½ feet ahead of your right leg. Soften your knees, keep your hips under your spine, and keep your torso tall.

Movement

2. Swing your right arm forward and your left arm back, the way you do when you're walking.

3. Without hesitating or changing the position of your legs, change directions, swinging your right arm back and your left arm forward. This completes 1 repetition. Shoot for a total of 10 to 15 repetitions, and then switch legs so your right leg is in front and repeat the exercise.

Tips and Precautions

Start with small swings to get the hang of moving the kettlebells without hitting your legs. As you feel more comfortable, increase the swinging motion to pump up the intensity of the exercise.

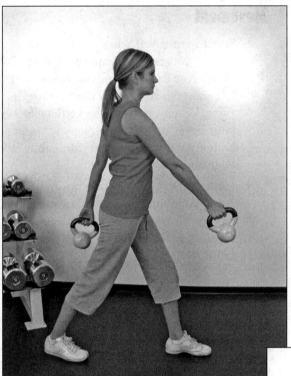

Starting/ending position.

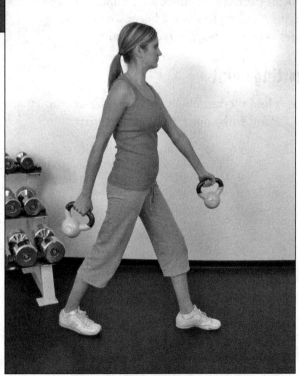

Midpoint position.

Partial Squat with Front-Back Arm Swings

Ready to squat and swing? Swinging the kettle-bells in front and behind you while you squat not only wakes up your abs, but also activates the muscles in your legs and butt. It sounds simple enough, but this move can be tricky. You'll need to use a good dose of brain power to keep your arms moving fluidly in opposite directions. I've found that when most people get the hang of it, they think this move is a lot of fun, and I love putting some "fun" in functional training.

Real-Life Activities It Helps You Do

This squat-and-swing exercise can facilitate some of the simplest tasks, such as rolling over in bed or turning to check your blind spot while driving. It also gives you a boost when dancing, water skiing, or playing racquet sports.

Starting Point

1. Hold the kettlebells by your sides as you stand with your feet hip-width apart.

Movement

2. Squat lightly as if you were going to sit on a high barstool as you swing your right arm across the front of your body to the left and your left arm behind you to the right. When swinging the kettlebells, keep your lower body still and let your upper body rotate, making sure your palms face your body.

3. Come back to the starting position, and swing your right arm behind you and your left arm in front of you. This completes 1 repetition. Do a total of 10 to 15 repetitions.

Tips and Precautions

Your arms have to come away from your body to swing without hitting your butt or your knees.

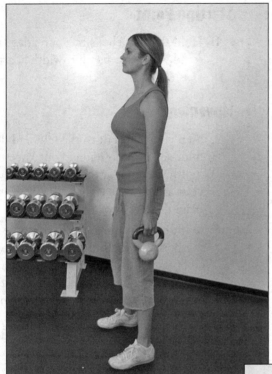

Starting/ending position.

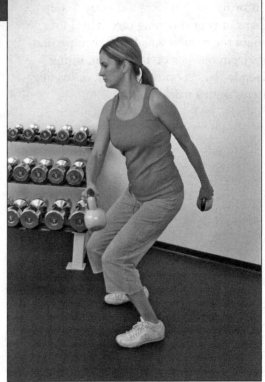

Midpoint position.

Side Step Two-Arm Opposite Swing

By now, you're probably turning into a real "swinger." Here's another chance to swing the kettlebells, only this time, you move them both in the same direction. Swinging both kettlebells to one side taxes your trunk's rotary and lateral muscles. In addition, your inner and outer thighs have to get involved for stabilization. These are the same muscles you use every time you pick up something on one side and put it back down on the other side—a functional movement you probably do every single day.

Real-Life Activities It Helps You Do

The next time you go to the grocery store or the hardware store, notice how you swing your arms to one side to pick up items off the shelf and then swing them the opposite way to put those items in your shopping cart. This move also mimics the motion you'd use when passing sandbags from one person to another, lifting a heavy laundry basket onto a counter, or loading heavy items onto a truck bed.

Starting Point

1. Hold the kettlebells by your sides as you stand with your feet hip-width apart.

Movement

2. Step your left foot to the left, and do a mini-squat by softening your knees and lightly bending at the hips. Swing both of your arms to the right, allowing them to bend if necessary.

3. Without pausing, come back to the starting position and immediately step to the right with your right foot as your arms swing in the opposite direction. Let your arms continue swinging back and forth like a pendulum as you step from side to side for a total of 10 to 15 back-and-forth swings.

Tips and Precautions

Start with a gentle swing, and hold the kettlebells far enough in front of you so you don't hit your knees with them.

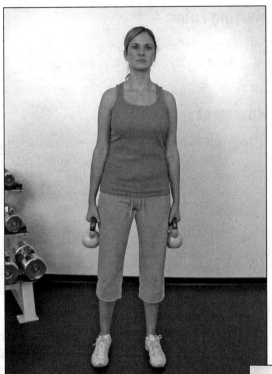

Starting/ending position.

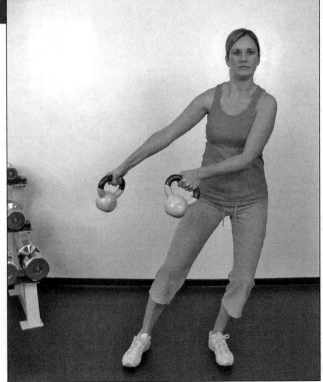

Midpoint position.

Squat

If you've done all the exercises to this point, you're already very familiar with the squat and how it targets the muscles in your legs and butt. Here, you add the weight of the kettlebells to this basic move to increase the intensity.

A lot of people tend to lean forward when performing a squat with the kettlebells. Don't! If you lean forward, your center of gravity shifts forward and you place more stress on your knees. By keeping your spine upright, you can keep the exercise focused on your legs and butt. This keeps your knees happy.

Real-Life Activities It Helps You Do

Anytime you scoop up a toddler off the ground, pick up a case of water bottles, or move furniture, you'll be grateful you practiced this kettlebell squat.

Starting Point

1. Hold the kettlebells by your sides as you stand with your feet hip-width apart.

Movement

2. Squat as if you were going to sit back into a chair. Keep your weight on your heels, and keep the kettlebells in line with your heels rather than letting them swing forward.

3. Push into your heels to come back to standing and then repeat the squat 10 to 15 times.

Tips and Precautions

The lower you squat, the tougher it is to keep your spine erect.

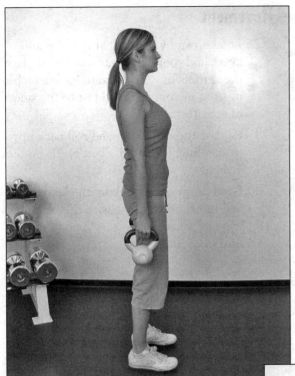

Starting/ending position.

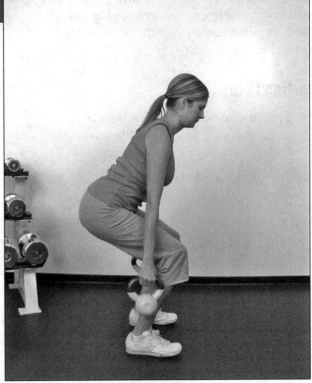

Midpoint position.

Pick Up, Put Down

Bending down to pick up or put down something is something we all have to do on a daily basis. For many people, though, this common movement isn't easy. A tight or achy back often prevents people from wanting to bend down this way.

Here, you train the muscles in your back as you round your spine to reach the ground. This increases your strength and improves your flexibility so you can place heavy objects on the ground or pick them up with greater ease. The next time you're faced with a heavy box that needs to be moved, you won't have to ask someone else to do it for you.

Real-Life Activities It Helps You Do

Pick up, put down helps you when lifting heavy objects off the floor, moving furniture, getting down low to tackle an opponent playing football, or bending down to get the ropes or open the hatches when sailing.

Starting Point

1. Hold the kettlebells by your sides as you stand with your feet hip-width apart.

Movement

2. Bend down by bending at the hips and knees and rounding your spine, and place the kettlebells on the ground a few inches in front of your toes and just to the sides of your feet.

3. Release the kettlebells and roll back up to standing, leaving the kettlebells on the ground.

4. Bend down again, pick up the kettlebells, and return to standing with the kettlebells by your sides. Repeat this series 8 to 12 times.

Tips and Precautions

Move slowly and gently at first, and gradually begin speeding up the transition from one position to the other.

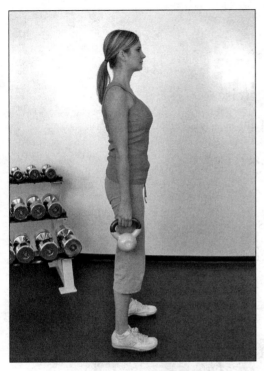

Starting/ending position.

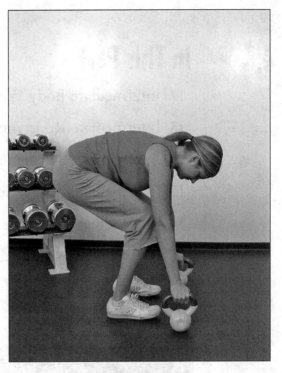

First position.

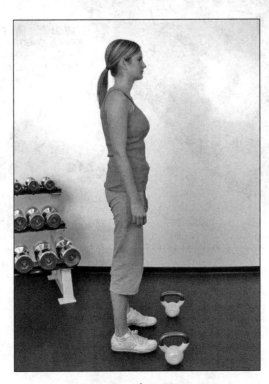

Second position.

In This Part

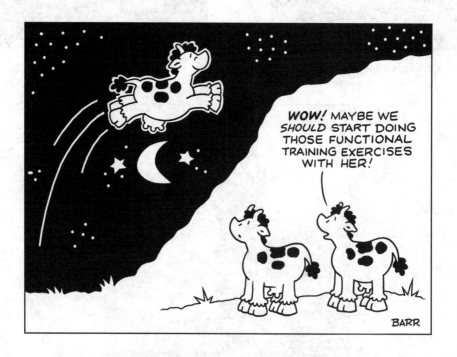

Part 4

Intermediate Functional Exercises

Now that you've been introduced to the basics of functional training, it's time to step it up with more challenging exercises. Part 4 promises to wake up muscles you never knew you had and test your balance and coordination.

When you're able to perform these exercises, you'll know you're on the road to functional fitness!

In This Chapter

- ◆ Creating more body resistance
- ◆ Moving in more than one direction at the same time
- ◆ Ramping up the speed
- ◆ Bending and extending your spine
- ◆ Softening your impact with the ground

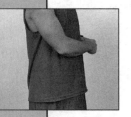 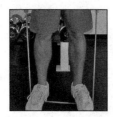 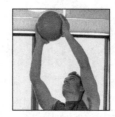 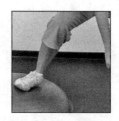 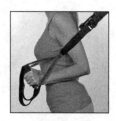 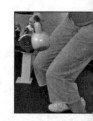

Chapter 12

Intermediate Body Weight Exercises

If you've mastered the beginner body weight exercises in Chapter 6, try these intermediate exercises. Being able to perform the beginner movements using the proper form ensures that you're functionally fit enough to tackle these exercises, which are more physically demanding.

To do the exercises in this chapter, you won't need any equipment—just your body weight working against gravity. What makes these exercises more complex than the beginner body weight movements? First, they require your body to move more dynamically in multiple directions. Second, they add speed to the equation. Third, they involve moving your limbs farther away from your center of gravity, which adds to the resistance.

Thanks to these new elements, your body has to work harder against gravity. Because of this, you'll begin to learn one of the most important secrets of functional training—how to react softly with the ground while moving so there's less impact on your body. Less impact equals less stress on the joints and, ultimately, less chance of pain or injury. When you don't have any pain or injuries, your body moves better and more freely, and that's the main goal of functional training.

Forward Crawl

The forward crawl mimics one of our most primal movement patterns: using the opposite arm and leg while moving. This pattern is so basic, even babies do it naturally when they first start crawling. The action teaches babies how to coordinate movement, and this exercise does the same for you.

Using both your upper and lower body, the forward crawl forces you to integrate coordination into your movement. Although it's a whole-body exercise that works nearly every muscle you've got, you'll feel it more in your upper body, especially in your arms and shoulders.

Real-Life Activities It Helps You Do

This exercise helps with walking and running whether you amble at a leisurely pace or run a 6-minute mile. It also simulates a climbing motion, which can come in handy if you have to climb a ladder to fix a leaky roof or if you're a rock climber.

Starting Point

1. Start down on the ground on all fours with the palms of your hands and the balls of your feet on the floor. Your arms should be about shoulder-width apart, and your feet should be about hip-width apart. Your butt should be up in the air, and your knees should be bent, but don't let them touch the floor.

2. Keep your eyes facing down at the ground rather than looking up, which can strain your neck.

Movement

3. Start to crawl just like you did when you were a baby, only don't let your knees touch the ground. Simultaneously move your right arm and left foot forward as far as is comfortable. As soon as they touch the ground, shift your left arm and your right foot forward.

4. Keep crawling on your hands and feet for 20 to 30 yards, or about 15 steps.

Tips and Precautions

If you're like most people when you first try this exercise, you'll probably take bigger steps with your feet than with your arms, which will make your knees hit your arms. Shorten your footsteps so they match your arm movements. Also, avoid swaying your hips from side to side to prevent irritating your hip and knee joints. A great trick you can use to keep your hips from swaying is to pretend you're crawling on a plank and that you'll fall off if you don't move in a straight line. If you don't have enough space to go 20 to 30 yards in a straight line, crawl in a circle.

Variations

If this exercise is too difficult for you, crawl on your hands and knees on a carpeted floor. Do this until you work up to crawling on your hands and feet.

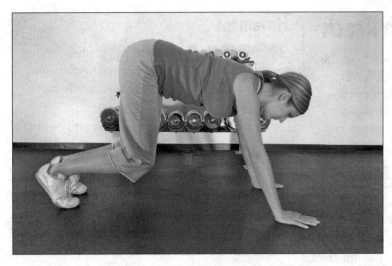

Starting/ending position.

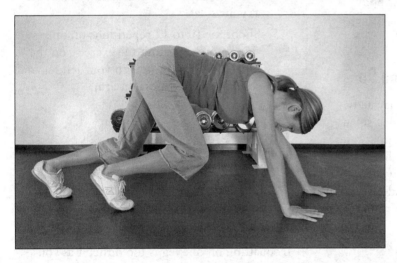

First position.

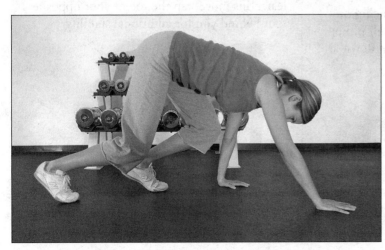

Second position.

Single-Leg Squat with Reach

The single-leg squat with reach starts where the one-leg stand you tried in Chapter 6 left off. Be sure you've mastered that move before trying this more challenging exercise, which adds a squat and a reach to pump up the balance and coordination required.

The good news is you're in charge of just how tough it gets by controlling how far down you squat and how far out you reach. The deeper you squat and farther you reach, the more intensity you'll add.

Although this exercise works both the upper and lower body, it's primarily a lower body movement that targets the glutes, quadriceps, hamstrings, and calves.

Real-Life Activities It Helps You Do

You'd be surprised how many everyday activities require you to perform a single-leg squat with reach, such as filling your glass at a water cooler and reaching for a pan at the back of a low kitchen cupboard. More active types might use this motion to lunge forward and hit a volley in tennis.

Starting Point

1. Start in a one-leg stand by balancing on your right leg and hiking your left hip up slightly. Hold your arms straight down at your sides.

Movement

2. Squat with your right leg, pushing your butt back as if you were trying to sit in a chair. Your left leg will naturally move behind your right leg.

3. As you squat, reach your left arm out in front of you and bring it across and down your body as if you were reaching out to pick up an overnight bag. Your left arm in front of you and your left leg behind you work as counterbalances to help keep you steady on your right leg.

4. Push off your right leg to come back to your one-leg stand with your arms down at your sides.

5. Shoot for 10 to 12 repetitions on one side before repeating the exercise on the other side, squatting with your left leg and reaching with your right arm.

Tips and Precautions

To avoid stressing your knee, be sure to sit back into your hips as you squat.

Variations

If squatting on one leg is too difficult as you learn this move, tap the toe of your opposite foot behind you for additional stability.

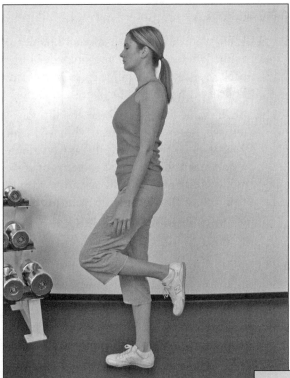

Starting/ending position.

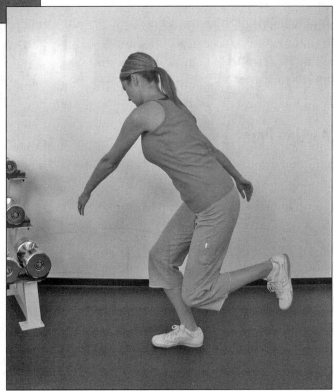

Midpoint position.

Side-to-Side Squat with Overhead Reach

Similar to the beginner partial side squat with lateral reach, this intermediate exercise combines side-to-side movement with an upper body reach. Some of my clients have a tough time getting the hang of this exercise because it really gets your body moving in different directions. That means you've got to exercise your brain, too, to be sure each part of your body is moving in the right direction. When you perform this exercise correctly, you'll feel it working all the way down the sides of your body from your arms to your feet.

Real-Life Activities It Helps You Do

Have you ever run a broom along the ceiling from one side of a room to the other to remove cobwebs? Have you ever hung curtains or taken them down to get them cleaned? While playing baseball, have you ever moved to the side and reached up to catch a high ball? Then you've probably used the very muscles involved in the side-to-side squat with overhead reach.

Starting Point

1. Stand with your feet facing forward about shoulder-width apart.

2. Hold your arms up so your elbows are at shoulder height and your forearms are bent up at 90 degrees with your palms facing forward, kind of as if a burglar had just told you "Hands up!"

Movement

3. Using your left leg, step about 18 inches to the left and squat so you sink your hips back the same way you do to sit in a chair. Your right leg should be almost straight.

4. At the same time, straighten and lift your left arm out over your head while you lean your body to the right as if you were doing a simple side bend. Don't rotate your torso or tilt your body forward or backward as you lean to the right. Relax your other hand down at your side. You'll feel a nice stretch along the side of your torso when you do this properly.

5. Return to the starting position and then squat to the right using the right leg while your right arm reaches over to the left. Keep alternating sides until you're done. A total of about 16 to 20 repetitions is a good goal.

Tips and Precautions

Keep your spine tall while you lean, and don't round your shoulders. Also, keep your eyes fixed forward. A lot of my clients try to look up while doing this exercise, which can strain the neck.

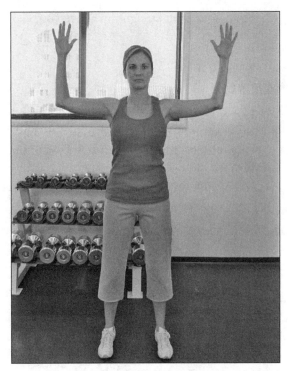

Starting/ending position.

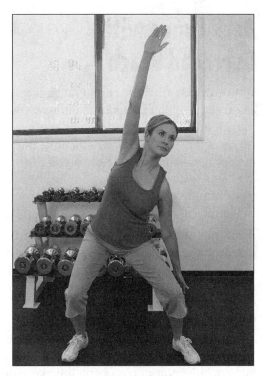

First position.

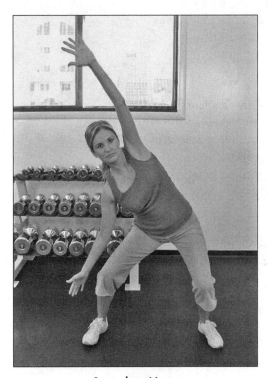

Second position.

Back Lunge with Overhead Reach

You've already tried the partial lunge (with crossover reach) in Chapter 6, and now you get to try a full lunge. Lunges are one of the best exercises you can do to strengthen the muscles in your legs and butt. And when you add an overhead reach, you engage your back muscles, too.

What makes this exercise such a winner is that it not only strengthens your legs and back, but also increases mobility in your hips and shoulders. Just try to find a single machine at the gym that can do all that at the same time!

Real-Life Activities It Helps You Do

Hooray for this exercise! Thanks to the back lunge with overhead reach, you'll find it easier to cheer at a football game or paint the ceiling. If you're more athletic, you'll improve your ability to jump up to catch a ball or field a goal in soccer.

Starting Point

1. Stand in a split stance—that's a fancy fitness term for standing with one leg ahead of the other. In this stance, your feet face forward about shoulder-width apart with your left leg about 18 inches behind your right leg. Bend your knees slightly, transfer your weight to your left leg, and tilt your pelvis under. This activates your left glute, increases the stretch in front of your left hip and makes the muscles in your upper back kick in.

2. Hold your arms straight up above your shoulders.

Movement

3. Lower yourself down into a lunge as if you were going to kneel on one knee, but don't let your knee touch the ground. Don't lean forward with your upper body or let your arms come forward.

4. Push yourself back up to standing, and repeat the exercise, taking your right foot back. Keep alternating sides until you've done 6 to 8 lunges on each side.

Tips and Precautions

As you take your arms overhead, don't shrug your shoulders. Keep pulling them down away from your neck the way you did in beginner movements like the lying wave good-bye and the lying straight-arm raise (see Chapter 6).

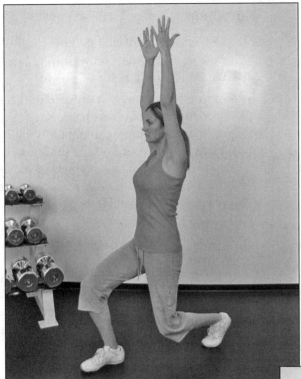

Starting/ending position.

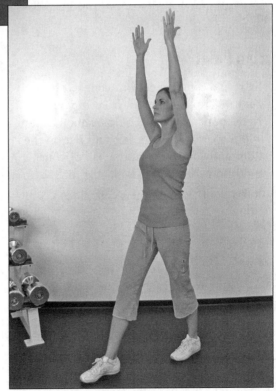

Midpoint position.

Lunge with Rotation

Did you know your obliques have about 36 separate functions? Traditional abdominal crunches and sit-ups only get the obliques to perform a handful of these functions. With the multi-muscle lunge with rotation, however, your obliques will be operating at full force, incorporating nearly every single one of those vital functions. That's thanks to the twist I've added to a basic lunge, another powerhouse exercise that targets several muscle groups at once.

Mastering this exercise strengthens your lower body while helping you learn to bend and rotate more efficiently.

Real-Life Activities It Helps You Do

This exercise helps you with activities that require you to twist your torso while your legs are moving forward, such as walking, running, or dancing.

Starting Point

1. Start in a split stance with your left foot about 18 to 24 inches in front of your right foot. Your feet should be about hip-width apart, with your left foot flat on the floor and your right on the ball of your foot. Both feet should be facing forward.
2. Relax your arms down at your sides.

Movement

3. Lower your body straight down as if you were going to kneel on your right knee, but don't let it touch the ground.
4. As you lunge, rotate your torso to the left, keeping your shoulders level. Reach your right arm out almost straight at shoulder height across your body to the left as if you were reaching out to pick up something off a counter. Only reach your arm as far as is comfortable.
5. Rotate back so you're facing forward as you simultaneously push with your left leg to raise your body back up to your split stance. Repeat 8 to 12 times with your left leg forward, and do another set of repetitions with your right leg forward as you twist your torso to the right and reach to the right with your left arm.

Tips and Precautions

Don't lean forward as you lunge because it will stress everything incorrectly. When you rotate, don't bend to the side or round your shoulders. Keep your torso erect and your shoulders level. It's better to rotate only a little rather than bend to try to increase the twist. If it's too hard for you to rotate with your arm outstretched, bring your arm in closer to your body.

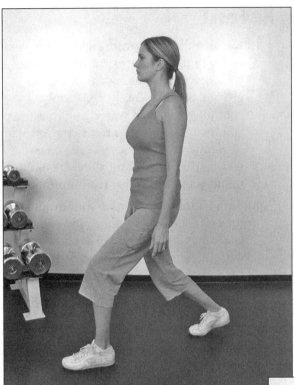

Starting/ending position.

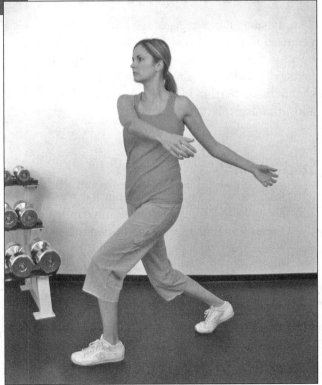

Midpoint position.

Lunge to Hip Stretch

This exercise adds speed and a dynamic up-and-down motion to your workout repertoire. Like so many functional training exercises, this movement gets your entire body working to strengthen and add flexibility to your ankles, knees, hips, spine, trunk, and shoulders.

You'll have to work extra hard against gravity in this exercise because it requires you to lean forward as if you were trying to pick up something off the floor. When you lean your body weight forward, your leg muscles have to fire to prevent you from falling forward. Getting back up to the starting position requires almost as much effort. Go slowly at first with this exercise until you get comfortable with the motion, and gradually add speed for a more explosive movement.

Real-Life Activities It Helps You Do

This dynamic move engages the same muscles you need to pull weeds in your garden or pick up a toddler off the floor and lift her overhead. It can also facilitate a simple game of catch, simulating the action of reaching down to field a low ball and then reaching up to catch a high ball.

Starting Point

1. Begin in a split stance with your left foot about 18 to 24 inches in front of your right foot. Your feet should be about hip-width apart, with your left foot flat on the floor and your right on the ball of your foot. Both feet should be facing forward.

2. Hold your arms down at your sides.

Movement

3. Keeping the ball of your right foot in contact with the floor, lower your body until your right knee is almost touching the ground. Simultaneously, bend forward at your hips and reach your right arm across your body toward the floor to the left side of your left foot as if you were going to pick up a quarter off the floor. It's okay to round your back as you reach for the floor.

4. Push up through your left foot to come back to a standing position, and swing your right arm straight up overhead, the way you might if you were saying, "Look! I found a quarter!"

5. With your arm up high, rotate your torso to the right as you push the heel of your right foot into the ground. At the same time, clench your right glute to press your right hip forward. This helps keep your hips aligned and gives you a good stretch through your hips and obliques.

6. As soon as you reach your highest point with your arm, swoop it back down and lunge to repeat the exercise. Aim for 6 to 10 repetitions on this side, and switch to the other side. Ideally, you want to make the transition quickly, but you might have to work up to that.

Tips and Precautions

Yes, this exercise is all about transitioning from low to high quickly, but don't trade proper form for speed. Extend your body fully as you reach up, and try to come close to touching the floor on each repetition. If you shorten the movements, you're just cheating yourself out of the true benefits of this exercise.

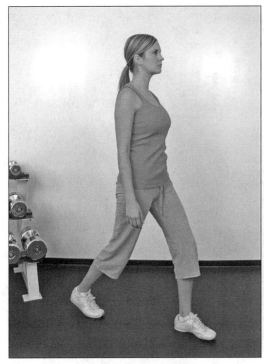

Starting/ending position.

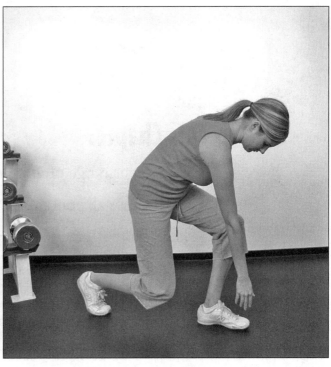

First position.

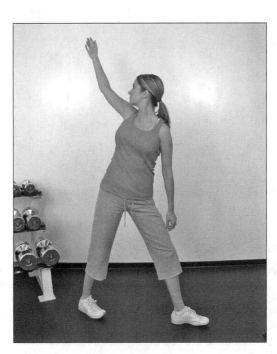

Second position.

In This Chapter

- ◆ Upping your range of motion
- ◆ Coordinating all your joints
- ◆ Adding more balance to the resistance
- ◆ Revealing one-sided weaknesses
- ◆ Changing directions

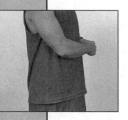
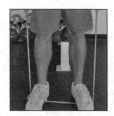
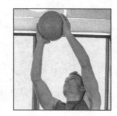
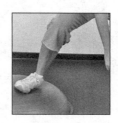
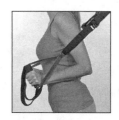
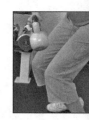

Intermediate Resistance Band Exercises

By now, you've realized that resistance bands can really make your muscles burn—in a good way. The beginner resistance band exercises in Chapter 7 showed you the basics of working against resistance. Many of my clients rave that they feel improvement in their movement and less tightness in their bodies after practicing those basic moves. That's good because you'll need a little extra mobility to perform the exercises in this chapter!

You'll soon discover that every exercise in this chapter works your legs and arms at the same time, which goes against the traditional weight training philosophy that says you should train legs one day and arms the next. But your body isn't divided into two separate halves. In real life, you use your legs and arms every day in just about everything you do.

Some of these moves also introduce you to a real-world situation that's notorious for causing injuries: changing direction. By teaching your body how to react when you have to zig and then zag, you have a much better chance of avoiding getting hurt.

Single-Leg Squat with Row

Remember the one-leg stand with row from Chapter 7? Like that move, this exercise targets the chain of muscles that runs from your hand all the way down to your opposite foot. What makes this exercise more intense is the squat, which really fires up the muscles in your standing leg. By making your glutes and quads work harder, your body learns to stabilize your knee in addition to strengthening your legs and butt. When your legs are strong and your knees feel stable, you'll feel like you can do just about any activity.

Real-Life Activities It Helps You Do

Water skiers and slalom skiers will love this exercise, which can also help you feel more stable anytime you need to reach out and grab something.

Starting Point

1. Secure the resistance band at knee height, and face the anchor point.

2. Grasp the handle with your right hand with your palm facing to the left. Pull it toward you the way you would pull open a door handle so there's no slack in the band, keeping your arm in close to your side and letting your elbow bend. Relax your left arm down at your side.

3. Balance on your left leg by lifting your right leg and raising your right knee out in front of you.

Movement

4. While maintaining tension on the band, lean forward and straighten your right arm as you reach toward the anchor point, as if you were still holding a door handle as the door swung shut.

5. At the same time, sit back into a squat with your left leg and swing your right leg behind you without putting your right foot on the floor. When you do this move, your right leg will naturally move behind you, helping keep you balanced.

6. Come back to the starting position by pulling the band back, keeping your shoulders back and down. Repeat 8 to 12 times on this side, and repeat the exercise using the left arm while standing on the right leg.

Tips and Precautions

Don't shrug your shoulder as you pull the resistance band toward you. When you squat, be sure the hip of your standing leg doesn't jut out to the side.

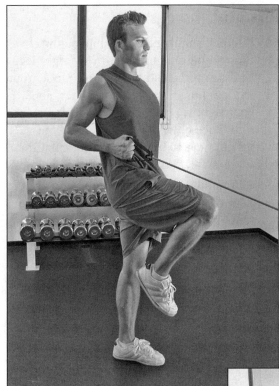

Starting/ending position.

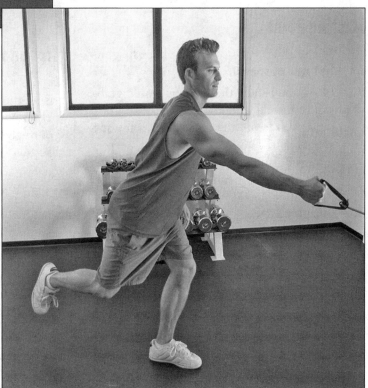

Midpoint position.

Lunge Row

By now, I'm sure you've learned to love lunges! Yes, they're real butt burners that strengthen the glutes, but they also open the hips to give you more flexibility there. In this version, I add an upper-body row to the mix. Thanks to the added resistance from the band, your body has to coordinate all the muscles in your legs, abs, back, shoulders, and arms to perform this exercise.

When a single move improves both strength and flexibility while targeting nearly every muscle in your body, you've gotta be a fan.

Real-Life Activities It Helps You Do

If you want to go power walking or running, you'll want to put this exercise on your to-do list.

Starting Point

1. Secure the resistance band at knee height, and face the anchor point.
2. Grasp the handle the way you would grab a door handle with your right hand with your palm facing to the left. Pull it toward you so there's no slack in the band, keeping your arm in close to your side and letting your elbow bend. Relax your left arm down at your side.
3. Balance on your left leg by lifting your right leg and raising your right knee out in front of you.

Movement

4. Keeping your torso erect, lunge down by taking a big step back with your right leg, landing on the ball of your right foot. Your left leg should be bent at the knee, and your right leg should be bent with your right knee nearing the floor. Tilt your pelvis under to increase the stretch at the front of the right hip and leg.
5. As you lunge back, reach forward with your right arm until it's straight, keeping tension on the band. Your right hand should end up at about waist height. Don't lean your upper body forward as you reach with your arm.
6. Use your left foot and glute to push off the floor to come back to your one-leg stand, and pull the band back toward you. Shoot for 8 to 12 repetitions and then change sides.

Tips and Precautions

If your back knee hurts when you tilt your pelvis on the lunge, simply back off on tilting your pelvis. As your fitness progresses, gently tilt your pelvis a little more each time you lunge back.

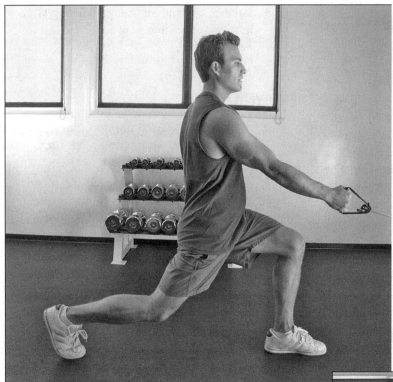

Starting/ending position.

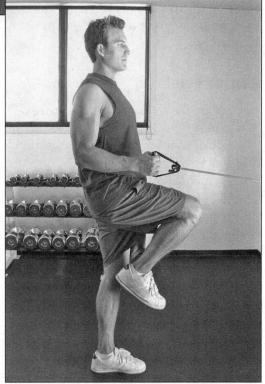

Midpoint position.

One-Leg Stand to Side Squat with Rotations

If you've been practicing the exercises in the previous chapters, you're probably getting to be a real pro at one-leg stands. Most likely, that means your balance has improved. In this exercise, I'm going to throw a few more movements at you to keep you on your toes—literally. The side squat intensifies the work in your lower body, while the rotations get your arms, abs, back, and shoulders engaged.

One of the best things about this full-body exercise is that you can control the intensity. As your functional fitness progresses, you can squat deeper and deeper to spike the intensity.

Real-Life Activities It Helps You Do

Swinging a baseball bat, moving boxes, even sitting on the toilet and reaching for the toilet paper will be a breeze for you if you practice this exercise.

Starting Point

1. Secure the resistance band at approximately chest height, and turn so the right side of your body is facing the anchor point.

2. Grasp the handle with both hands, and straighten your arms out in front of you at shoulder height the way a police officer would hold his arms out front at target practice. Scoot away from the anchor point until there's no slack in the band.

3. Balance on your right leg by lifting your left leg and raising your left knee out in front of you.

Movement

4. Step your left leg to the side, and squat down as if you were trying to sit back into a chair.

5. At the same time, rotate your torso and arms to the left, keeping your arms as straight as possible and your shoulders level. Don't bend your spine as you rotate. As you rotate, your right heel should naturally come off the ground, allowing your right foot to pivot.

6. Return to the starting position, and repeat 8 to 12 times before switching to the other leg.

Tips and Precautions

As you squat to the side with your left leg, let your right foot and knee do whatever feels comfortable for you. Depending on how flexible you are, your right knee may rotate inward and down toward the floor while you pivot on the ball of your right foot, or you may end up with both of your knees facing forward like a traditional squat.

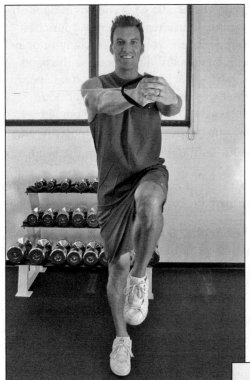

Starting/ending position.

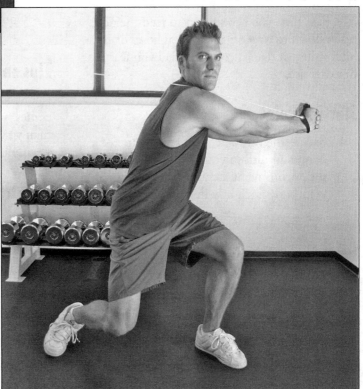

Midpoint position.

Squat with Diagonal High-to-Low Pulls

This exercise is a good reminder that the sum of your parts is a heckuva lot stronger than each individual part. Yes, it looks primarily like an arm move, but it also gets your abs, butt, and legs involved. That helps you create more power, which allows you to use a band with more resistance. If you tried this exercise doing just the arm movement without the squat element, you'd probably have to use a lighter resistance band.

This all-in-one exercise also gets your core working exactly the way it was designed to function—coordinating and linking the movements of your upper and lower body.

Real-Life Activities It Helps You Do

The next time you bend down to feed the dog, reach down to turn off the garden hose, or hit a high volley in tennis, you'll be glad you learned this exercise.

Starting Point

1. Secure the resistance band to the top of a door, and turn so your left side is facing the anchor point. Scoot forward a bit so your body is slightly in front of the band.

2. Grasp the handle with your right hand so your right arm reaches across your chest to the left as if you were reaching to open a high cupboard door. Because the band is anchored a bit behind you, rotate your chest slightly toward the anchor point. Relax your left arm down at your side.

3. Stand with your feet hip-width apart, and scoot until there's no slack in the band.

Movement

4. As you bend down into a squat, rotate your right arm, torso, and head down and to the right. Keep your arm straight as you rotate. Your right hand should end up to the right of your right knee.

5. Return to the starting position, and repeat the move 10 to 15 times using your right arm before moving on to do 10 to 15 more using your left arm.

Tips and Precautions

Remember that the power in this exercise comes from your torso and lower body rather than your arm, so don't rely on your arm strength to move the band.

Variations

Intensify the challenge by grasping the handle with both hands and rotating both arms.

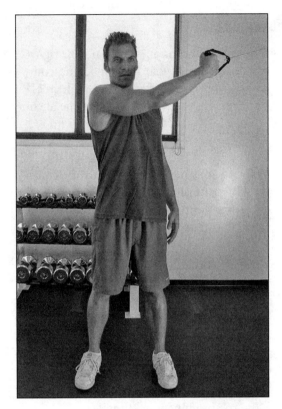

Starting/ending position.

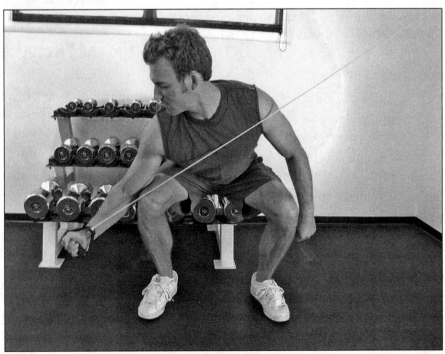

Midpoint position.

Transverse Step with Rear Fly

Get ready for some fancy footwork. This exercise gets you moving in every direction, which means you have to move your feet. Going from facing backward to facing forward and from standing tall to squatting down low—it's enough to make your head spin!

Actually, that's the whole idea of this exercise. In the real world, quick changes in direction can make you lose your balance and make you feel like you're falling. The first few times you try this exercise, you might lose your balance. With practice, you'll learn how to keep your body upright.

Real-Life Activities It Helps You Do

If someone calls out your name and you whirl around to see who it is, if you start to shut the front door behind you and then whip back around because you realized you forgot your keys inside, if you do pirouettes on the dance floor, or if you suddenly change direction for any reason, you'll benefit from this move.

Starting Point

1. Secure the resistance band at shoulder height, and turn so the left side of your body is facing the anchor point.

2. With your left arm out straight to your left side at shoulder height, grasp the handle with your left hand and scoot to the right until there's no slack in the band. Relax your right arm down at your side.

3. Stand with your feet shoulder-width apart.

Movement

4. In one swift motion, pivot on your right foot and rotate your left leg behind you until your body turns about 180 degrees so your right side is now facing the anchor point. As you rotate, bend down into a wide squat as if you were sitting back into a chair with your knees wide apart and your feet facing outward. Let your upper body rotate along with your lower body, keeping your left arm straight out to your left side at approximately shoulder height.

5. Return to your starting position by pushing off both legs as you pivot on your right foot and lift your left leg. You'll find that the big stretch in the resistance band will actually help pull you back to the starting position.

6. When you can do 10 to 12 of these on each side without taking any extra steps or losing your balance, you'll know you're on the road to functional fitness.

Tips and Precautions

If you find it too difficult to rotate all the way around in a single step at first, take an extra step in the middle. Doing this exercise on a surface that grips can make it tough to pivot. To make it easier to pivot, try this move on a carpeted floor.

Starting/ending position.

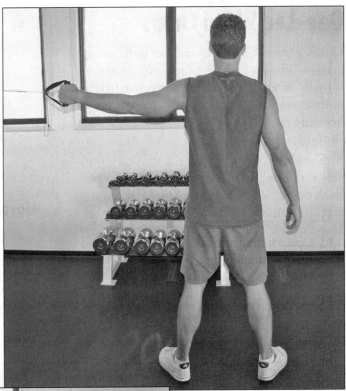

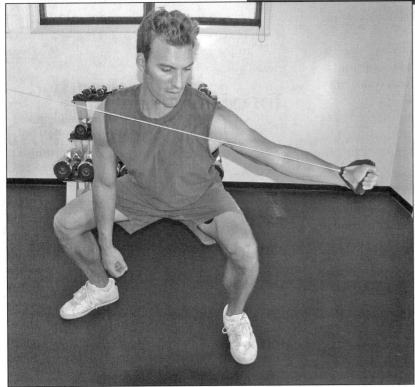

Midpoint position.

One-Leg Wood Chops

One-leg wood chops are all about overloading one side of your body at a time. Not only does this effectively strengthen and improve balance on your standing leg, but it also quickly lets you know if one side of your body is weaker than the other.

If you're like most of my clients, you'll probably find that you're able to do more repetitions on one leg than the other and that you feel more balanced on one side than the other. Don't worry. This is completely normal, but it does mean that you need to work your weaker side more to make your body more balanced.

Real-Life Activities It Helps You Do

As its name suggests, this exercise facilitates chopping wood, as well as simple tasks like placing heavy objects on the floor or even tying your shoes.

Starting Point

1. Secure the resistance band at about ear height, and turn your body so your left side is facing the anchor point.

2. Grasp the handle with both hands on your left side with your right arm straight across your body and your left elbow bent the same way you would hold an ax. Scoot to the right until there's no slack in the band. Keep your torso erect, and don't lean to either side.

3. Balance on your right leg by lifting your left leg and bringing your knee forward.

Movement

4. Bend down into a squat on your right leg while your left leg swings behind you without touching the ground.

5. As you squat, rotate your torso and arms down and to the right as if you were going to swing an ax to chop down a tree. Your hands should end up to the right of and at about the same height as your right knee.

6. The stretch in the band will help pull you back to the standing position. Do 8 to 12 repetitions on the right leg, then switch to the left leg.

Tips and Precautions

Tap your back foot on the ground if you can't keep your balance.

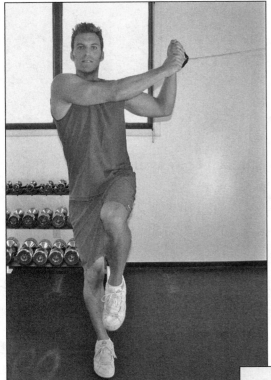

Starting/ending position.

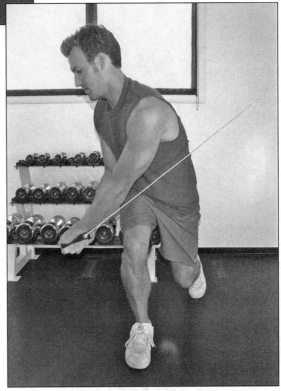

Midpoint position.

In This Chapter

- ◆ Moving the medicine ball farther away from your body

- ◆ Picking up the pace

- ◆ Slowing down the ball

- ◆ Using every muscle, from head to toe

- ◆ Adding more movement in different directions

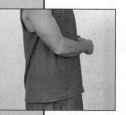 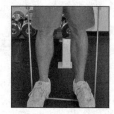 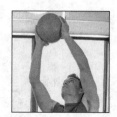 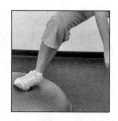 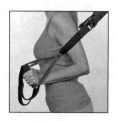 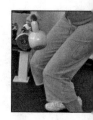

Intermediate Medicine Ball Exercises

I know the medicine ball movements look like a lot of fun—and they are—but don't jump straight into these intermediate exercises unless you've already perfected the beginner and intermediate body weight and resistance band exercises in Chapters 6, 7, 12, and 13. If you bypass those movements, your muscles won't know how to react when you maneuver the ball away from your body, and that can cause stress or even injury to your joints and back.

But with the proper foundation, you'll be prepared to tackle this chapter's exercises, which involve pushing the ball to the outer limits. These exercises also require you to move the ball with speed while you twist and turn through different planes of motion. When you add speed to the equation, your muscles have to work extra hard to slow down the ball to keep you balanced and to prevent it from flying out of your hands. If you think you're ready to try, let's get started!

One-Leg Squat with Two-Arm Rotation

Although this exercise may look similar to some of the moves you did in the earlier body weight and resistance band chapters, it adds the dynamic movement of the ball to increase your range of motion. Thanks to the added weight of the ball, your body will rotate farther and get more of a prestretch, which gives you more power so you can reach up higher.

Get ready for a bigger balance challenge, too, as you try to follow the ball with your eyes as you move up and down and twist right and left.

Real-Life Activities It Helps You Do

After practicing this exercise, it will seem a lot easier for you to secure your little one in a child seat in the backseat of your car or pick up heavy objects while off balance. It will also improve more athletic maneuvers, such as hiking a football.

Starting Point

1. Balance on your left leg by raising your right foot off the ground so your shin is parallel to the ground.
2. Hold the medicine ball at belly button height with your arms slightly bent.

Movement

3. Squat down into your left leg as you rotate your torso to the left and reach the ball down toward the ground as if you were putting something on the floor to the outside of your left foot. Don't let the ball actually touch the ground, though.
4. In one smooth motion, push off your left leg to come back to your one-leg stand as your torso twists to the right, and you swing the ball up over your right shoulder as if you were going to throw it up into the air. Remember to follow the ball with your eyes to increase the balance challenge.
5. Repeat 10 to 12 times on your left leg, and switch to your right leg.

Tips and Precautions

A lot of people have trouble keeping their eye on the ball when it's up over their shoulder. If you lose your balance here, just tap your other foot down momentarily. You can also keep your eyes facing forward or down at a fixed point until you're able to track the ball without losing your balance.

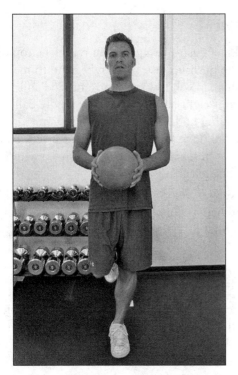

Starting/ending position.

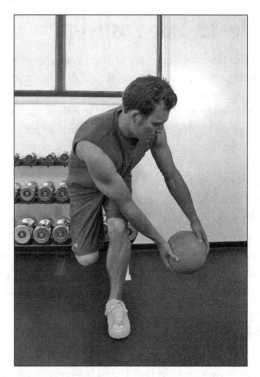

First position.

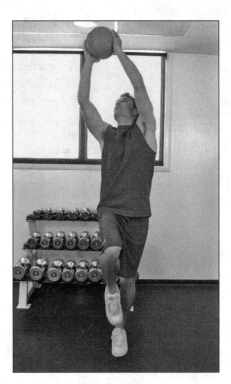

Second position.

Side-to-Side Push-Ups

Simple push-ups are one of the best exercises ever invented, and when you add the medicine ball into the mix, they're even more amazing. This version targets your rotator cuff muscles as well as all the muscles that stabilize your shoulder blades, pelvis, and spine. But that's not all. This super move is great for improving your hand-eye coordination, which can pay off big-time in daily activities and sports.

Plus, because real life doesn't always happen on flat, carpeted floors, it's good to practice moving on uneven surfaces. In this case, the ball creates an uneven foundation for your push-ups to make them more functional than ever.

Real-Life Activities It Helps You Do

Ever drop something off your desk and have to balance one arm on the desk while you reach down to retrieve the item? Ever have to open a heavy fire door? Ever seen a football linesman fending off an opponent? All these activities involve the muscles trained in this exercise.

Starting Point

1. Get down on the floor in a push-up position with your left hand on the floor and your right hand on the medicine ball. Because the ball is higher than the ground, the arm that's on the ball has to bend more to keep your body even.

Movement

2. Do a push-up, and as you reach the top of the push-up, use your right hand to make the ball roll toward your left hand and take your right hand off the ball. As the ball is rolling under your chest, place your right hand on the ground and lift your left hand onto the ball. Do another push-up with your left hand on the ball.

3. Keep passing the ball from hand to hand in between each push-up until you've done a total of 12 to 20 push-ups.

Tips and Precautions

Start very slowly and keep your hand stable on the ball before attempting a push-up. Also, be aware that having one hand higher than the other can make your hips sag, which you don't want.

Variations

To make this exercise easier, do your push-ups on your knees rather than your toes. If that's still too difficult, you can eliminate the push-ups altogether and just hold your body in a plank position while you roll the ball back and forth.

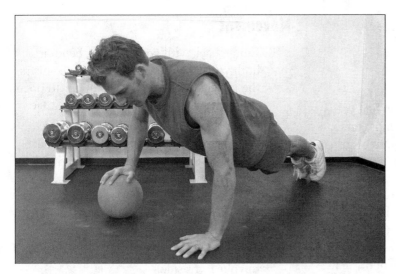

Starting/ending position.

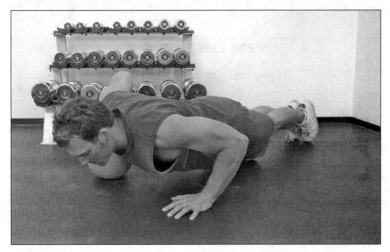

First position.

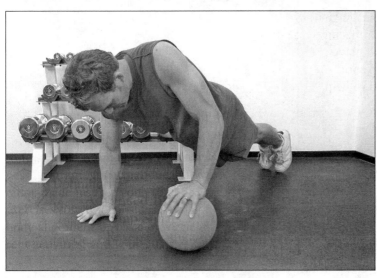

Second position.

Reverse Lunge to Shoulder Press

If you're a desk jockey, here's a full-body strengthening exercise just for you. When you hunker down at a desk all day, your hips, torso, abs, and shoulders get crunched together. To combat that, this exercise encourages you to open up those muscles known as the *anterior chain*. Doing so actually helps you breathe better, and what's more functional than breathing? It also increases the blood supply to your organs and your brain to help keep you mentally sharp. Combined with the strengthening benefit, that should be enough motivation to add this move to your workout repertoire.

Real-Life Activities It Helps You Do

Stepping down a ladder with a box in your hands, getting off a boat while holding a heavy tackle box, or going up for a spike in volleyball will all seem more natural if you practice this exercise.

Starting Point

1. Stand with your feet hip-width apart and your spine erect.
2. Hold the medicine ball at shoulder height with your left hand with your palm facing up, similar to the way a basketball player might hold a ball to shoot a jump shot. Tap the ball with your right hand to help you balance it.

Movement

3. Lunge back with your left leg, bending both your knees until your left knee nears the ground. Tilt your pelvis under to open your left hip, and keep your left foot facing forward and your torso erect.
4. At the same time, press the ball overhead with your left arm, letting your right arm fall away from the ball.
5. Push off of your left leg to come back to standing as you bring the ball back down to shoulder height. Shoot for 10 to 12 repetitions on your left side before switching to your right side.

Tips and Precautions

If you feel any discomfort when extending your arm all the way up, keep both hands on the ball and press it directly overhead instead of over your shoulder.

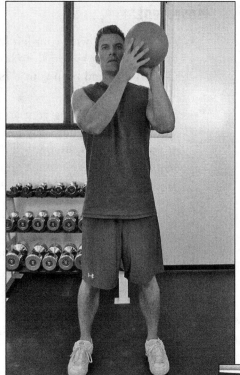

Starting/ending position.

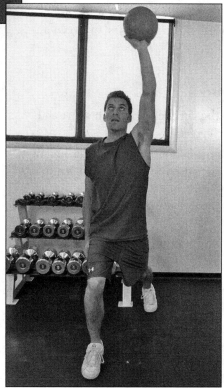

Midpoint position.

Forward Lunge with Rotation

This head-to-toe body-blaster makes your muscles work against gravity, your body weight, and the weight of the medicine ball while you're moving forward and twisting your torso. That means your lower body muscles—especially your quads, calves, hamstrings, and glutes—have to learn to slow down all that weight so your foot can land softly on the ground when it lunges forward rather than hitting it with a jarring thud. Plus, your upper body needs to keep that moving ball under control to avoid dropping it. That's a lot to ask from one exercise, but with practice, you should be able to handle it.

Real-Life Activities It Helps You Do

This movement mimics the act of walking or running downhill, down the stairs, or down a trail.

Starting Point

1. Stand with your feet hip-width apart and your torso erect.
2. Hold the medicine ball at shoulder height on your right side with your right hand under the ball with your fingers pointing to the right and your left hand on top.

Movement

3. Lunge forward with your left leg as you bend both your knees. Keep both feet facing forward, and keep your torso straight as you lunge.
4. Simultaneously, swing your arms down like an ax across your body to the left side of your left thigh, stopping at about belly button height. Keep your eyes on the ball as you move it up and down to test your balance.
5. Push into your left leg to come back to standing as you raise the ball back to shoulder height. Switch the ball to your left shoulder, and lunge forward with your right leg. Keep going from side to side until you reach a total of 20 to 30 repetitions.

Tips and Precautions

If you find it too difficult to coordinate your movements when alternating sides, you can do a series of 10 to 15 on one side first and then do the other side.

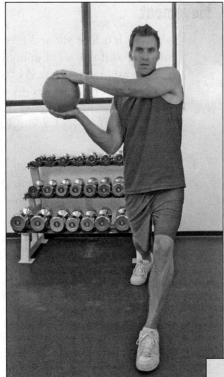

Starting/ending position.

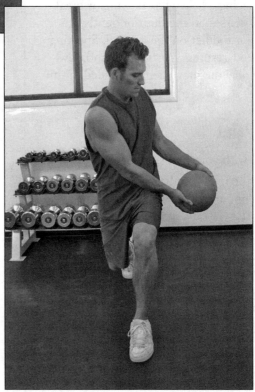

Midpoint position.

Side Squat with Floor Touch

I like to call this exercise "the great distracter" because it gets you to focus on doing a side-to-side squat so you won't notice that you're rounding your spine as you try to touch the medicine ball to the ground. Many people are afraid of getting injured when rounding the spine, so they tense up in this position. Unfortunately, that makes you more likely to hurt yourself. When you bend over without tensing up, your nervous system relaxes and your muscles do what they're supposed to, which helps protect your back. Learning to use your butt muscles as you bend down and reach up is another key to protecting your back when it's rounded.

Real-Life Activities It Helps You Do

Think of placing a heavy box of wine or breakable crystal glasses on the floor or gently setting a baby or toddler on the ground. Sporting activities like wrestling, martial arts, and bowling also involve the movements included in this exercise.

Starting Point

1. Stand with your feet shoulder-width apart.
2. Hold the medicine ball with both hands with your arms extended straight overhead.

Movement

3. Step your left foot about 2 feet to the left and squat as if you were going to sit on a chair slightly to your left. As you squat, slowly rotate your torso and bend your spine to bring the ball down and touch it on the ground to the left side of your left foot.
4. In a smooth and swift motion, use your glutes, torso, and legs to push yourself back to standing as you reach the ball back overhead.
5. Repeat the exercise on the right side, and continue alternating sides for a total of 16 to 20 times.

Tips and Precautions

Don't reach the ball all the way down to the floor if it doesn't feel comfortable.

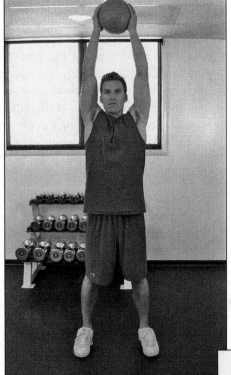

Starting/ending position.

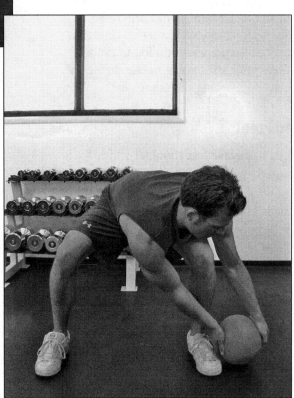

Midpoint position.

Lateral Lunge with Opposite Rotation

Here we go with another zigzag move that gets you twisting in opposite directions. By adding the weighted medicine ball to the picture, you have to fire up your outer thigh and butt muscles to slow it down as you push it farther away from your body. That increases your lower body strength while the twist helps create lots of flexibility in your abs and back. When you've got strength and flexibility on your side, quick changes in direction in real life won't throw you for a loop.

Real-Life Activities It Helps You Do

Anyone who's ever walked a dog knows he can bolt in the opposite direction to go after a passing cat or squirrel, yanking your arm one way while your body's heading in another direction. This exercise also prepares you for any sport that involves your arms going in one direction while your body's facing the other way.

Starting Point

1. Stand with your feet shoulder-width apart.
2. Hold the medicine ball with both hands with your arms reached out in front of you at belly button height.

Movement

3. Step your left foot to the left so your feet are about 2 feet apart as you squat down. While squatting, rotate your torso and arms to the right, allowing your left arm to bend slightly and your right arm to straighten. Keep the ball at the same height on your torso as your body shifts up and down.
4. Push off using your glutes and legs to return to standing with the ball in front of you, and then squat and rotate to the opposite side. Keep going from side to side until you reach 16 to 20 repetitions.

Tips and Precautions

Keep your movement small when you first try this exercise and gradually progress to squatting deeper and rotating farther.

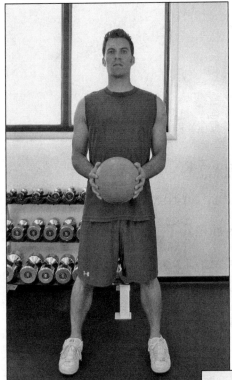

Starting/ending position.

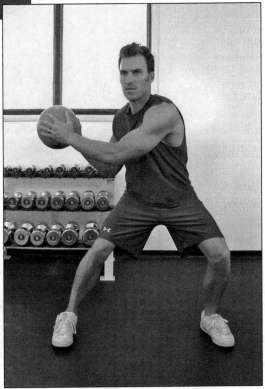

Midpoint position.

In This Chapter

- ◆ Building strength with the TRX
- ◆ Creating your own stability on the TRX
- ◆ Working with multidirectional TRX exercises
- ◆ Judging the proper distance of your movements

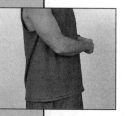
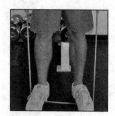
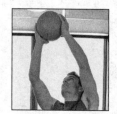
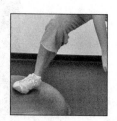
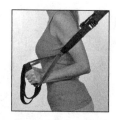
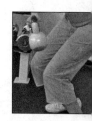

15

Intermediate TRX Exercises

The beginner TRX moves in Chapter 9 were designed to help you become familiar with the way the system reacts when you move. The exercises in this chapter begin to show you the limitless possibilities of this functional fitness tool. Here, you start working against more of your own body weight to build up your strength. The added weight also introduces an element of instability, which is what makes these exercises ideal for functional training.

Because the TRX handles move freely, you have to activate the muscles throughout your body to keep the handles still as you do the exercises. If you don't, the handles will start swinging all over the place, making it very difficult or even impossible to perform the movements.

Chest Press

This move is similar to a push-up or a bench press. Even if you're new to working out, you've probably seen images of bodybuilders or professional athletes doing a bench press, lying on a bench and using both hands to hoist a heavy barbell over their chest.

Because the person is lying on a smooth, flat bench, this traditional move works the muscles in the chest and shoulders but not much else. A push-up works more upper body muscles, but it involves working against a fixed object, in this case, the floor. When you try this same motion with the free-flowing TRX, you have to use nearly every muscle you have to stabilize your body before you can do the chest press. Maybe I should have called this exercise "chest press plus"!

Real-Life Activities It Helps You Do

Learning to create a stable platform so you can produce power with your upper body helps with opening a heavy door, popping up to standing on a surfboard, or boogie boarding. It also improves your ability to prevent someone from pushing you off balance, such as fending off an opponent in any type of martial arts or wrestling.

Starting Point

1. Face away from the anchor point, and grasp the handles. Hold your arms straight out in front of you wider than shoulder-width apart at shoulder height with your palms facing down. Scoot away from the anchor point until there's no slack in the system.

2. Walk your feet back toward the system so your body is leaning slightly forward. Your body should resemble a traditional push-up or plank position with your arms and body straight. The angle of your body depends on your fitness level. In the beginning, try remaining closer to standing. As you progress, lean farther forward by moving your feet back toward the anchor point.

Movement

3. Keeping your torso rigid at all times to help keep the handles as still as possible, bend your elbows and lower your body as if you were performing a push-up.

4. Use your strength and power to push your body back up to the starting position. A good goal for this exercise is 10 to 15 repetitions.

Tips and Precautions

Expect your arms to wobble like crazy during this exercise. To prevent the handles from swinging away from you, keep your movements smaller at first until you get the hang of it.

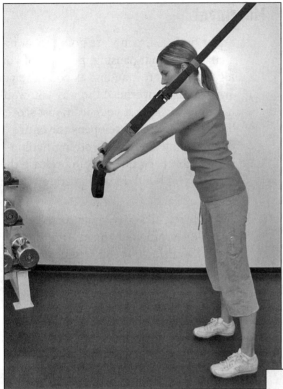

Starting/ending position.

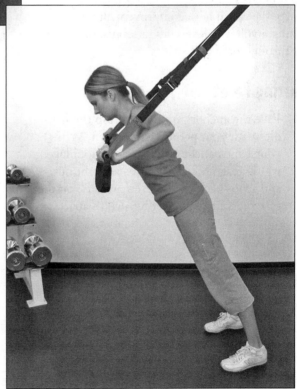

Midpoint position.

Isolated I with Squat

I love the I, and so will you! It's a whole-body strengthening exercise that also improves your posture. Learning to stand up straight can work wonders for your functional fitness. The more upright you are as you move, the less your body has to work against gravity to keep you upright.

Think of a water bottle: it stands up all day long until you tip it. Then it wobbles around until it either rights itself or falls down. Your body follows the same pattern throughout the day—smooth as silk when it's upright and then kicking into action when it's off balance. By adopting good posture, you'll notice more fluid movement in everything you do.

Real-Life Activities It Helps You Do

Every time you stand up or get out of a chair, you'll be glad you practiced the isolated I. Sporty types will notice improvement when spiking a volleyball, serving in tennis, or following through on a golf swing.

Starting Point

1. Face the anchor point, and grasp the handles with your palms facing down. With your hands at chest height and shoulder-width apart, hold your arms straight out and scoot back until there's no slack on the system. Keep your feet hip-width apart.

Movement

2. Squat back as if you were going to sit into a chair. Without pausing, push off of your legs to return to standing as you raise your arms straight overhead the way you would jump up to cheer if your team just scored. This part of the move opens the entire front of your body while strengthening your entire back side, helping release the tension you build up while sitting at your desk.

3. Immediately lower your arms, and sink back down into your squat. Aim for 10 to 12 repetitions. If you're squatting low enough, you'll feel your heart rate jump after that many reps.

Tips and Precautions

For severely tight shoulders, keep your arms in the isolated W position from Chapter 9's beginner TRX moves rather than lifting them overhead.

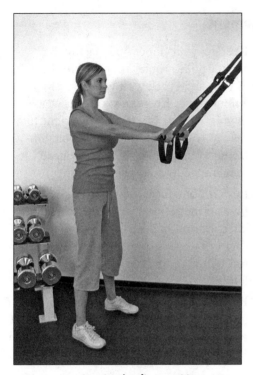

Starting/ending position.

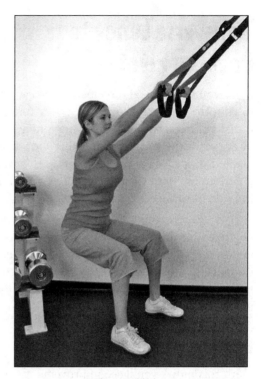

First position.

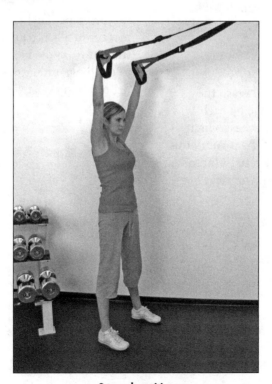

Second position.

Transverse Lunge to One-Leg Pivot

Have you ever parked too close to the car next to you? To get out of your car, you have to rotate your body around and swing one leg out of the car while keeping your other foot firmly planted inside. Many people can't do this without grabbing onto the door handle or clutching the side of the door. Not anymore!

This exercise trains the lower body muscles you need for this type of maneuver, in which one foot remains fixed while you change directions. With a little practice, you'll be able to shimmy out of that car without having to hold on for dear life.

Real-Life Activities It Helps You Do

With this move, you'll see improvement when getting out of a car, taking a backswing in golf, using a forehand in tennis, or swinging a baseball bat.

Starting Point

1. Face the anchor point, and grasp the handles with your palms facing each other. With your hands at chest height and shoulder-width apart, hold your arms straight out and scoot back until there's no slack on the system. Keep your feet hip-width apart.

Movement

2. Keeping your upper body facing the anchor point, rotate your hips to the right as you lunge back with your right foot into a mini-squat. Keep most of your weight in your left leg as you put your right foot behind you. Your right foot should end up facing toward the right while your left foot remains facing forward.

3. Push off of your left leg to lift your right foot off the ground, and raise your right knee in front of you. In the same motion, rotate your hips to the left and let your right knee continue to rotate across your left leg.

4. Bring your right foot back down to the ground in the starting position, and do 10 to 12 repetitions. Repeat on the other side.

Tips and Precautions

As your functional fitness improves, turn this move into a heart-pumping exercise by going straight from the knee-up position back down to the lunge rather than returning to the starting position in between.

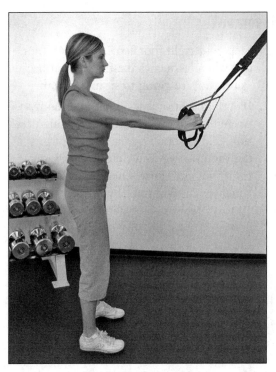

Starting/ending position.

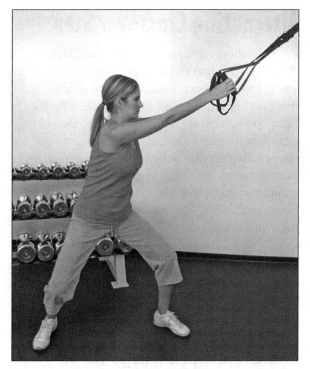

First position.

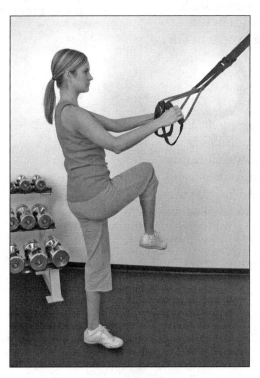

Second position.

Alternating Crossover Step

Put your thinking cap on for this one! While targeting your inner and outer thighs, the alternating crossover step requires you to do one thing on one side of your body and then do the exact opposite on the other side a split second later. Coordinating this side-to-side "dance" places heavy demand on your nervous system, forcing you to time your steps correctly and to accurately judge how big your steps should be. For example, take too big a step, and the TRX tugs your upper body uncomfortably.

In this exercise, think of the TRX as your dance partner and coordinate your movements together to create a smooth, rhythmic motion. When you get into the flow, you could be ready for *Dancing With the Stars*.

Real-Life Activities It Helps You Do

Learning to time your movements and judge distances while moving can be tremendously beneficial for dancing, playing any kind of sporting activity, or just getting in or out of the shower.

Starting Point

1. Face the anchor point, and grasp the handles in front of you with your palms facing each other. With your elbows slightly bent at shoulder height and your feet hip-width apart, bend your knees so you're in a mini-squat. Be sure there's no slack in the system.

Movement

2. Step your right foot across your left foot, and when it touches the floor, squat back as if you were going to sit into a chair.

3. In a fluid motion, use your lower body strength to come back to the starting position, and as soon as your right foot hits the ground, step your left foot past your right foot and squat. One step to each side equals one repetition. If you can perform 10 to 15 repetitions without stopping or getting tangled up, give yourself a pat on the back.

Tips and Precautions

Maintain tension on the TRX throughout this exercise by keeping your movements within a certain range of motion. For example, if you stand up too high, you can create slack in the system, which might cause a jolt when you shift into your squat position.

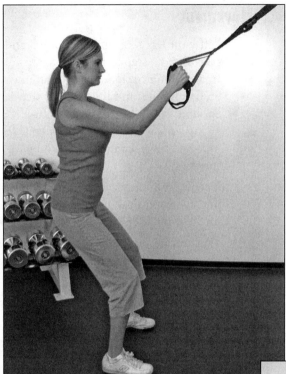

Starting/ending position.

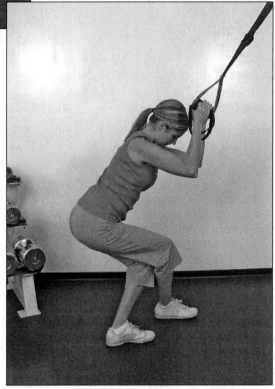

Midpoint position.

Side Squat

Similar to the alternating crossover step you just did, the side squat also gets you moving from side to side. What's different here is that you take bigger steps to each side, which takes you farther away from your center of gravity. This makes your inner and outer thighs work even harder to slow you down so your foot can land softly rather than with a thud.

Learning to land gently as you move helps protect your joints. Your knees and hips will thank you for this one!

Real-Life Activities It Helps You Do

Washing your car, painting a fence, trimming the hedges, dancing, and all sports—any activity where you're moving side to side—will feel more natural after this exercise.

Starting Point

1. Face the anchor point, grasp the handles in front of you with your palms facing each other, and bend your elbows at about shoulder height. Soften your knees, and keep your feet hip-width apart. Be sure there's no slack in the system.

Movement

2. Lift your left foot off the ground, and take as big a step as possible to the left. Imagine you're standing over an uncovered manhole, and if you don't step far enough, you'll fall in. Keep both feet facing forward, and as soon as your foot touches the ground, sink down into a squat.

3. Use the muscles in your legs and butt to push yourself back up to standing, and return your foot to the starting position.

4. Without hesitation, repeat the move on the right side. Continue going side to side 20 to 30 times.

Tips and Precautions

Be aware that when you take a large step to the side, the TRX pulls your torso in the opposite direction, creating some rotation on the spine. If it's too much rotation for you, take smaller steps.

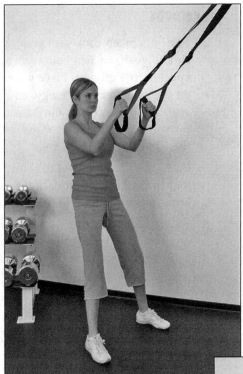

Starting/ending position.

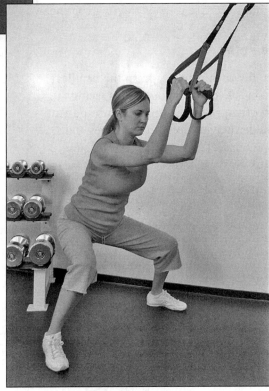

Midpoint position.

Back Lunge with Knee-Up

If you want to climb your way to the highest level of functional fitness, this exercise helps you get there. Similar to a climbing motion, it trains the muscles in your hips and butt to accelerate to create the power you need to go uphill, but it also trains those areas to decelerate to soften your landing. That way, you won't be pounding your joints as you walk, hike, or run uphill.

If you've been avoiding hills and stairs because they seem too challenging for you, this exercise gives you the power you need to motor up these obstacles.

Real-Life Activities It Helps You Do

Climbing hills, going up stairs, and climbing ladders won't seem like as much of a challenge if you add this exercise to your training routine.

Starting Point

1. Face the anchor point, grasp the handles in front of you with your palms facing each other, and bend your elbows at about shoulder height. Soften your knees and keep your feet hip-width apart. Be sure there's no slack in the system.

Movement

2. Take a big step back with your right foot, and lunge down as if you were going to kneel on the ground. Place your right foot on the ground as you lunge, and use your arms to help hold you up. As you lunge, tilt your pelvis to increase the stretch on the front of your right hip.

3. Push into your left foot to return to standing. In the same motion, bring your right knee forward and up in front of you.

4. Return to the starting position. Do a total of 10 to 15 repetitions on your left leg, and then do the same on the other side.

Tips and Precautions

Try to create a fluid motion throughout this exercise rather than pausing at the bottom of the lunge or in the knee-up position.

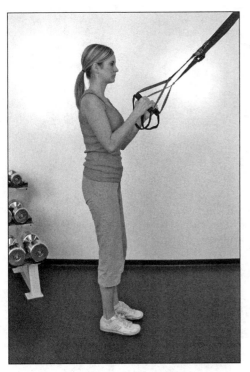

Starting/ending position.

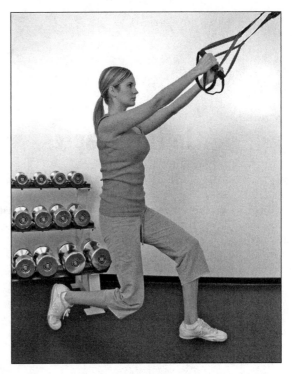

First position.

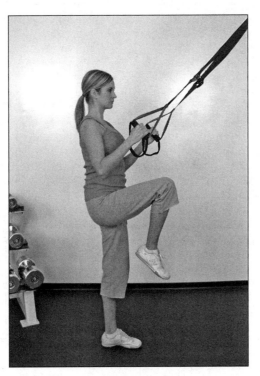

Second position.

In This Chapter

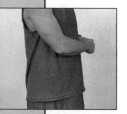
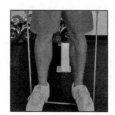
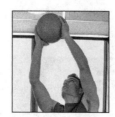
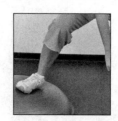
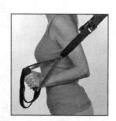
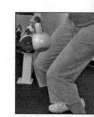

Chapter 16

Intermediate BOSU Exercises

By now, you're either having a blast bouncing around on the BOSU, or you think it's the toughest piece of equipment you've ever come across. Either way, you have to admit that it has a huge impact on your functional training. The beginner moves gave you just a hint of what you can do with this amazing tool. Now it's time to expand your repertoire to include movements you probably thought were impossible when you first stepped on the BOSU.

Only if you're feeling comfortable performing the beginner BOSU moves from Chapter 10 should you step it up with these intermediate exercises. The added jumps, bigger movements, and changes in your center of gravity in this chapter make those beginner moves look like a piece of cake. When you get the hang of these exercises, your functional movement will sky-rocket.

Squat to Side Leg Lift

Standing on the BOSU without flailing around is hard enough for some people. Imagine what it will feel like when you start moving your legs and arms away from your center of gravity as you try to balance on top of the dome. That's exactly what you'll find out with this exercise that involves a leg lift out to the side while you balance and squat on one leg.

This movement is a perfect example of a functional exercise that increases strength in the major muscles of your lower body while improving your balance.

Real-Life Activities It Helps You Do

When you master this move, you should feel a lot more confident walking up stairs, standing on a boat, ice skating, or dancing.

Starting Point

1. Stand on the BOSU with your feet hip-width apart. Let your arms hang down at your sides, and keep your eyes facing forward.

Movement

2. Squat back as if you were going to sit in a chair, and keep your upper body erect rather than leaning forward. Bringing your arms out in front of your body the way you might reach out to pick up a child off the ground can help keep you balanced as you squat.

3. Push off both legs to come back to standing, and as you do so, lift your right leg out to your right side as high as is comfortable, keeping it straight. Think of it as if your right leg were a drawbridge and you were raising it up to let a car or boat pass under it. Your arms can do whatever's necessary to keep you balanced. Expect to feel your left foot going crazy in this position.

4. Lower your right leg so you're back to the starting position, and repeat the exercise by squatting and then lifting your left leg out to the side. Alternate from side to side until you've done a total of 10 to 12 repetitions on each leg.

Tips and Precautions

As always, stand near a wall or countertop if you need a balance aid. Also, don't try to raise your leg up too high at first. It's better to start small and gradually increase the height.

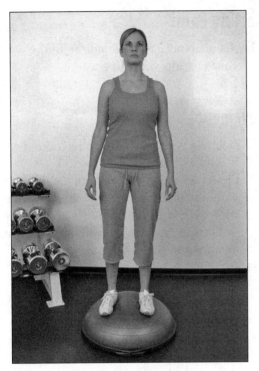

Starting/ending position.

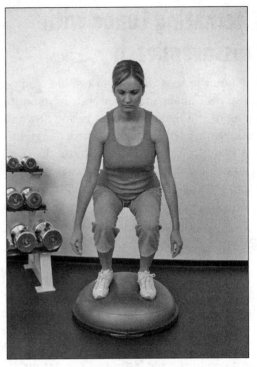

Midpoint position.

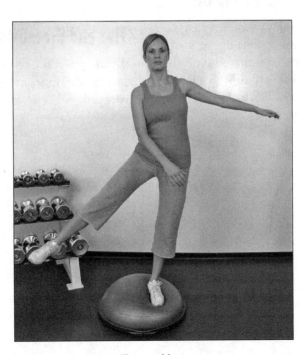

First position.

Alternating Lunge with Crossover Reach

Anytime you have to move fast in life, you need to use your upper and lower body in opposition. Think of an Olympic sprinter racing down the track—as her left leg flies forward, her right arm swings ahead while her left arm reaches behind. Of course, you probably won't be racing in the Olympics anytime soon, but you can benefit from this basic principle, which is one of the things your body will learn from this exercise.

Not only that, the BOSU's height means you can lunge lower than you could with both feet on the floor. This deeper lunge activates your glutes, quads, calves, and hamstrings even more than a regular lunge, which makes it easier for you to get back up. Yep, that's right. The farther down you lunge, the faster you can get up. If you don't believe me, try it.

Real-Life Activities It Helps You Do

You'll feel the benefits of this exercise when you're slalom skiing, running, fencing, or just bending down low to pick up something off the floor. You might even be able to dip your dance partner with such ease, you'll think you're ready for *Dancing with the Stars!*

Starting Point

1. Stand about 2 feet behind the BOSU with your feet hip-width apart.

Movement

2. Keeping your torso erect, step onto the BOSU with your left foot so it's just shy of the top of the dome, and lunge down as if you were going to kneel down. Don't let your right knee touch the ground, though. In the same motion, reach your right arm forward and across your body to the left as far as you can without tipping over. Ideally, your right hand should end up about 6 inches ahead of and 12 to 18 inches to the left of your left foot.

3. Push off of your left leg to come back to standing behind the BOSU, and repeat the exercise with your other leg. Continue alternating sides until you've lunged a total of 20 to 30 times.

Tips and Precautions

As you progress, try to touch your hand to the ground out in front of the BOSU as you lunge forward.

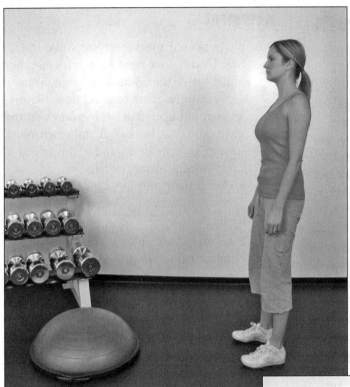

Starting/ending position.

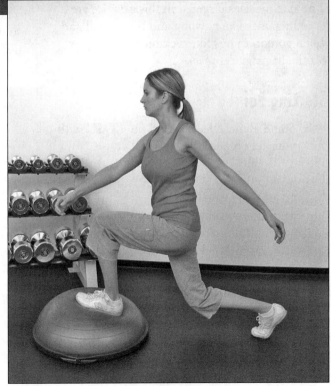

Midpoint position.

Lunge with Open Side Reach

In this version of the lunge, you reach your arm out to the side of your body rather than across it like you did in the preceding exercise. This seemingly small change makes a huge difference in your body dynamics. Here, you're working the sides of your butt, hips, and thighs rather than just focusing on your quads and hamstrings. With today's sedentary lifestyle, we don't use these side muscles often, which makes this exercise more difficult than the last one.

You'll find that you're far more likely to lose your balance when you reach out to the side. In part, that's because when you're going forward, you've got those five toes as your last defense to keep you from falling down. When moving to the side, your toes can't help you.

Real-Life Activities It Helps You Do

The side muscles targeted in this exercise are used in games like bowling and boccie ball and when you do things like pick up your luggage off the baggage carousel.

Starting Point

1. Stand about 2 feet behind the BOSU with your feet hip-width apart.

Movement

2. Keeping your torso erect, step onto the BOSU with your right foot so it's just shy of the top of the dome, and lunge down as if you were going to kneel down. Don't let your left knee touch the ground. At the same time, lean to the left and reach your left arm directly down and to the side as far as you can. Your left hand should end up lower than your hip. Do whatever you need to with your right arm to help you balance.

3. Push off of your right leg to come back to standing behind the BOSU. Then lunge forward with your left leg, and lean to the right. Keep switching sides, and aim for 20 to 30 lunges.

Tips and Precautions

This exercise challenges the arch of your foot, so if you typically wear orthotics or arch supports, be sure to wear them for this move.

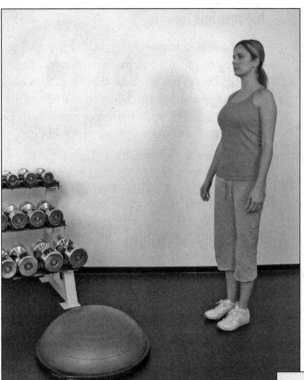

Starting/ending position.

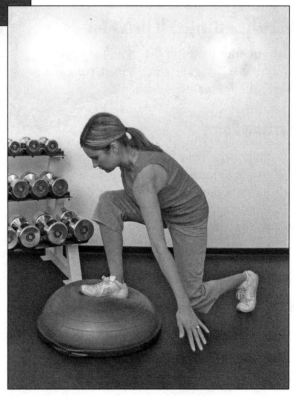

Midpoint position.

Side-to-Side Jump

Ready to jump for joy? Jumping requires you to use more muscles to accelerate upward and then to decelerate as you land. The act of jumping also pumps up the amount of force your body experiences, which can improve your bone density. Because you have one foot on solid ground while the other is on the unstable dome throughout this exercise, it also confuses your nervous system, making it work harder to coordinate your movements.

With all this going on, jumping on the BOSU will probably feel weird at first. As you progress, the squishy dome will eventually act like a mini-trampoline and help propel you from side to side to make the move easier. When you start having fun flying from side to side, you'll know your functional fitness level is starting to soar.

Real-Life Activities It Helps You Do

Mastering this dynamic move can help you if you're playing tennis, racquetball, squash, dodgeball, or even hopscotch.

Starting Point

1. Stand with your feet together about 2 feet to the right of the BOSU, and step your left foot onto the center of the dome. Bend your left leg slightly while keeping your hands down at your sides and your torso erect. Squat down as if you were going to sit on a barstool or a chair. The deeper you squat, the more you'll load your muscles, which will help you jump higher, faster, and farther to the side.

Movement

2. In one dynamic move, push off your left leg to jump up in the air and over the BOSU. Your left foot should end up on the ground about 2 feet to the left of the BOSU, and your right foot should land on top of it where your left foot had been.

3. As you land, immediately squat down again to prepare to jump back to the other side. Jump back and forth 20 to 30 times.

Tips and Precautions

Let your arms do whatever feels natural to you as you jump. You might want to swing them behind you as you squat, and then reach forward as you jump to help create momentum to jump higher.

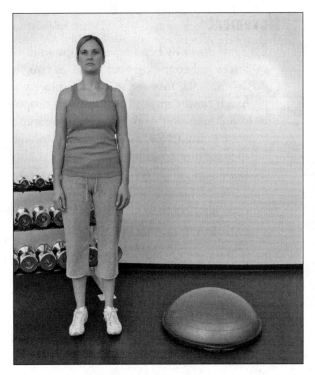

Starting/ending position.

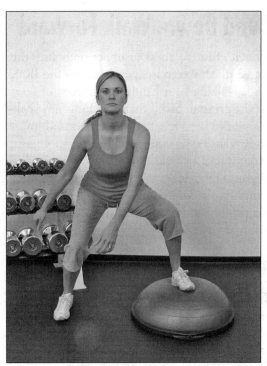

First position.

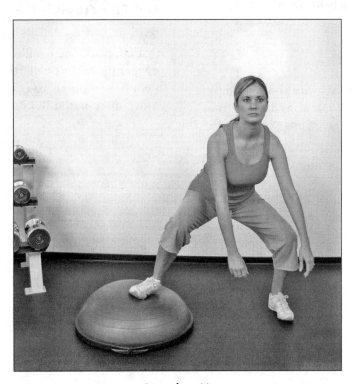

Second position.

Bend Down, Walk Forward

Now it's time to get your upper body into the act. With this exercise, you stand on the BOSU while walking your hands out in front of you on the ground. So all that twitching and shaking you've been feeling in your feet and lower body transfers to your hands, arms, shoulders, and chest. This wakes up the stabilizing muscles in your upper body, which helps protect your joints. At the same time, supporting your body weight on your hands makes you stronger. Strong and stable—it's a beautiful combination.

Real-Life Activities It Helps You Do

Thanks to the bend down, walk forward, you'll feel more secure whenever you need to get down on the ground, such as getting under the car to retrieve something, crawling under your desk to pick up something you dropped, shimmying under a low fence, or doing a military-style obstacle course where you have to crawl under a series of ropes.

Starting Point

1. Stand on the BOSU with your feet hip-width apart with your arms down at your sides, your torso erect, and your eyes facing forward.

Movement

2. Bend down by bending your hips and knees and rounding your back. As you curl down, reach forward so you can place your hands on the ground as if you had dropped something on the ground in the dark and were going to feel around with your hands to see if you could find it.

3. Start walking your hands forward one at a time as far as you can without letting your hips sag toward the floor. When your hips start to drop, that's where you stop. Depending on your strength and flexibility, you may reach a push-up position or even farther.

4. At this point, put it in reverse and walk your hands one at a time back toward the BOSU, and roll back up to standing. Work your way up to 10 to 15 repetitions.

Tips and Precautions

If your body just doesn't want to bend down that far, place one hand on the ground first and stagger the other one farther ahead, similar to a crawling motion. You can also place your feet wider apart on the BOSU to facilitate the bend.

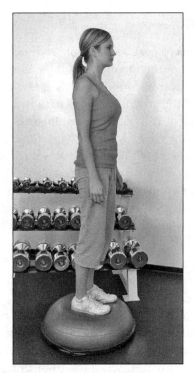

Starting/ending position.

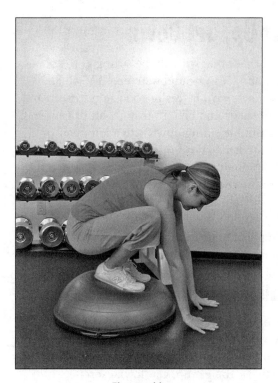

First position.

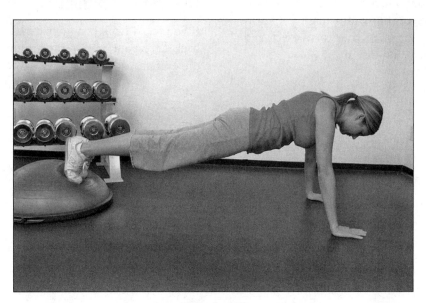

Second position.

Get Up, Get Down

You'd think that with all the sitting at the computer and lying around watching TV we do these days, we'd be really good at getting in and out of chairs and bed. In truth, a lot of people have trouble sitting down into a low chair or onto the bed and need to use their hands to avoid plopping down with a thud. This exercise shores up the strength in your lower body, especially in your abs, to help you take a seat without having to use your hands. This is another example of a functional ab exercise that doesn't require you to do a traditional crunch.

Real-Life Activities It Helps You Do

Anytime you need to sit down onto a low surface while you're holding packages, a baby, or any other object, you'll be glad you've been practicing the get up, get down exercise.

Starting Point

1. Stand about 6 inches in front of the BOSU with your feet hip-width apart, your arms down at your sides, your torso erect, and your eyes facing forward.

Movement

2. Do a deep squat so your butt ends up a bit forward of the top of the BOSU. As soon as your rear end hits the BOSU, lift your feet off the ground and lean back with your torso as if you were leaning back in a La-Z-Boy recliner. Ideally, your torso and legs should both be straight so your body forms a V, but it's okay if your legs bend or your spine rounds a bit. Do whatever you want with your arms to help keep you steady, but try not to put them on the BOSU or the ground.

3. Hug your knees in close to your chest, rock forward, and put your feet on the ground and stand up. At first, you may need to put your hands on the BOSU to help push you up to standing. With time, you may be able to do so without any help from your hands. Shoot for 10 to 15 repetitions.

Tips and Precautions

If you feel a twinge in your back as you lean back, keep your feet on the ground throughout the exercise.

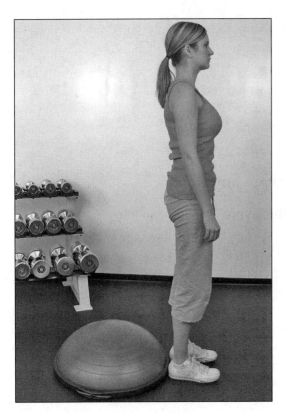

Starting/ending position.

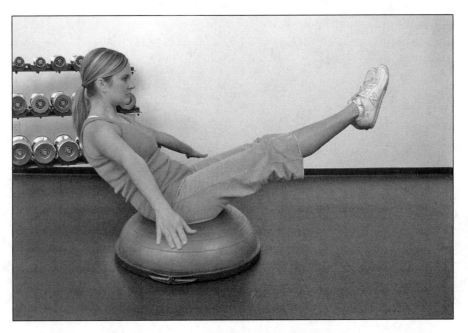

Midpoint position.

In This Chapter

- ◆ Your lower + upper body = more power
- ◆ Timing your movements effectively
- ◆ Keeping your movements under control
- ◆ Working your shoulders and wrists
- ◆ Adding footwork

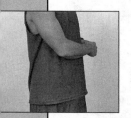
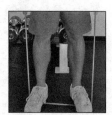
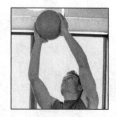
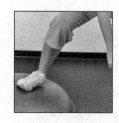
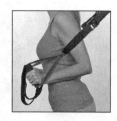
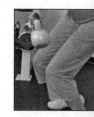

17

Intermediate Kettlebell Exercises

Remember those beginner kettlebell moves from Chapter 11? Of course you do! They were designed to introduce you to the concept of moving while carrying extra weight. Now that you're familiar with the kettlebells, it's time to start moving them more dynamically to increase the intensity.

These bigger movements require power, coordination, and control—functional skills you've already learned from the other intermediate exercises in Part 4. Here, you have to incorporate all those skills at the same time in each exercise. When you've conquered all the exercises in this chapter, you are ready to graduate to the advanced moves in Part 5. Now that's something to feel good about!

Pick Up and One-Arm Press

In a perfect world, you'd always be able to pick up heavy objects using both hands while keeping your body weight evenly distributed. Unfortunately, in the real world, that's not always the way it works. Doing heavy lifting with only one hand is a common occurrence in daily life. This action loads one side of the body and tips you off balance. Helping you gain the strength and stability you need to do single-handed lifting is what this exercise is all about.

Real-Life Activities It Helps You Do

Placing your suitcase in the overhead compartment or hoisting heavy equipment onto a high shelf won't seem so difficult after you do this move a few times. Plus, you'll feel the benefits when playing sports like golf where you load one side of your body on the backswing and then the other side on the follow-through.

Starting Point

1. Stand with your feet hip-width apart, and place two kettlebells on the floor in front of each foot with the handles facing your body. Relax your arms at your sides.

Movement

2. Squat down as if you were going to sit in a chair, and round your spine until you can reach the kettlebells.

3. Grasp the right kettlebell with your right hand and, using the muscles in your legs and butt, return to standing. In one motion, bend your elbow to lift the kettlebell off the ground and extend your arm straight up over your right shoulder.

4. Bend your elbow and lower the kettlebell as you squat and bend down, and place it back on the floor in front of your right foot. Pick up the left kettlebell, lift it overhead, and place it back on the floor to finish the first repetition. Do a total of 10 to 15 repetitions.

Tips and Precautions

Don't pause as you return to standing and hoist the kettlebell. If you hesitate, all that power you created with your lower body will be lost, and you won't be able to transfer that power to your upper body. That means you might not be able to lift the kettlebell overhead.

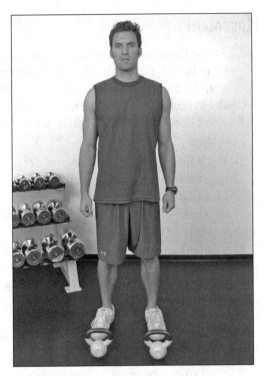

Starting/ending position.

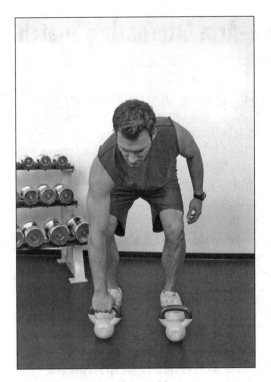

First position.

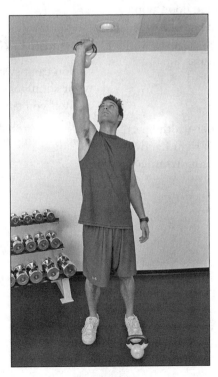

Second position.

One-Arm Alternating Snatch

Like the pick up and one-arm press, this exercise requires you to use your lower body to create the power needed to lift the kettlebell overhead. In this version, however, you swing the kettlebell overhead with your arm straight rather than lift it with a bent arm. Keeping your arm straight as you swoop the kettlebell upward is a lot like swinging a longer golf club—it's harder to control, but when done correctly, it creates more force for a longer drive.

If you don't swing that long club just right, though, the ball slices or hooks, and you can hurt your shoulder. It's the same idea here—you want to swing the kettlebell in a nice, smooth motion to build strength in your shoulder without tweaking anything.

Real-Life Activities It Helps You Do

Practice this exercise, and you'll breathe easier when you have to lift up the garage door, pop the hood of your car, or start the lawn mower. This move also benefits golfers, windsurfers, kite surfers, water skiers, and sailors.

Starting Point

1. Stand with your feet shoulder-width apart, and hold a kettlebell in your right hand at your side with your palm facing your leg.

Movement

2. Swing the kettlebell in front of you to belly button height, bend your knees into a squat, and round your spine as you swing the kettlebell back between your legs. Look down at the kettlebell as you swing it through your legs.

3. Without hesitation, use the muscles in your legs and butt to straighten up to standing, and swing the kettlebell over your right shoulder with your arm straight.

4. Swing the kettlebell back down as you bend down and swing it between your legs. Raise the kettlebell only to belly button height this time. In the same motion, grasp the kettlebell with your left hand and remove your right hand. Then swing the kettlebell down and up with your left hand to complete your first repetition. Try for 10 to 15 repetitions.

Tips and Precautions

If you can't swing the kettlebell all the way over your shoulder, just go as high as possible. It's okay if you can only bring it up to shoulder height at first. With practice, you should be able to swing it higher and higher.

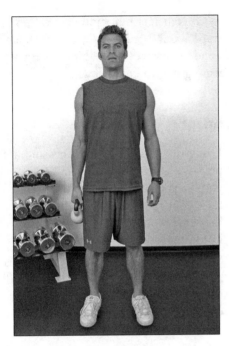

Starting/ending position.

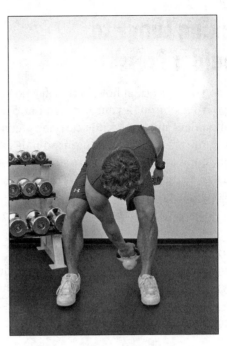

First position.

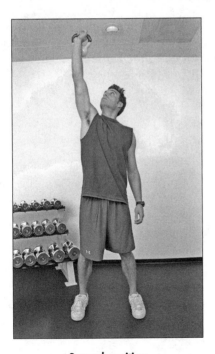

Second position.

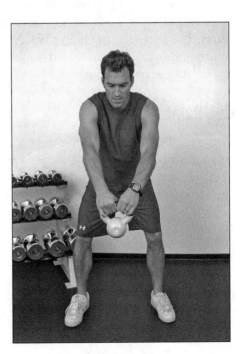

Third position.

Walking Lunge to Shoulder Press

Okay, so you've learned how to transfer power from your legs through your torso and into your shoulders and arms while carrying weight. Bravo! Now try it while walking. It sounds easy enough, but a lot of people don't step each foot forward in a straight line, and that can seriously limit your functional fitness. In this exercise, a wobbly walk can make the weights go up in a funny way, causing you to lose your balance.

With some effort, you learn to walk each foot in a straight line. This simple improvement gives you greater efficiency of movement, which means you're able to play sports or do chores for longer periods of time without getting tired.

Real-Life Activities It Helps You Do

You'll feel greater ease of motion whenever you walk while carrying a baby or toddler, hike while carrying a backpack, or climb a ladder while hoisting heavy objects overhead to place them in the attic or on the roof.

Starting Point

1. Grasp the kettlebells, and lift them up so your elbows are bent at 90 degrees at shoulder height and your palms are facing forward in a "hands-up" position. The kettlebells should be hanging behind your forearms.

2. With your feet hip-width apart, step forward about 2 feet with your left leg and bend your knees into a lunge as if you were going to kneel down.

Movement

3. Using the muscles in your legs and butt, push up to standing on your left leg while you lift your right foot off the floor and raise your right knee up in front of you. In the same motion, lift the kettlebells overhead.

4. Step your right foot about 2 feet forward, and go back down into a lunge as you lower the kettlebells to the starting position. Keep alternating sides until you've done 20 to 30 lunges.

Tips and Precautions

If you're having trouble coordinating the movement, start out by simply walking while raising and lowering the kettlebells. Then add the lunges when you're ready.

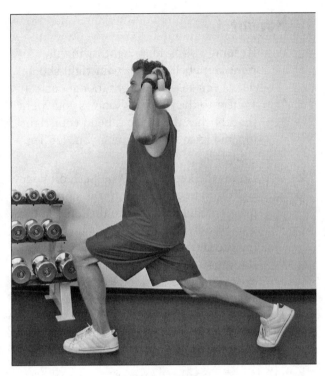

Starting/ending position.

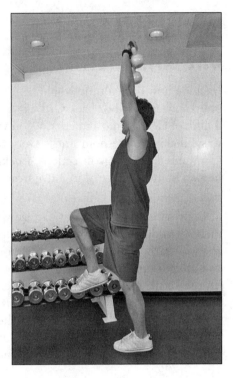

First position.

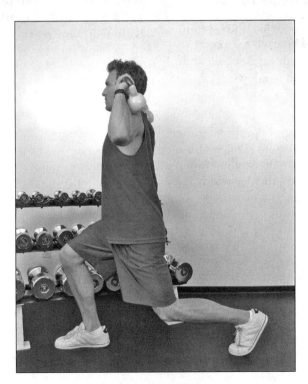

Second position.

Partial Side Squat to One-Arm Snatch

Imagine how difficult life would be if you could only move forward or backward like a car. Think of all the time and energy you would waste making three-point turns every time you wanted to change directions. Luckily, the human body is designed to move from side to side.

Improving this movement pattern while carrying added weight is what this exercise is all about. It targets the bigger muscles in the legs and obliques to produce the power you need to lift the kettlebell overhead on one side. Then you have to turn on the smaller stabilizing muscles in your side to help you shift to the other direction. If you don't activate those important stabilizers, you risk toppling over to the side.

Real-Life Activities It Helps You Do

Practicing side-to-side movements is great for anyone who wants to field goals in a soccer game, work on sails on a boat, catch a ball while shuffling to the side, or wash windows.

Starting Point

1. Hold the kettlebells down at your sides with your palms facing your thighs while standing with your feet shoulder-width apart.

Movement

2. Keeping your arm straight, swing the right kettlebell up over your right shoulder as you step your right foot about 1½ feet to the right. As soon as your right foot touches the ground, bend your right hip and knee while keeping your left leg straight.

3. Lower the kettlebell as you push off your right foot to come back to the starting position, and then step to the left and take a small squat with your left leg while lifting the kettlebell over your left shoulder. Repeat 10 to 15 times, noting that for this exercise, 1 side-to-side series equals 1 repetition.

Tips and Precautions

The heavier the kettlebell you use, the lower you'll have to squat to produce enough power to lift the kettlebell overhead. Try lighter kettlebells while you get the hang of this exercise.

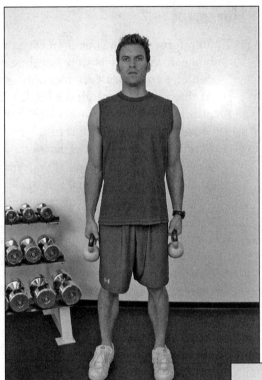

Starting/ending position.

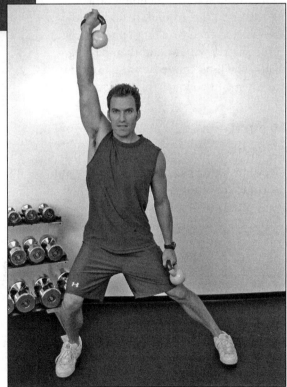

Midpoint position.

Walking Floor Touch to Snatch

When Aerosmith sang "Walk This Way," they probably didn't have the walking floor touch to snatch in mind, but maybe they should have. This walking exercise targets every muscle in your body while testing your powers of coordination. It also gets you moving through a full range of motion, from down low to up high while twisting in opposite directions, which really fires up the abs. Working your abs without crunches or sit-ups? That's something to sing about.

Real-Life Activities It Helps You Do

Walking, running, bending over to pick up laundry and then hanging it up to dry, picking fruit off a high tree and then bending down to put it in a basket on the ground, fielding a low ball in baseball and then reaching up to throw it, taking the snap down low and then passing the football—you'll be amazed how many things feel better when you conquer this exercise.

Starting Point

1. Hold the kettlebells in your hands with your palms facing your thighs as you stand with your feet hip-width apart.

Movement

2. Step forward with your right foot and lunge down as if you were kneeling, but don't let your back knee touch the ground. At the same time, reach the kettlebell in your left hand gently across the front of your body and touch it to the ground lightly in front of your right foot. As you're reaching forward, let your back round and keep the weight of the kettlebell in your hand rather than resting it on the floor.

3. Use the muscles in your legs and butt to push yourself back up to standing as you step your left leg forward. In the same motion, swing the left kettlebell up over your left shoulder, keeping your arm straight the entire time.

4. As soon as your left foot touches the ground, sink back down into a lunge, lower the left kettlebell down to your side, reach the right kettlebell across, and gently tap it on the ground in front of your left foot. Push yourself up to standing as you swing the right kettlebell overhead to complete your first repetition. Shoot for 8 to 10 repetitions.

Tips and Precautions

This exercise can be a real brain twister, so don't be surprised if it throws you for a loop at first. If you're having trouble coordinating the alternating movements, try doing one side at a time instead.

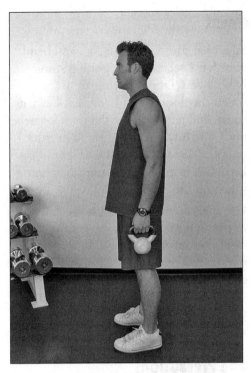

Starting/ending position.

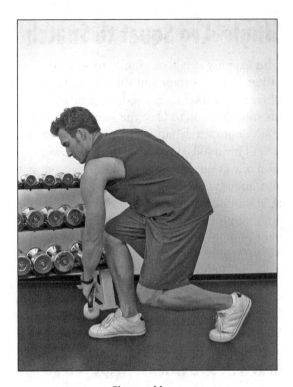

First position.

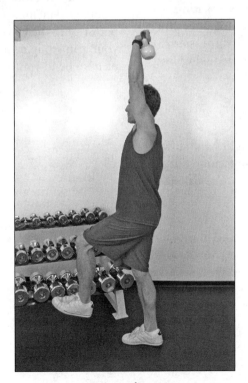

Second position.

Single-Leg Squat to Snatch

This exercise may look similar to some of the others in this chapter, but there's one big difference: rather than alternating sides, this one requires you to blast the same side until you've completely fatigued the muscles on that side. This builds more strength and power than any other exercise in this chapter, but it also leaves you feeling tired. That's why I put this exercise last. If you tried this move before attempting the other exercises in this chapter, your muscles would probably be too pooped out to perform them.

One thing that won't require as much effort here is the coordination factor. Your brain can take a vacation while you power through this repetitive move.

Real-Life Activities It Helps You Do

Sports that require a lot of leg strength—such as skiing, snowboarding, surfing, ice skating, and cycling—will seem far less taxing after you master this exercise. You'll also find it easier to do activities like changing a tire or looking into a low cupboard.

Starting Point

1. Hold a kettlebell in your right hand down at your side with your palm facing your leg. Lift your right foot so you're balancing on your left leg.

Movement

2. Squat back into your left hip, and bend your left knee as your right leg swings behind you. Don't let your right foot touch the floor. Round your back as you squat, and gently lower the right kettlebell until it lightly taps the ground in front of your left foot. Keep the weight of the kettlebell in your hand rather than letting it rest on the floor.

3. Use the muscles in your left leg and butt to push up to standing as you raise your right knee in front of you. In the same motion, keep your right arm straight and swing the kettlebell up over your right shoulder. Repeat the exercise 10 to 15 times before switching to the left side.

Tips and Precautions

Tap your back foot down lightly if you have trouble balancing. If you become fatigued while performing the repetitions, and you can't keep your arm straight in the overhead position, it's okay to bend your elbow.

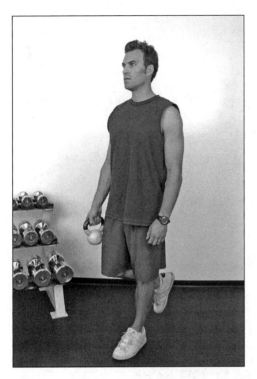

Starting/ending position.

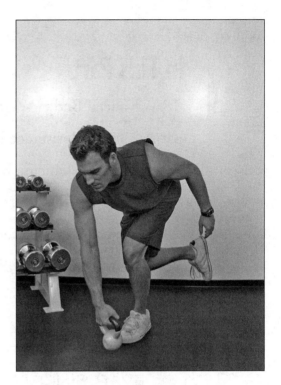

First position.

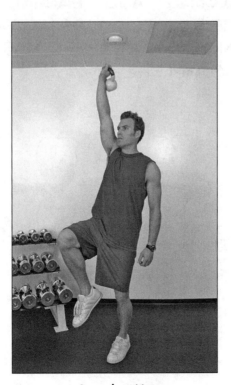

Second position.

In This Part

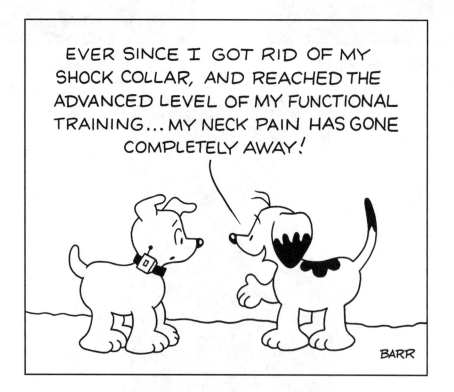

Advanced Functional Exercises

You've made it! If you're ready to tackle these advanced exercises, you've probably already noticed big improvements in your functional fitness. Way to go! The complex exercises in Part 5 take your training further than you ever thought possible.

With the ability to do these exercises, you'll perform better in sports, your everyday movements will feel more fluid, and your body will be ready to react to any unexpected physical challenges life throws at you. Now that's functional fitness!

In This Chapter

- ◆ Moving faster to get your heart pumping
- ◆ Going from low to high and high to low
- ◆ Increasing your coordination
- ◆ Strengthening the major muscle groups

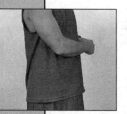 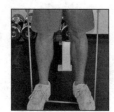 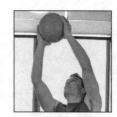 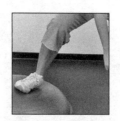 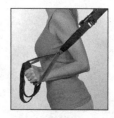 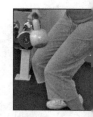

Chapter 18

Advanced Body Weight Exercises

You won't need any equipment to perform the advanced exercises in this chapter, just your body weight. You will need a solid foundation in functional fitness, though, so don't attempt these exercises until after you've gotten comfortable with the beginner and intermediate moves in Chapters 6 and 12.

The exercises in this chapter can be surprisingly challenging. Many of my clients are amazed to discover just how much of a workout they get with these advanced body weight exercises. They will tax your sense of balance and seriously test your coordination.

I tell my clients to practice these exercises slowly at first to pick up the proper form and then start cranking up the speed. By transitioning rapidly through these movements, you'll get your heart rate up, which will add a healthful cardio element to your workout. Plus, many of them are designed to teach your body how to react properly to those unpredictable real-life situations that require you to move quickly in unexpected ways—and to do so without getting hurt.

One-Leg Reverse Rotational Lunge

This exceptionally helpful exercise teaches your body how to move and respond to sudden changes in direction. It gets your whole body moving but focuses mainly on strengthening and mobilizing your legs, hips, butt, and torso. Learning how to use the muscles in your lower body to maintain your balance while rotating and lunging can be a real-world life-saver, or at least a knee-saver. In a perfect environment, your knees would always be perfectly aligned, but in unpredictable situations, they may rotate inward, which can cause an injury if your body doesn't know how to react. This exercise teaches you to use your hips, butt, legs, and feet to take the stress off your knees. Plus, its high-to-low-to-high movement kicks up your heart rate.

Real-Life Activities It Helps You Do

This exercise will help you handle unpredictable surfaces and situations—for example, if you're rock hopping or hiking on an uneven surface or walking on a slick sidewalk and your foot slips out from under you and your knee twists inward. It's also great for any sport in which you have to react quickly, such as when you're lunging for a volleyball and it hits the top of the net and changes direction.

Starting Point

1. Balance on your left leg by raising your right foot behind you so your right shin is parallel to the ground.
2. Raise your left arm straight up overhead while keeping your right arm down at your side.

Movement

3. Step your right leg behind you about 18 inches, and sit back so you're in a deep squat with your knees out wide and your feet angled outward. Your left knee will rotate slightly inward.
4. Keeping your back straight, rotate your torso and swing your left arm down near your right shoe, as if you were going to reach into the back of your shoe to remove a pebble.
5. Swing your left arm back up into the air as you return to balance on your left leg with your left arm straight overhead. Perform 10 to 12 repetitions on the left leg, and then switch to balance on the right leg with your right arm overhead.

Tips and Precautions

Do this exercise slowly at first to avoid over-rotating your knee. If you feel a twinge in the knee that rotates inward, push down on the big toe of that foot. This helps the muscles of your foot work, which helps take stress off your knee.

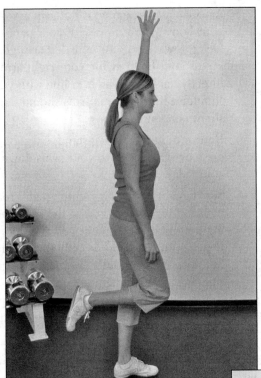

Starting/ending position.

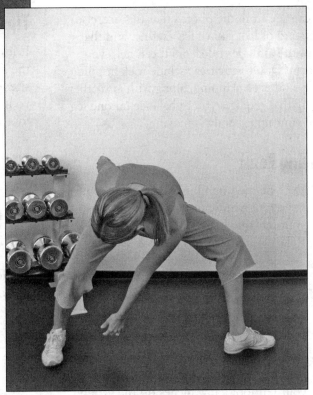

Midpoint position.

One-Leg Side Squat with Reach

The one-leg side squat with reach builds on the single-leg squat with reach you did in the intermediate body weight exercises in Chapter 12. By adding a side squat to this move, your standing leg has to do overtime to keep you balanced. Because it targets the big muscle groups of the glutes, legs, and trunk, this exercise gets your heart pumping, too.

When my clients first see this move, they think they won't be able to do it, but with practice, they succeed. Eventually, the movement pattern becomes ingrained, and they can use it naturally in their daily lives without having to think about it.

Real-Life Activities It Helps You Do

You can see from the photos that this exercise looks kind of like you're ice-skating, and that's one of the athletic endeavors it can help you perform. Other activities include rock hopping, skiing, and even skipping, along with any other activity that requires you to balance on one leg while your upper body is moving.

Starting Point

1. Do a one-leg stand by balancing on your right foot with your left leg raised up so your left shin is parallel to the ground. Relax your arms down at your sides.

Movement

2. Squat with your right leg, pushing your butt back as if you were trying to sit back in a chair. Your left leg will naturally move behind you to help you balance. Keep your left foot a few inches off the ground.

3. As you squat, reach your left arm across your body to the right with your palm facing toward you. As your left arm goes across your body, swing your right arm directly back, keeping it in line with your shoulder. Both of your arms should have a slight bend at the elbow.

4. Return to your one-leg stand, balancing on your right leg with your arms down at your sides.

5. Squat again with your right leg, and reach your left leg directly out to the side, keeping it at least 2 or 3 inches off the floor. Reach your left hand directly forward in line with your shoulder, and swing your right arm directly behind you again. Repeat the series 6 to 10 times, balancing on the right leg and then switching to the left leg.

Tips and Precautions

If it's too difficult for you to hold your foot off the ground in the squat, you can tap your opposite foot on the ground. If you feel any pain in your knee, it's probably because your hips or foot isn't positioned correctly. Be sure to sit way back in your hips, push down with the big toe of your standing leg, and spread the toes of your standing foot.

Variations

Add intensity to this move by jumping each time you come out of the squat. This adds more cardio to the move and makes your muscles work harder.

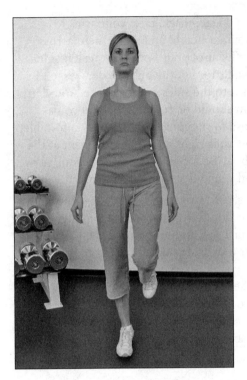

Starting/ending position.

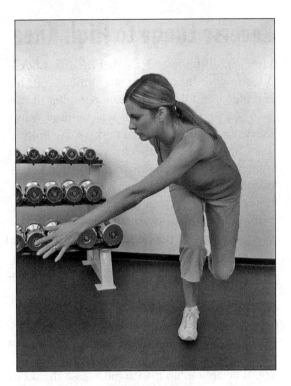

First position.

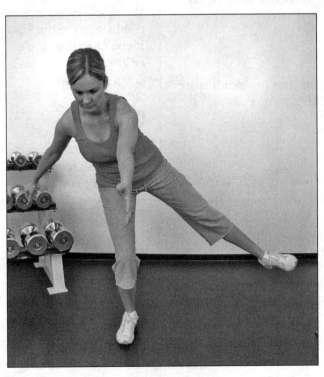

Second position.

Reverse Lunge to High Knee

Here's a full-body exercise that increases flexibility in your hips while it strengthens your legs and glutes and gets your heart pumping. It can help you perform powerful athletic moves, but that's not all. If you sit at a desk all day long at work, this exercise is also for you. Sitting all day tightens your hips, and if your hips aren't flexible enough to move properly, your lower back has to take over, which can lead to lower back pain. By learning how to open your hips with this exercise, you can help prevent that dreaded aching in your back. That alone should be motivation to add this exercise to your routine.

Real-Life Activities It Helps You Do

Anytime you need to take a step backward, like climbing down a ladder or stepping off a boat, you'll be able to do it with more ease thanks to this exercise. It also helps with more dynamic moves, like jumping up to make a layup in basketball.

Starting Point

1. Stand erect with your feet hip-width apart and your arms down at your sides.

Movement

2. Step back as far as possible with your right leg, and lunge down so your right knee almost touches the ground. Your left knee should be bent and in line with your left ankle. Be sure your right foot is still facing forward, and keep your torso erect rather than leaning forward or backward. Tilt your pelvis under to increase the stretch in the front of your right hip.

3. As you step back, raise your arms to shoulder height and move them across the front of your body to your left side similar to the way hula dancers wave their arms to the sides as they dance. Your left arm should be reaching behind you as close to shoulder height as is comfortable, and your right arm should be bent at the elbow. Be sure you rotate only your arms and keep your hips facing forward.

4. Push off with both feet, and as your body rises up, lift your right knee up high to your chest and lift up onto the ball of your left foot as if you were going to hop up. As you do so, swing your arms over to the other side of your body. When you can do 8 to 12 repetitions on each side in rapid succession, you'll know you're on the road to excellent functional fitness.

Tips and Precautions

When you're in the lunge, you should feel a good stretch in the hip flexor of your back leg. If you're feeling discomfort in your lower back or knee, don't step back as far and don't bend down as deeply.

Variations

Make this exercise even more challenging by standing on an unstable surface, such as a rolled-up towel, or take it outside and stand on sand or grass in your bare feet.

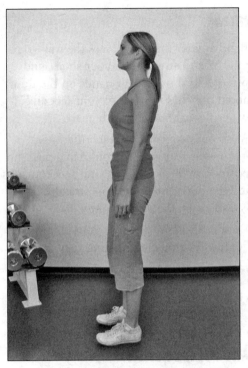

Starting/ending position.

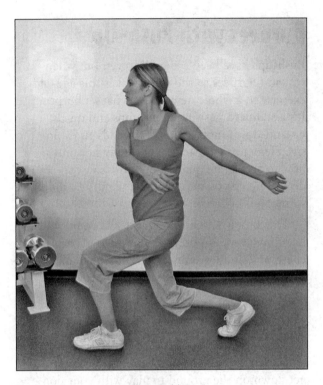

First position.

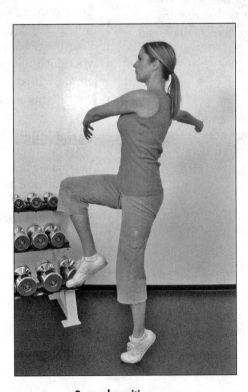

Second position.

Burpees with Push-Up

Push-ups have been around forever, but when you add burpees to the mix, it takes this age-old exercise to a whole new level. What's a burpee? It's a standard push-up plus jumps and quick up-and-down movements. This adds an explosive element that teaches your body not only how to accelerate quickly, but also how to decelerate so you make contact with the ground softly.

This heart-pumping exercise gets your whole body involved, targeting your shoulders, arms, chest, abs, and legs. Yes, it will be a challenge at first, but that's the best way to improve your functional fitness.

Real-Life Activities It Helps You Do

This exercise will come in handy if you want to get down on the ground to play with your dog or your kids and you need to hop up quickly. It also prepares you for sports that require explosive movement, like soccer, baseball, and basketball.

Starting Point

1. Stand with your feet hip-width apart and your arms down at your sides.

Movement

2. Bend at your hips and knees the way you might bend down to tie your shoes, and place the palms of your hands on the floor about 6 inches in front of your feet and wider than shoulder-width apart.

3. As soon as your hands reach the floor, jump your feet back so you're in a push-up position with the balls of your feet touching the floor and your arms straight. This is also called the *plank position*.

4. Do a push-up by bending your elbows to 90 degrees and straightening them again.

5. Jump your feet back to about 6 inches from your hands, and return to standing. Work your way up to 10 to 15 repetitions.

Tips and Precautions

If you feel a twinge in your lower back as you go into the push-up, you may be dropping your hips and arching your lower back. To prevent your lower back from sagging when you do your push-up, push your butt up slightly in the air and tilt your pelvis under rather than making your body completely straight.

Variations

When you're first trying this move, you can eliminate the jumps and move your feet one at a time instead. To intensify the move, add a jump as you come back to standing.

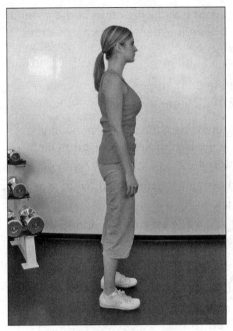

Starting/ending position.

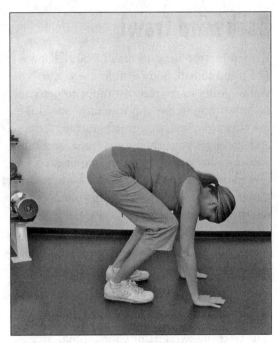

First position.

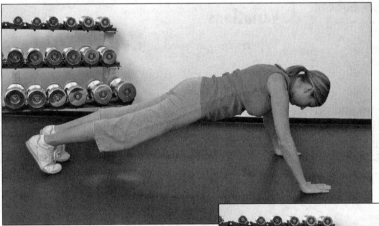

Second position.

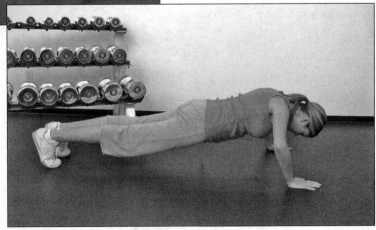

Third position.

Backward Crawl

Remember the forward crawl from Chapter 12's intermediate body weight exercises? Now you're going to rewind that move to get your body heading in the opposite direction. Like the forward crawl, this exercise strengthens and stabilizes your shoulders, spine, and hips. Crawling backward, however, requires you to rely more heavily on your upper body to create power. You can't cheat by using your legs to initiate the movement.

Plus, you'll discover that getting your body to move in reverse can be a bit of a brain teaser that requires a healthy dose of coordination!

Real-Life Activities It Helps You Do

The next time you paint your ceiling, lift objects over your head as you walk backward, clean your carpet on all fours, or play a game of football or rugby, you'll be glad you practiced this exercise.

Starting Point

1. Start with the palms of your hands and the balls of your feet on the floor. Your arms should be about shoulder-width apart, and your feet should be about hip-width apart. Your butt should be up in the air, and your knees should be bent, but don't let them touch the floor.

2. Keep your eyes facing down at the ground rather than looking up, which can strain your neck.

Movement

3. Start crawling backward by moving your left arm and right leg backward as far as is comfortable.

4. Without resting, move your right arm and left leg backward.

5. Keep crawling on your hands and feet for 20 to 30 yards, or 10 to 15 steps.

Tips and Precautions

Avoid shrugging your shoulders or swaying your hips back and forth as you crawl backward.

Variations

When you get good at it, try crawling backward up stairs.

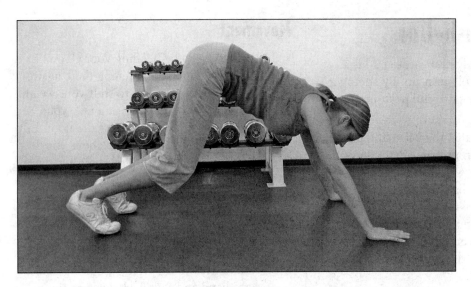

Starting/ending position.

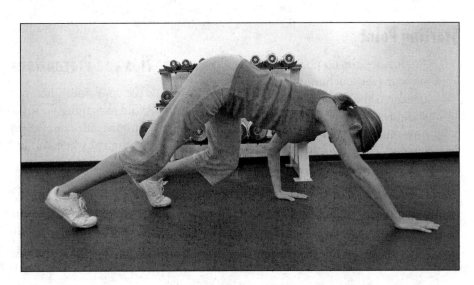

Midpoint position.

Rotational Push-Ups

Here's another full-body exercise that adds a new twist to the good ol' push-up. By adding a rotational element, the powerful push-up turns into a balancing act.

Take note, though, that the balancing portion of this exercise is different from what you've seen in the other body weight exercises. Those movements all involve balancing on your feet. This gem shifts the balance to your upper body and fires up all those muscles that stabilize your shoulders. It also targets your abs and the muscles that stabilize your ribs and pelvis.

Real-Life Activities It Helps You Do

If you need to push a heavy door, or if you're ever unfortunate enough to have to fend off an attacker, you'll be glad you practiced this exercise. It's also great for swimming and can help prevent injuries to your wrists and shoulders if you fall.

Starting Point

1. Assume a push-up position with the balls of your feet touching the floor and your hands on the floor slightly wider than shoulder-width apart. Keep your body in a straight line, and focus your eyes on the ground without dropping your head down.

Movement

2. Do a push-up by bending your elbows to 90 degrees and straightening them again. As you push up, rotate to shift your weight to your left arm and leg, and take your right hand and right foot off the floor. Lift your right hand straight up above your shoulder as if you were reaching for the ceiling. Simultaneously, lift your right leg away from your left as high as you can take it while keeping it straight. Your silhouette will look like you're getting ready to make a snow angel in this position.

3. Rotate back to the right, and bring your right hand and foot back down to the ground so you're back in the push-up position.

4. Do another push-up, and shift your weight to your right arm and right leg, lifting your left hand and leg into the air. Come back to the push-up position. Keep alternating sides for a total of 10 to 16 repetitions.

Tips and Precautions

Take your time when performing this exercise. Avoid shrugging your shoulders while rotating onto one side, and keep your head, torso, and hip aligned when you're on one side.

Variations

If this expert move is too tough for you, don't lift your leg and foot into the air when you rotate to the side. Let your foot rest on top of the foot that's touching the ground.

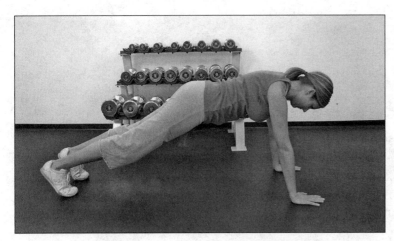

Starting/ending position.

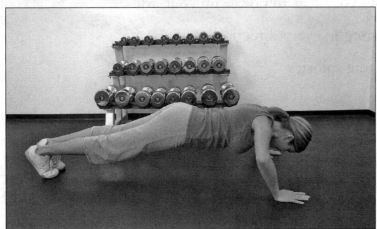

First position.

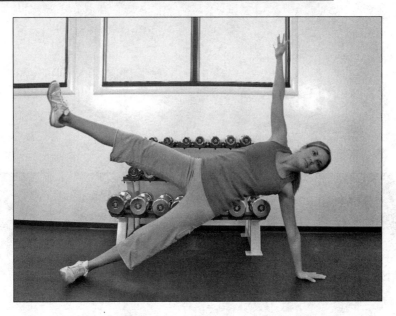

Second position.

In This Chapter

- ◆ Using your entire body
- ◆ Getting your feet moving
- ◆ Using your legs to power up your arms
- ◆ Twisting in every direction
- ◆ Burning calories

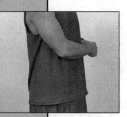
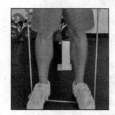
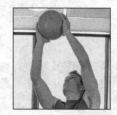
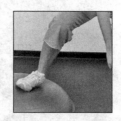
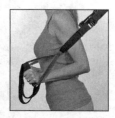
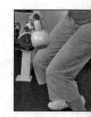

19

Advanced Resistance Band Exercises

I'd like to borrow a title from The Beatles and call this chapter "Twist and Shout" because the exercises here get your body twisting in every direction, and you'll be shouting "I did it!" when you finally master them. I have to admit that when my clients first see some of these exercises demonstrated, a lot of them say, "No way, I can't do that." With practice, though, they end up doing far more than they ever thought possible. I'm sure you will, too.

Many of these complex moves get you moving up and down, forward and backward, and side to side—all in the same exercise. Plus, they test your balance and your ability to coordinate all the muscles throughout your body. The key here is to take it slow and make adjustments as you learn the moves. For example, you can always use a lighter resistance band in the beginning to make an exercise easier. Or you can tap your other foot down on the ground until you're able to stand on one leg throughout an entire exercise.

When you feel comfortable, start going through the moves more rapidly. Because many of them get you going from down low to up high, they'll get your heart pumping so you can burn some serious calories.

One-Leg Ice Skater with One-Arm Chest Fly

Remember that 1980s exercise gadget called the ThighMaster? It targeted the inner thighs and turned out to be one of the best-selling pieces of exercise equipment of all time. With that old-school product, you could be sitting at your desk while squeezing away with your inner thighs. That's great, but unfortunately, that isn't how you use your inner thighs in real life.

Your inner thighs are designed to stabilize your body as you're standing, walking, moving, balancing, or transferring weight from one foot to the other. That's the way the one-leg ice skater works, and that's why it's one of the best moves you can do to target those inner—and outer—thigh muscles. Thanks to the added chest fly, your upper body muscles get a workout, too.

Real-Life Activities It Helps You Do

When you get out of a car, get off a bike, get off a horse, or deboard a boat, you have to put one leg on the ground and push off of that leg to lift your other leg. That's what this exercise teaches you to do.

Starting Point

1. Secure the resistance band at belly button height, and turn your body so your right side is facing the anchor point.

2. Grasp the handle with your right hand, and scoot to the left until there's no slack in the band. Then with a slight bend in your right arm, pull the band all the way across your chest to the left as if you were opening a sliding glass door. You should feel a good amount of tension in the band. Relax your left arm down at your side.

3. Balance on your left leg by lifting your right foot off the floor and raising your right knee in front of you.

Movement

4. Squat down into your left leg so your left hip is sitting back as if you were going to sit in a chair. As you squat, straighten your right leg out in the direction of the anchor point, and keep it suspended without touching the ground.

5. As you straighten your right leg, bring your right arm across your chest until it's straight out to your right side at about belly button height. Do whatever feels comfortable with your left arm to help you balance.

6. Return to the starting position, and repeat 8 to 12 times on the left leg before doing the same number of repetitions on the right leg with the band in your left hand.

Tips and Precautions

Don't let the hip of your standing leg jut out to the side as you squat. If you can't maintain your balance with your leg straight out to the side, tap your foot down.

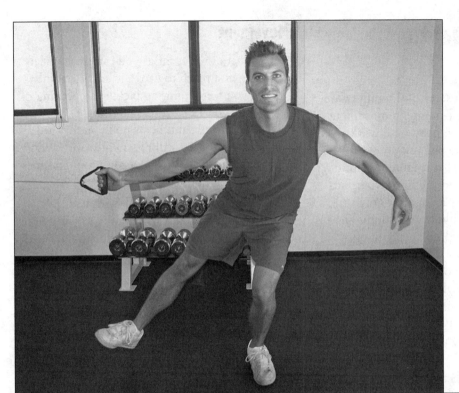

Starting/ending position.

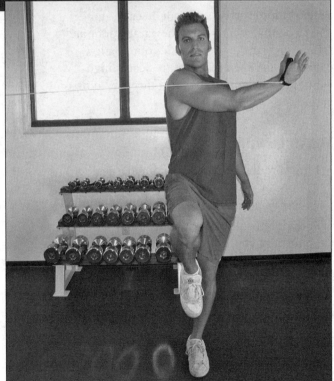

Midpoint position.

Single-Leg Squat to High Pull

You'll really fall for this exercise—literally! One part of this dynamic heart-pumping movement takes you from standing to bending down so low that you may feel like you're falling forward, and that's exactly what it's intended to do. As your body gets closer to the floor, your butt and legs have to work harder against gravity to keep you from tumbling. If your glutes and quads aren't strong enough to keep you upright, your feet and toes have to kick in to help out. Luckily, your feet have more than 150 muscles and ligaments at your service to help get the job done. By activating all those muscles, your body learns how to fend off gravity to help you avoid falling in real-life situations.

Real-Life Activities It Helps You Do

Practice this exercise so it will be easier for you to bend down to open the garage door and raise it up, get the glass cleaner out of a low cupboard and then reach up to clean a high window, or field a baseball and throw it to first base.

Starting Point

1. Secure the resistance band underneath a door or under a heavy object, such as the foot of a bed. Face the anchor point.

2. Grasp the handle with your right hand the way you would put your hand on the handle of a baby stroller, and scoot back until there's no slack in the band. Relax your left arm down at your side.

3. Balance on your left leg by lifting your right foot off the floor so your shin is parallel to the floor.

Movement

4. Squat down as far as you can on your left leg, and reach toward the anchor point as if you were going to pick up something off the floor. Let your spine round as the tension in the band helps pull you forward. Your right leg will naturally swing behind you, and you'll feel your left foot and toes working hard to keep you balanced.

5. In a single motion, push with your left leg to come back to standing as you raise the band up over your right shoulder with your right arm straight and your palm facing forward the way you would open a garage door. At the same time, raise your right knee as high as you can in front of you.

6. Lower your right arm and leg back to the starting position, and perform the movement 8 to 12 times before switching to your other side.

Tips and Precautions

If your shoulders are tight, you can bend your elbow a little as you reach overhead. Tap your back foot down if you have trouble balancing.

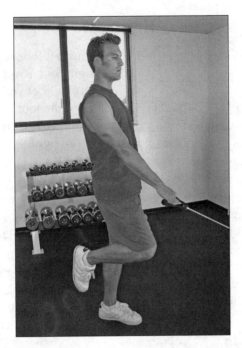

Starting/ending position.

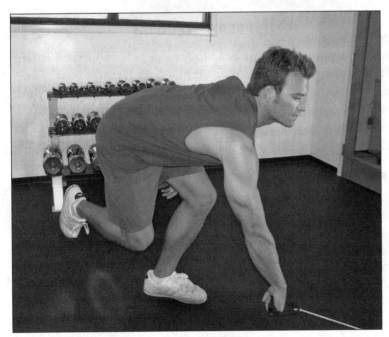

First position.

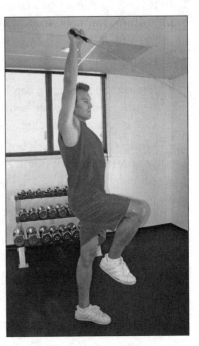

Second position.

Crossover Squat with Opposite Pull

Can you say "pretzel"? Here's one of those twisting exercises I warned you about. This superb full-body move will have you stepping one way while your arms, shoulders, and torso swing the opposite way. That causes your spine to rotate, which is one of the body's key functional movements. If you're like a lot of people, though, you may avoid twisting your back as you age for fear of injuring it. Remember the old adage "use it or lose it"? It applies here, and if you don't practice rotating your spine, you start to lose the ability to do so, which can lead to spinal degeneration and back pain. Ouch!

Real-Life Activities It Helps You Do

Golfers love this move because the extra spinal rotation makes it possible to get a bigger backswing (translation: longer drive) without tweaking the lower back or shoulders. It can also help if you're a dancer or a baseball player, or if you're simply getting out of the shower.

Starting Point

1. Secure the resistance band at shoulder height, and turn your body so your right side is facing the anchor point.
2. Grasp the handle with both hands with your arms straight out in front of you at shoulder height like a police officer at target practice, and scoot to the left until there's no slack in the band.
3. Stand with your feet shoulder-width apart.

Movement

4. Step your left foot across and in front of your right foot as you squat down into your left leg. Let your right foot pivot on the ball of the foot and your right knee bend closer to the ground as your left leg crosses the right.
5. At the same time, keeping your torso erect and your shoulders fairly level, rotate your arms to the left. Your left arm will bend as you twist, but try to keep your right arm as straight as possible.
6. Push down into your left foot to propel you back to standing, and bring your arms back to shoulder height in front of you. Do 10 to 15 repetitions on one side before switching to the other side.

Tips and Precautions

Don't bend to the side or lean forward during the movement phase, and be sure to take a big enough step to avoid getting your legs tangled up.

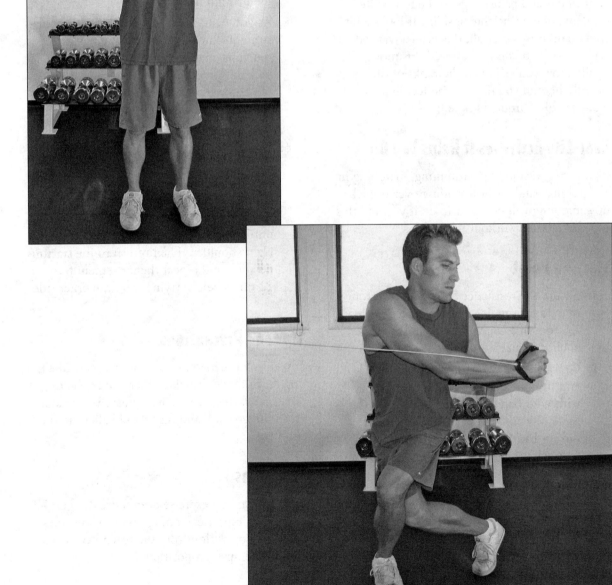

Starting/ending position.

Midpoint position.

Stork Stance with Shoulder Flexion

A lot of people keep their legs straight when bending over. That's why I've included the stork stance, which gets you reaching down without bending your standing leg. This exercise puts your glutes and hamstrings to the test while challenging your balancing skills. It looks a bit tricky, and it is—after all, this is an advanced exercise. When you've mastered this move, you'll know you've joined the ranks of the functionally fit, and you might even feel like you're ready to join Cirque du Soleil!

Real-Life Activities It Helps You Do

Gardening, vacuuming, swimming, marching in a marching band, or just bending over to pick up something will be easier to do if you add this exercise to your workout routine.

Starting Point

1. Secure the resistance band at the bottom of a door or under a heavy object, such as the foot of a couch or bed, and face the anchor point.

2. Grasp the handle with your right hand, and stretch your right arm out straight with your hand at about waist height the same way you would grab onto a lawn mower handle. Scoot back until there's no slack in the band. Relax your left hand down at your side.

3. Balance on your left leg by lifting your right foot off the ground so your right shin is parallel to the ground.

Movement

4. Keeping your standing leg and spine straight, bend forward at your hip and swing your right leg behind you as high and as straight as is comfortable. You might feel like a gymnast on a balance beam in this position, which activates your inner thigh muscles.

5. As you bend forward, reach your right arm straight down until your hand is almost touching the ground as if you wanted to pick up something you dropped. A lot of people have a tendency to rotate their torso in the direction of the leg that's lifted, but keep it parallel to the ground.

6. Use the power in your left hamstring and glute to bring you back to your one-leg stand while you swing your right leg in front of you and raise your knee up high. Simultaneously, swoop the band overhead until your right arm is straight over your right shoulder. Then return to the starting position and repeat the movement 8 to 12 times before trying it on the other side.

Tips and Precautions

If you feel a twinge in your lower back while you reach down, it's likely that you're rotating your torso. Keep your torso squared and parallel to the ground, and that should alleviate the problem.

Variations

Make this tricky exercise even more difficult by adding a jump or extending up onto your toes when you transition from the reach-down position to the up-high position.

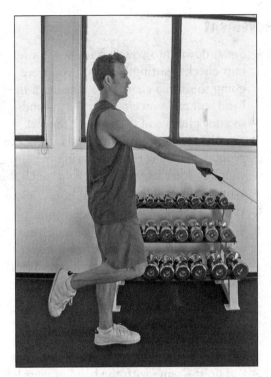

Starting/ending position.

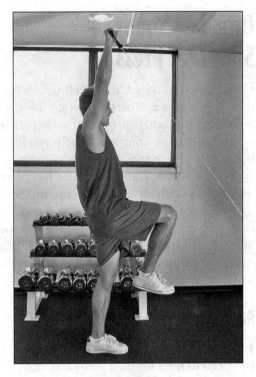

First position.

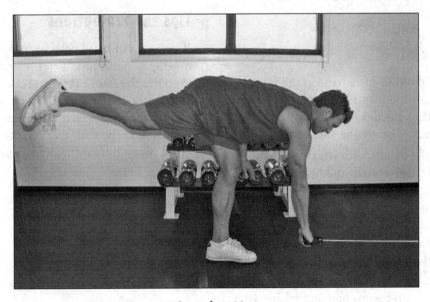

Second position.

One-Leg Squat to Shoulder Press

Have you ever noticed how weightlifters use their legs to power a barbell up into the air? Your body can benefit from that same motion by learning to use your legs to help you lift heavy objects—or resistance bands—with your arms. As you learn to transfer force from the large lower body muscles to the smaller upper body muscles, you'll also get a good cardio blast, thanks to the up-and-down movement. Getting your heart pumping while you strengthen your entire body—it's like an entire workout in one single exercise.

Real-Life Activities It Helps You Do

You'll be glad you did this exercise the next time you need to lift a kayak, a surfboard, or skis onto the roof of your car. The next time you go bowling, notice how you transfer force from your legs to your arms to roll the bowling ball down the lane.

Starting Point

1. Secure the resistance band at the bottom of a door or under a heavy object, such as the foot of a bed, and turn your body so your back is facing the anchor point.

2. Grasp the handle with your right hand, palm facing forward, and bring it up to shoulder level with your elbow bent the way you might hold a duffel bag over your shoulder. Scoot forward until there's no slack in the band. Relax your left hand down at your side.

3. Balance on your left leg by lifting your right foot off the ground and raising your knee in front of you.

Movement

4. Squat down into your left leg so your left butt cheek is sitting back as if you were going to sit in a chair. The tension in the band will pull you closer to the ground so your glutes and thighs have to work extra hard to prevent you from hitting the ground. Let your right leg swing behind you, but don't let your right foot touch the ground, if possible.

5. With a swift movement, extend your body upward and reach your right hand up above your head and in front of you like you're reaching for a high cupboard. Simultaneously, sweep your right leg forward and raise your knee as high as is comfortable.

6. Return to the starting position, and go from high to low to high 8 to 12 times, and do the same with the band in your left hand while balancing on your right leg.

Tips and Precautions

If you get confused with so many body parts moving at once, just keep the band at your shoulder the entire time and concentrate on getting the leg movement down first. When you're comfortable with that, add the arm extension at the end. You can also tap your foot down if you have difficulty balancing.

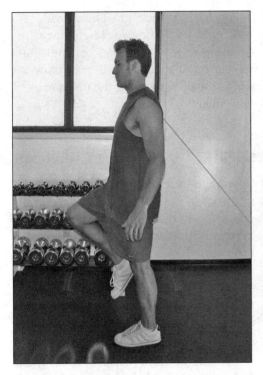

Starting/ending position.

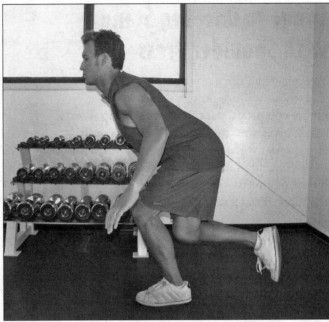

First position.

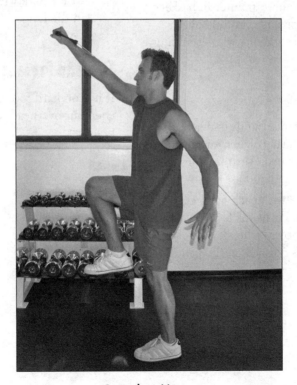

Second position.

Lunge to One-Leg Stand with Shoulder Press

You could call this exercise "TNT" because it gives you explosive power. By starting in a deep lunge, you prestretch the glutes and hip flexors, which gives you the ability to spring upward and transfer force to your upper body. It's the same concept used by runners in the starting blocks of a race—the farther down they crouch, the more they can explode out of the starting blocks.

Like some of the other exercises in this chapter, this exercise teaches your body an important functional lesson: if you want to do something forceful with your arms up high, you need to get your legs down low first.

Real-Life Activities It Helps You Do

This exercise gives you more power in your whole body to shoot a three-pointer in basketball, play on the offensive line in football, or toss heavy boxes up to someone who's standing on a truck or boat.

Starting Point

1. Secure two resistance bands underneath a door or under a heavy object, such as the foot of a couch or bed. Turn so your back is facing the anchor point.
2. Grasp one handle with each hand at shoulder height with your palms facing forward, allowing your elbows to bend. Scoot forward until there's no slack in the band.

3. Take a big step back into a lunge with your right leg, letting your right knee come close to the floor and keeping your torso erect. The lunge gives your body a big base of support for the upcoming movement.

Movement

4. In an explosive movement, push down into your left heel and right toes to spring upward and press both arms straight overhead as if you were cheering after your team scored a touchdown. Your goal is to go up onto the toes of your left foot and raise your right knee as high as you can in front of you. This helps drive your whole body upward and gives your arms more power.
5. Come back down to the starting position, and repeat 10 to 12 times before doing 10 to 12 more with your left leg behind you in the lunge.

Tips and Precautions

If it's too hard for you to get both arms straightened out overhead, you can alternate arms at first.

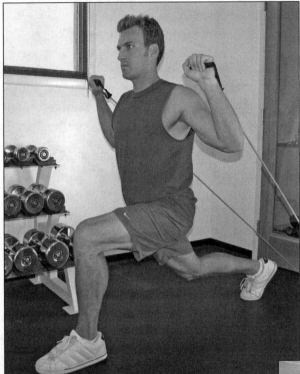

Starting/ending position.

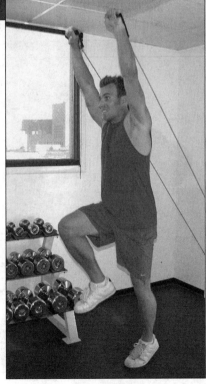

Midpoint position.

In This Chapter

- Having fun with hopping and jumping
- Adding more force
- Throwing you off balance
- Using combo moves

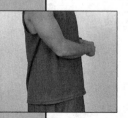
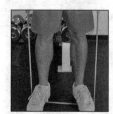
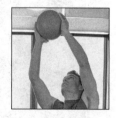
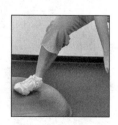
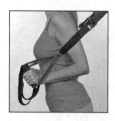
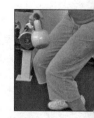

Chapter 20

Advanced Medicine Ball Exercises

If you've been doing all the exercises up to this point, you've probably reached new heights of functional fitness you never thought possible. Congratulations! As always, there's even more you can do to improve the way your body moves. This chapter introduces you to medicine ball exercises that take your training to the limit.

Remember how I mentioned that people love the medicine ball because it reminds them of being a kid? This chapter will really take you back to those days, thanks to the addition of dynamic moves such as hopping and jumping. Not only does this add to the fun, but it also kicks up the intensity of your workout and pushes your muscles harder than ever.

Athletes, weekend warriors, and recreational sports lovers will get the most out of these challenging exercises. The creative combo moves are designed to help you perform better on the field, on the court, or on the golf course. Naturally, when you can handle athletic activities with ease, you'll find that everyday movements are a breeze.

Push-Up to Pike with Feet on the Ball

We're going to try something a little different here and use the medicine ball *under* your feet rather than have you pick it up. The wobbly ball engages a lot of the little muscles that provide stabilization for your hips, spine, and shoulders. At the same time, the powerful push-up to pike focuses on the large muscles in your upper body and torso, including your chest, shoulders, and abs. After all, that's how your body works in real life—your large and small muscles engaging at the same time. Even better, this move looks really impressive and will wow your friends and family!

Real-Life Activities It Helps You Do

Whether you're hoisting a bicycle or luggage on top of your car, diving off a springboard, jumping up from paddling to standing on a surfboard, or push-starting a car, you've got something to gain from this exercise.

Starting Point

1. Get down on the floor in a push-up stance with your hands on the ground and your toes balanced on the medicine ball. Don't let your hips sag or your head tilt downward.

Movement

2. While working to keep your feet from rolling off the ball, lower yourself down into a push-up.

3. As you rise out of the push-up, lift your hips up into the air and use your feet to roll the ball toward your hands to form the shape of an inverted V. Only raise your hips as far as is comfortable, and try to keep your back and legs straight. Your knees might bend and go out to the sides a bit to help keep you balanced.

4. Lower yourself back down to the push-up position, and repeat 8 to 12 times.

Tips and Precautions

On your first few attempts, you can place just one foot on the ball and the other on the ground to help you stabilize. You can also start with just the push-up portion of the exercise and gradually work up to the pike.

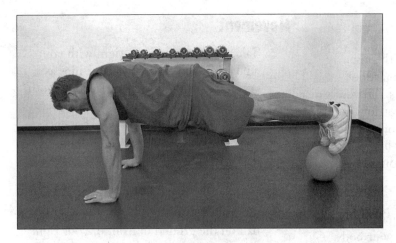

Starting/ending position.

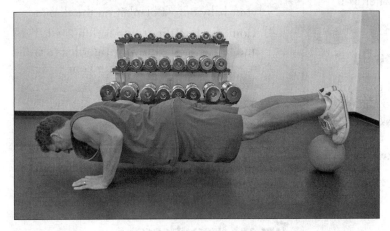

First position.

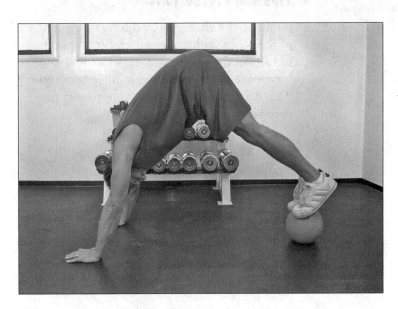

Second position.

Multiplanar Lunge

In the real world, you rarely repeat the same movement over and over the way you're instructed to perform most exercises. That's why the multiplanar lunge is ideal for functional training. It involves a matrix of six moves, including different combinations of lunges, rotations, and reaches, to get you going in all directions.

Sound confusing? It can be, but that's okay because that just adds more unpredictability to the exercise, which mimics the way your body has to make adjustments on the fly when you play sports.

Real-Life Activities It Helps You Do

This exercise gets you in gear for all types of sporting activities that require you to change directions quickly—think soccer, basketball, football, or tennis. You'll also notice the benefit if you need to pick up and move heavy boxes or chase after a toddler.

Starting Point

1. Start with your feet shoulder-width apart while holding the medicine ball in front of you at belly button height.

Movement

2. Take a large step to the right with your right foot, and sit back in your hips as if you were sitting in a chair. Keeping both hands on the ball, reach down to touch the ball to the ground about 18 inches past your right foot the way you might set down a heavy bag of groceries. It's okay if your back rounds as you reach down.

3. Return to standing, and then lunge forward with your right leg as you tap the ball on the ground in front of your right foot the way you might lean down to place your baby onto a blanket on the floor.

4. Come back to the start position again, and lunge back with your right leg as you reach the ball overhead with your arms extended straight.

5. Tilt your pelvis under to increase the stretch at the front of your hip.

6. Go back to standing, and repeat the series 10 to 15 times before switching to the other side.

Tips and Precautions

Ramp up the challenge by mixing up the order of the series. Enlist a friend or workout buddy to call out the movements at random: "Lunge forward left, lunge side right, lunge back right." This will really keep you on your toes to prepare you for sports activities.

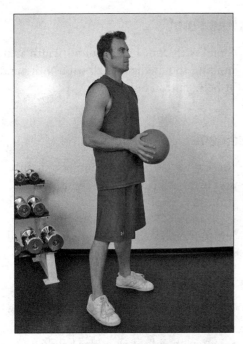

Starting/ending position.

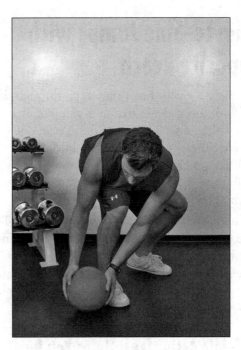

First position.

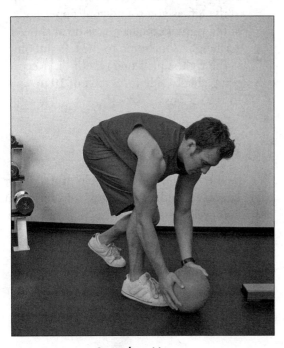

Second position.

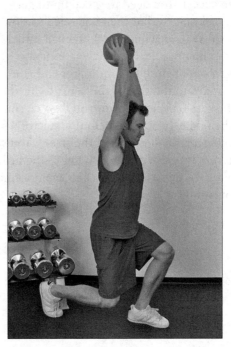

Third position.

Side-to-Side Jumps with Opposite Reach

Get ready for your heart rate to go through the roof with this exercise that gets you jumping from side to side. The major muscles in one leg provide the power to propel you into the air while the other leg has to kick in to dissipate those forces and bring you back down to the ground gently.

This exercise also teaches you how to accelerate quickly and decelerate just as fast to bring your body to a halt. These are some of the most basic movement patterns required when playing sports, and they can also come in handy in your daily routine.

Real-Life Activities It Helps You Do

Think about racing across the field to kick a goal in soccer. You need to speed up to get to the ball quickly, but then you need to slow down so you can actually kick the ball rather than running past it. It's the same in tennis when an opponent hits a wide shot and you have to race to the side of the court to hit the ball. If you don't slow down, you'll go crashing into the fence. It can also help if you have to chase down a toddler toward the street. You've got to run as fast as possible to get to the little one but then put on the brakes to avoid running into oncoming traffic.

Starting Point

1. Stand with your feet shoulder-width apart holding the medicine ball with both hands at belly button height.

Movement

2. Raise your left foot off the floor slightly and bring it over to your right foot. As it nears your right foot, push off of your right foot and jump to the right so your left foot lands where your right foot had been.

3. As you land, squat down as if you were sitting back into a chair and rotate your upper body to the left. Keep both hands on the medicine ball as you bring it out to your left side at shoulder height.

4. Without resting or returning to the starting position, push off both feet and jump to the left as you rotate your upper body to the right so the ball ends up at shoulder height. One jump to the left and one to the right equals one repetition. Keep going side to side for a total of 10 to 15 repetitions.

Tips and Precautions

The muscles in your butt will help protect your back, knees, and ankles during this exercise, but only if you really sit back—like you're going to sit in a chair—as you squat.

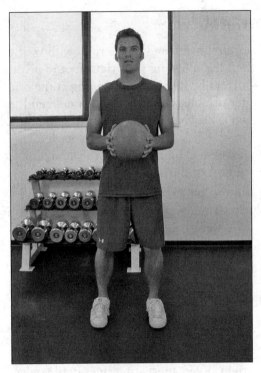

Starting/ending position.

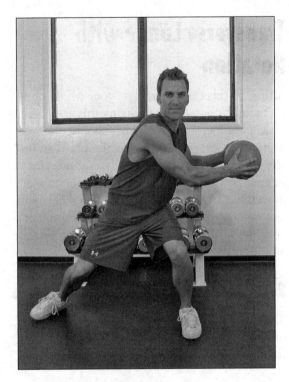

First position.

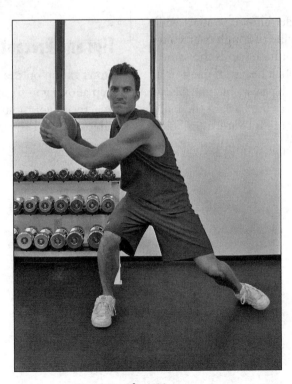

Second position.

Transverse Lunge with Rotation

Although this exercise targets your whole body, it's mainly a butt-burner. Giving this area a little extra focus is a great idea because your derriere is designed for so much more than just sitting. In fact, your glutes and other muscles in your rear end play a huge role in functional movement and safeguard your knees, back, and ankles from getting tweaked. They're some of your hardest-working muscles, so give them the attention they deserve.

Real-Life Activities It Helps You Do

The transverse lunge with rotation really pays off when you're running uphill, sprinting on a flat track, or playing golf or racquetball.

Starting Point

1. Stand with your feet hip-width apart while holding the medicine ball high over your right shoulder with both hands the same way you might hold a heavy sandbag or a shot put. Bend both arms a bit, and place your right hand near the back of the ball with your palm facing forward.

Movement

2. Step forward and to the right with your left leg, allowing your right foot to pivot naturally. If you were standing at the center of a clock, your left foot would end up somewhere in between the 1 and the 2 on the dial. Lunge down as your left leg crosses in front, and lower your right knee almost to the ground.

3. In the same motion, swing your arms down and across your body to the left as if you were swinging an ax. The ball should end up to the side of your left hip. While swinging the ball, keep your torso straight rather than bending your upper back.

4. Come back to standing, and lift the ball over your left shoulder so you can repeat the exercise with your right leg lunging forward and your torso twisting to the right. Keep alternating sides until you've done the exercise 20 to 30 times.

Tips and Precautions

Don't skimp on the step forward. Taking a big step allows you to sink down into the lunge to activate your glutes, hamstrings, quads, and calves, which helps protect your knees.

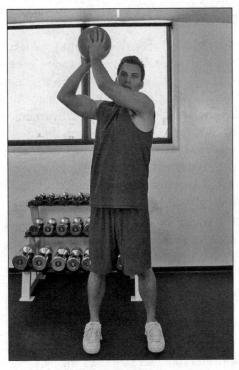

Starting/ending position.

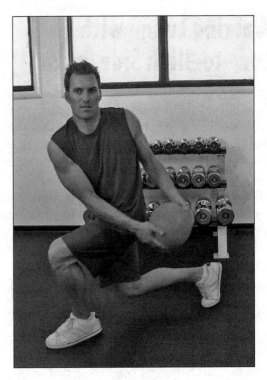

First position.

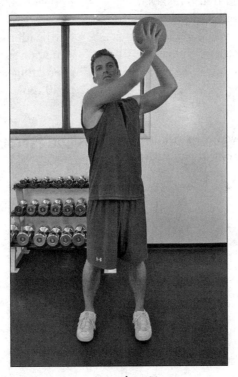

Second position.

Walking Lunge with Low-to-High Side Reach

I like to think of this exercise as "The Destabilizer." With most exercises, you have a solid base of support, but not here. In fact, the goal is to throw you off balance as you reach down and then up over your head so your muscles have to figure out how to keep you from falling over. Don't be surprised if you do lose your balance at first; it may take some time for you to feel comfortable in these positions.

You'll be glad you took the time to perfect these moves, and being able to right yourself when you're about to fall flat on your face will pay big dividends in real life and in sports.

Real-Life Activities It Helps You Do

This exercise helps you bend down and scoop up a dropped cell phone or car keys without missing a step as you're walking. It also makes it easier to crouch down low to walk and paint the baseboards in your home. Plus, you'll get better at playing any sport that requires you to bend down low and then reach up high.

Starting Point

1. Stand with your feet hip-width apart holding the medicine ball in front of you with both hands at belly button height.

Movement

2. Step forward about 2 feet with your left leg, and lunge down as if you were kneeling, but don't let your right knee come in contact with the ground. At the same time, reach the ball down toward the ground to the right with your arms extended as if you were going to place a heavy box on the ground. The ball should end up about 1 foot away from your right knee. It's okay if your back rounds as you reach down.

3. Without shifting your feet, push yourself upright, twist your torso so you're facing to the right, and swing the ball up overhead. In this position, your hips and upper body are facing to the right while your feet remain facing forward. To be sure you're in the right position, practice doing this move against a wall so your left foot, hip, and shoulder as well as the ball touch the wall next to you.

4. Return to the starting position, and repeat the exercise on the other side. Lunge forward with the other leg, and do exactly the same movement on the other side. Keep alternating sides until you've completed 30 to 40 repetitions.

Tips and Precautions

Be sure both feet continue to face forward as you lunge and reach overhead. Bend your hips, not just your back, when you lunge and reach down.

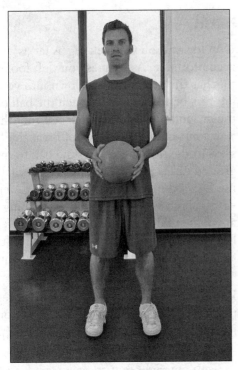

Starting/ending position.

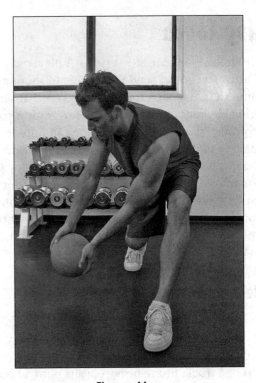

First position.

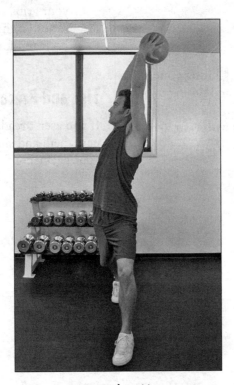

Second position.

Hop Touch

He shoots! He scores! Every NBA player knows that you've got to bend your knees to shoot a jump shot. The hop touch is based on that same principle but takes it even further—getting you to crouch down really low so you can hop or jump as high as possible as you reach up with the medicine ball. Targeting the leg muscles as you move forward and reach up, this dynamic exercise can send your heart rate to the moon if you do it rapidly. When you get the hang of this one, you'll be feeling like a functional training MVP.

Real-Life Activities It Helps You Do

Practice the hop touch, and you'll feel more at ease doing all sporting activities, especially shooting a basketball; tossing a bale of hay on top of a truck; lifting heavy objects onto a high shelf; or jumping onto a boat or a high platform such as a stage.

Starting Point

1. Balance on your left leg by lifting your right foot off the ground and raising your right knee in front of you. Hold the medicine ball with both hands with your arms extended overhead.

Movement

2. Hop forward on your left leg as far as is comfortable. As soon as your left foot touches the ground, squat down into your left hip, bend down, and touch the ball on the ground to the left of your left foot the way you would lower a box of breakable glass to the floor. Touching the ball to the ground can actually prevent you from falling forward in this deep bend. Don't even worry about what your right leg is doing as you bend down—it will naturally shift behind you to help keep you balanced. It's also okay if your back rounds as you bend down.

3. In one swift motion, push off your left leg to jump up and hop forward again on your left leg while you reach up with the ball as if you were going to shoot a basketball.

4. Lower your right foot to the ground, and raise your left knee forward as you extend your arms straight overhead to repeat the series on the other side. Keep switching back and forth 20 to 30 times.

Tips and Precautions

If you aren't ready for the hops, you can eliminate them and simply raise up onto the toe of your balancing foot instead.

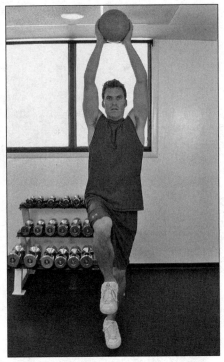

Starting/ending position.

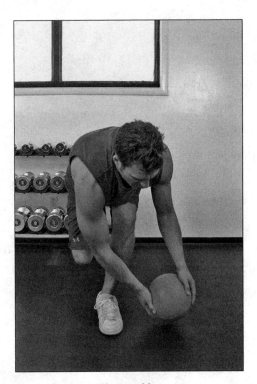

First position.

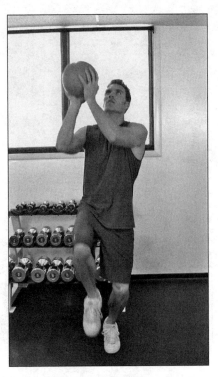

Second position.

In This Chapter

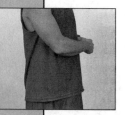
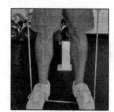
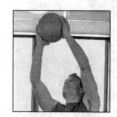
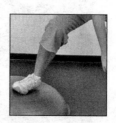
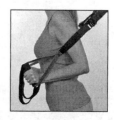
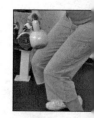

Chapter **21**

Advanced TRX Exercises

If you've made it this far, you're ready for the big leagues. Like hundreds of professional football players, United States Army Rangers, United States Marines, and mixed martial arts fighters who choose the TRX for their most extreme workouts, you'll be tackling some very demanding, heart-pumping moves in this chapter.

Get ready to blast your midsection with the most intense ab workout ever. You're definitely going to feel the muscles in your torso working at maximum capacity with some of these exercises. In the following pages, we target the fast-twitch muscles in your trunk used to create power, which means you'll do big movements with fewer reps. Although you do fewer reps, you can expect your body to fatigue very quickly.

When your body can't take it anymore, your technique may slacken, which can result in aches and pains. To protect your body from injury, it's better to stop when you can no longer do the move properly rather than trying to eke out a few more reps.

Single-Leg High-to-Low Reach

Strength, balance, flexibility—you'll work it all in this exercise. While balancing on one leg and shifting from high to low, you'll also get your heart rate up. Pretty good for a single exercise, huh?

For many people, the hardest part about this exercise is balancing. If there's any slack in the system, the TRX will throw you off balance. If you don't want to topple over, maintain constant tension on the system as you flow from high to low.

Real-Life Activities It Helps You Do

Whether you're reaching down to field a baseball and then throwing it, leaning down to scoop up a low volley and then hitting an overhead smash in tennis, or simply reaching down to pick up something and then placing it up on a high shelf, you'll do it with more ease thanks to this exercise.

Starting Point

1. Face the anchor point and grasp the foot cradles (not the handles) in your right hand. Scoot back until there's no slack in the system, and place your right hand in front of you at belly button height.

2. Lift up your right foot so you're balancing on your left leg. Let your left arm do whatever it needs to do to help you balance.

3. Extend your right hand overhead, and stand straight up while still balancing on your left leg. Maintaining tension on the system while you reach your hand overhead is crucial to keep you from tipping over.

Movement

4. Squat back as if you were going to rest the left side of your butt on a high barstool. As you squat, reach your right arm forward and across your left foot as if you were reaching out to open a car door. Be sure to keep tension on the system as you reach forward. As you squat, your right leg will naturally shift back to help you balance.

5. Continue squatting and reaching overhead without resting until you've done a total of 12 to 15 repetitions. Switch to the other side, and balance on your right leg with the foot cradles in your left hand.

Tips and Precautions

To help keep your balance, keep constant tension on the system throughout the exercise or tap your foot down if necessary.

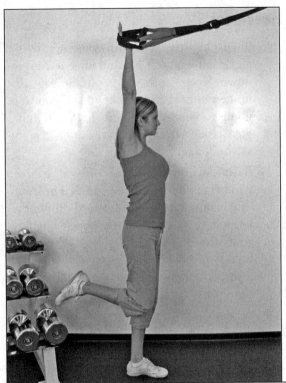

Starting/ending position.

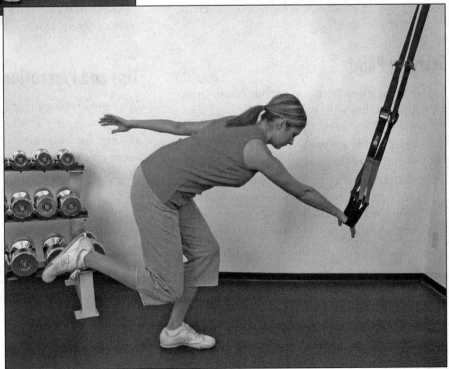

Midpoint position.

Sprinter's Start

Wanna feel like an Olympic sprinter? This leg blaster will let you experience what it's like to explode out of the starting blocks. Like a sprinter, you'll get down really low to help create a powerful burst of energy to propel you forward.

Learning how to move with explosive power will improve your performance in any sport you choose. You'll be quicker off the mark, quicker getting to the ball, and quicker to the finish line. When you can move like that, you'll always feel like a winner.

Real-Life Activities It Helps You Do

Anytime you need to bolt quickly—running in a race, playing sports, chasing after your dog when it runs into the street, racing up the stairs two at a time, or even running away from a mugger—your muscles will know how to create the power you need.

Starting Point

1. Facing away from the anchor point, grasp the handles with your palms facing each other. Bend your elbows at your sides so your hands are at about waist height, as if you were pulling open a pair of double doors. Scoot away from the anchor point until there's no slack in the system, and lean forward while keeping your body straight.

Movement

2. Take a big step back with your right leg, and bend your left hip and knee to lunge down. Keep your right leg straight for this lunge rather than bending it as if you were going to kneel down. The TRX will pull your elbows back toward the anchor point as you lunge.

3. In one swift motion, push off your legs as you bring your right knee up and in front of you and try to jump forward off your left leg, the way you might shoot a half-court shot in basketball. The TRX will hold you back, the same way it might feel if someone was blocking you from taking the shot.

4. As soon as your left foot touches back down on the ground, sink back down into your lunge again without pausing. Shoot for 12 to 15 repetitions to make your legs burn like crazy, and then switch to the other side.

Tips and Precautions

Your goal is to go from lunging as low as possible to jumping as high as possible without resting. Be aware that the higher you jump, the more the TRX will hold you back, increasing the intensity of the exercise.

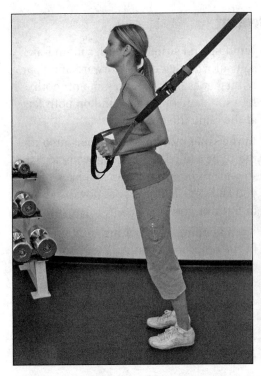

Starting/ending position.

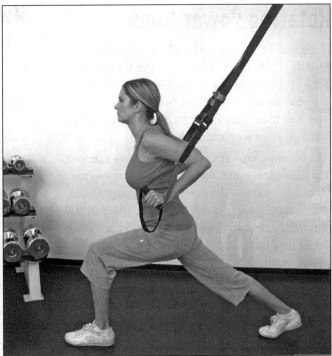

First position.

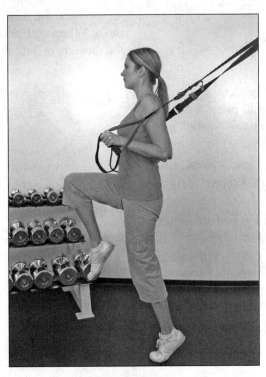

Second position.

Rotating Power Jump

Have you ever swung a baseball bat and hit the ball? If so, then you know that the force reverberates through your body. The same thing happens when you walk or run; every time your foot hits the ground, the force travels back up through your legs and body.

The same concept is at work in this exercise, but the forces come from both your arms (the "rotating" part of the exercise) and your legs (the "jump" part of the exercise) to meet in the middle, giving your abs and torso a killer workout. This is the way your abs were designed to work, and once you get a feel for it, you'll never want to go back to those dysfunctional crunches on the floor.

Real-Life Activities It Helps You Do

The rotating power jump will boost your performance when swinging a baseball bat, golf club, or racquet; slalom skiing; running; jumping; or walking.

Starting Point

1. Facing the anchor point, grasp the handles with your arms straight and palms facing down. Scoot back until there's no slack in the system.

2. Step your right foot back into a lunge, and bend forward at your hips, keeping your back straight.

3. Rotate your torso to the left and straighten your right arm out and down in front of you while your left arm goes straight up and back behind you. This should create the shape of a T.

Movement

4. Jump up and switch your legs in mid-air so your right leg comes forward and your left leg goes back. Try to jump off both legs simultaneously and land on both feet at the same time.

5. In the same motion, rotate your torso to the right while keeping your arms straight so your right arm goes up and back behind you and your left arm goes down and out in front of you.

6. Keep jumping and rotating from one side to the other until you've done a total of 20 to 30 jumps. The faster you go, the higher your heart rate will climb, making this an excellent heart-pounding exercise.

Tips and Precautions

You might want to try this move without the jump at first. In this case, simply step one foot forward and the other back as you rotate your torso. When you feel more comfortable with the movement, add the jump.

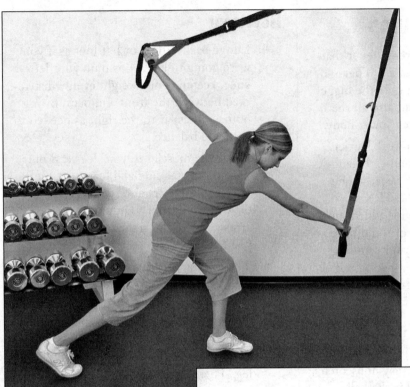

Starting/ending position.

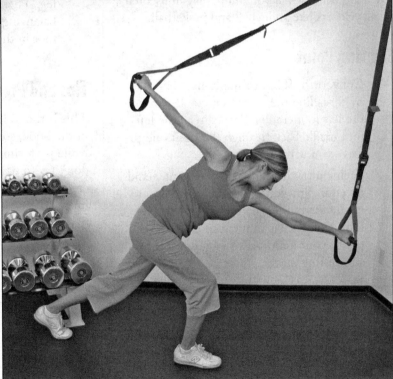

Midpoint position.

Suspended Lunge Jump

Here's an intense lower body strengthener that also challenges your sense of balance. That means you'll have to engage not only the bigger muscles in your legs and butt, but also all the smaller stabilizing muscles in your lower body.

In fact, the stabilizers have to work harder here than for any of the other one-leg balancing exercises in this book. That's because one of your feet will be secured in the TRX so you can't tap it down on the ground for added support if you're losing your balance. You'll have to rely solely on the muscles in your standing leg. When you've mastered this move, you'll be ready to take your balancing act on the road.

Real-Life Activities It Helps You Do

Thanks to the suspended lunge jump, you'll feel like a kid again when you jump, play hopscotch, or play sports like volleyball and basketball.

Starting Point

1. Convert the TRX to single-handle mode by threading the right foot cradle through the left foot cradle. Then thread the left foot cradle back through the right one to leave you with a single strap.

2. Facing away from the anchor point, stand on your right leg while holding the foot cradle in your left hand. Lift up your left foot, and place it in the foot cradle so the top of your midfoot is facing downward and resting on the cradle.

3. Hop forward on your right foot until there's no slack in the system.

Movement

4. Lunge back with your left foot as if you were going to kneel down on your left knee, keeping your weight evenly distributed between the front and back. Swing both arms as far to the right as needed to help you balance.

5. Using the muscles in your legs and butt, push up to standing and bring your left knee up and in front of you as you push off your right foot to jump up. Swing your arms as far to the right as needed to help you balance.

6. The instant your right foot makes contact with the floor after the jump, drop back down into your lunge in a fluid motion.

7. In one continuous motion, keep going from the lunge to the jump until you've done 10 to 15 repetitions on your right leg. Then switch and do 10 to 15 more balancing on your left leg with your right foot in the foot cradle.

Tips and Precautions

This is the toughest balance challenge exercise in the book, so don't be surprised if you tip over while performing it. If you're about to fall over, don't try to wriggle your foot out of the foot cradle; just put your hands down on the ground for support.

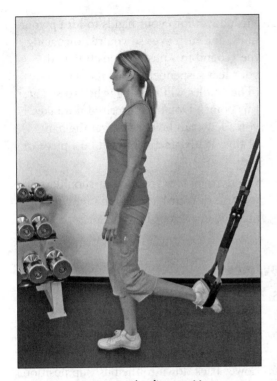

Starting/ending position.

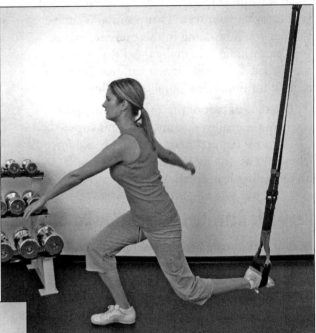

First position.

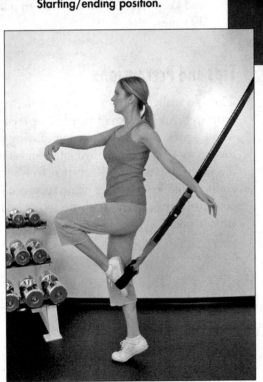

Second position.

Seesaw to Pike

Remember doing wheelbarrow races when you were a kid? You'd put both hands on the ground and a friend would pick up your feet so you could walk on your hands while they ran behind you, carrying your feet. That position is similar to what you'll be doing in this exercise, except your feet will be held up by the TRX. You probably didn't realize it as a kid, but this move is great for improving shoulder stability.

The second part of this exercise—the pike—is where the real work comes in. This super-tough move requires a lot of strength and force from your abs, shoulders, and hip flexors. It isn't easy, but it is worth the effort.

Real-Life Activities It Helps You Do

Diving off a diving board into a pool, sledding face first down a mountain, boogie boarding, and surfing are only some of the many things you'll be able to do with greater ease after trying this exercise.

Starting Point

1. Face the anchor point, and sit on the ground with your knees bent. Grab the foot cradles, and cross the left foot cradle over the right one. Lift up your right foot, and put it in the foot cradle on the left. Push your right foot down so it won't slip out. Then place your left foot in the right cradle and push your foot down.

2. Rotate your torso to the right, and place both hands on the ground to your right side so your right hand is farther behind your left hand.

3. Push down into your hands to lift up your body, and turn over so you're now facing the ground in a push-up position with your feet suspended in the foot cradles. (The cradles will no longer be crossed at this point.) Don't be surprised if it takes you a few tries before you get the hang of this. With practice, it will be a piece of pie.

4. Gently rock forward so your shoulders are forward of your hands. Don't let your hips sag, and keep your body rigid.

Movement

5. Push into your hands, and lift your hips into the air to form an inverted V. Only raise your hips as far as is comfortable, and try to keep your back and legs straight.

6. Lower back down to the push-up position, and keep going from push-up to pike 15 to 20 times.

Tips and Precautions

This is a really tough exercise, so you might want to break it down at first before trying the whole series. Start by practicing moving your torso forward and back through your hands in the push-up position. When that feels more comfortable, try the pike while balanced on your forearms. Then, graduate to the pike on your hands.

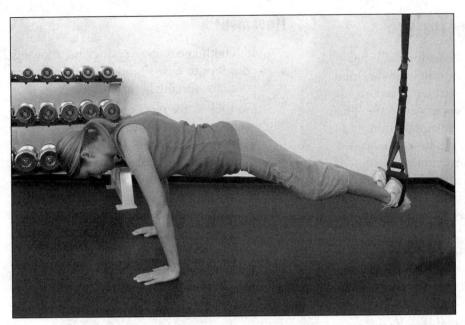

Starting/ending position.

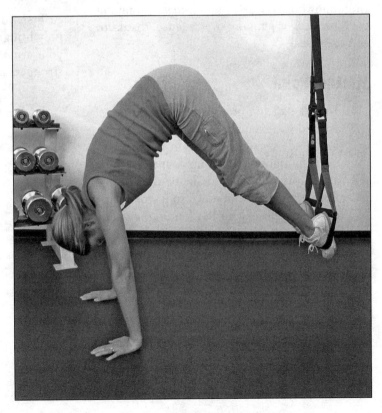

Midpoint position.

Suspended Hip Twist

This exercise may be called a hip twist, but you're really going to feel it in your abs. Like the seesaw to pike, you start out in a push-up position with your feet suspended in the TRX. To keep your hips from sinking down to the ground in this position, you have to engage your abs, and that isn't even the ab portion of the movement yet. When you do start moving, you work your abs in a completely functional way—extending one side while contracting the other side.

With a stronger midsection, all your movements in everyday life or in the most extreme sports will be more fluid.

Real-Life Activities It Helps You Do

You'll feel like you can glide through the air while snowboarding, skiing on moguls, jumping over hurdles, or jumping over a fence, thanks to this exercise.

Starting Point

1. Face the anchor point, and sit on the ground with your knees bent. Grab the foot cradles, and cross the left foot cradle over the right one. Lift up your right foot, and put it in the foot cradle on the left. Push your right foot down so it won't slip out. Then place your left foot in the cradle on the right, and push your foot down.

2. Rotate your torso to the right, and place both hands on the ground to your right side so your right hand is farther behind your left hand.

3. Push down into your hands to lift your body, and turn over so you're now facing the ground in a push-up position with your feet suspended in the foot cradles.

Movement

4. Pull both knees up to your chest, allowing your hips to raise slightly. You'll really feel your abs working here.

5. Go back to the push-up position, and then rotate your hips to the left as you bring your knees up to your left side and try to touch them to your left elbow. You should feel this working the left side of your torso.

6. Return to the starting position, and bring your knees out to the right side to target the right side of your trunk. With this move, you will have completed 1 repetition. A good goal for this exercise is 6 repetitions.

Tips and Precautions

At first, you may want to skip the side work and only bring your knees up to your chest between your arms. As your abs and shoulders become stronger, add the side moves.

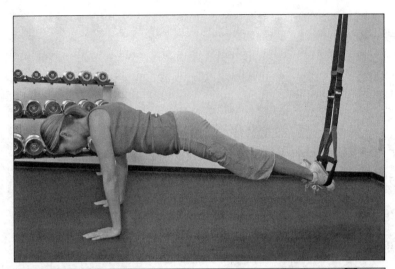

Starting/ending position.

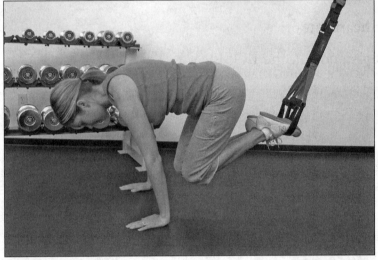

First position.

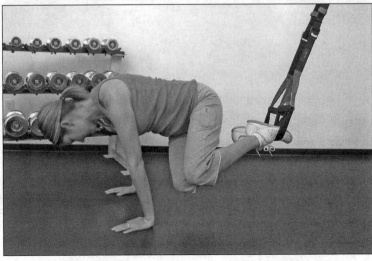

Second position.

In This Chapter

- Pumping up your power
- Coordinating both sides of your body
- Transitioning quickly from one movement to the next
- Spiking your heart rate
- Doing one-leg stands on the BOSU

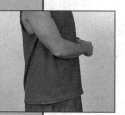
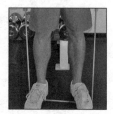
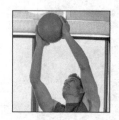
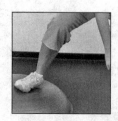
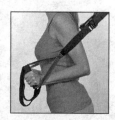
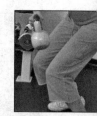

Chapter 22

Advanced BOSU Exercises

Now that you've made it to the advanced exercises, it's time to try more athletic movements on the BOSU. If you're still struggling with the intermediate or even the beginner BOSU moves in Chapters 10 and 16, keep practicing them and return to this chapter when you're feeling more confident about your "BOSU-bility." If you've successfully conquered all the BOSU moves in the previous chapters, get ready to step up the challenge!

Here, you'll be adding more explosive jumps on the BOSU that increase your power while challenging your coordination and sending your heart rate through the roof. Like athletes who have the ability to shoot a basketball right- or left-handed or kick a soccer ball equally well using either foot, you'll also learn how to improve the movement of both sides of your body with these moves. That helps eliminate imbalances, which is one of the best ways to increase your functional fitness.

Jump Squats

In this exercise, you'll be jumping up and down on the BOSU without letting your feet touch the ground. Similar to a trampoline, the BOSU provides some extra bounce, so you'll be able to soar higher than if you were jumping off the floor. In addition, the BOSU gives a little so it cushions your landing to help absorb the shock to your ankles, knees, and hips.

The act of jumping requires a combination of strength and power, and no, they aren't the same thing. Strength is the amount of weight you can lift, while power is how fast you can lift that same weight. Let's use your own body weight as an example. You may have the strength to walk 100 yards, but you would need power to run that same distance at break-neck speed. Athletes possess both strength and power, and that should be your goal, too.

Real-Life Activities It Helps You Do

Jump squats can make a big difference when diving, blocking a spike in volleyball, shooting a three-pointer in basketball, jumping onto the monkey bars in a playground, or climbing over a wall.

Starting Point

1. Stand on the BOSU with your feet hip-width apart with your arms down at your sides and your torso erect.

Movement

2. Squat down as deep as you can as if you were going to sit in a low chair. Reach your arms straight behind you as if you were reaching for the arms of that imaginary chair you're sitting back into.

3. In a dynamic motion, push off of both feet, swing your arms up high, and jump into the air with both feet coming off the BOSU.

4. As you land back on the BOSU, immediately bend your knees, hips, and ankles and return to your deep squat. Bending your knees helps soften your landing to keep your joints happy. Keep jumping and squatting 10 to 15 times.

Tips and Precautions

It's best to start with small hops and work up to bigger jumps as you feel more confident.

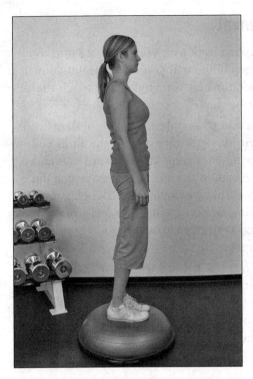

Starting/ending position.

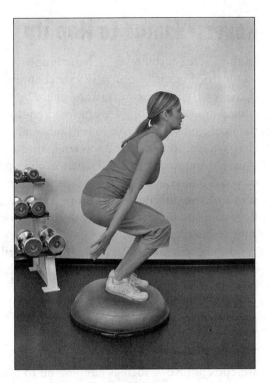

First position.

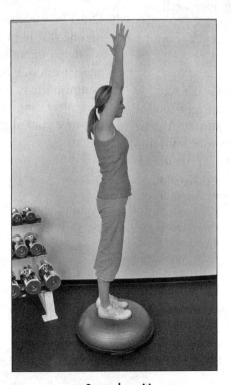

Second position.

Reverse Lunge to Hop Up

In this exercise, you take the basic lunge you learned in the beginner BOSU chapter (Chapter 10) into the next stratosphere by adding a powerful hop. This move strengthens the major muscles in your lower body and also requires some precision to land your foot squarely on top of the BOSU after each hop, or you'll lose your balance and have to step off the dome. Of course, the more you have to fight to maintain your balance, the more work your stabilizing muscles are doing, and that's a good thing. So don't worry that if you're flailing around you aren't getting anything out of the exercise. You are!

Real-Life Activities It Helps You Do

This exercise provides heaps of benefits for athletic endeavors, such as jumping up to spike a volleyball, hopping over a fence, doing the high jump or long jump, playing hopscotch, or skipping.

Starting Point

1. Stand on the BOSU with your left foot on top of the dome with your right foot lightly tapping the dome next to it. Almost all your weight should be in your left foot while your right foot is merely providing balance. Relax your arms down at your sides, and as always, keep your torso erect.

Movement

2. Lunge back with your right leg into a deep lunge as if you were kneeling down, but don't let your right knee touch the ground.

3. In one powerful movement, push off your left foot to spring up into the air as you swing your right knee forward as high as you can in front of you the way you did as a child when you were skipping. In the same motion, swing your left arm forward and your right arm back to help you jump higher.

4. Come back down with your left foot directly on top of the BOSU, and immediately dip down into a deep lunge again. Aim for 10 to 15 reps on your left foot, and switch to your right foot.

Tips and Precautions

Don't be surprised if you feel pretty smooth on one side but have to flap your arms around wildly on the other side. These types of imbalances from side to side are very common. To diminish them, focus on keeping your feet and hips facing forward as you jump. This will improve your alignment and balance.

Starting/ending position.

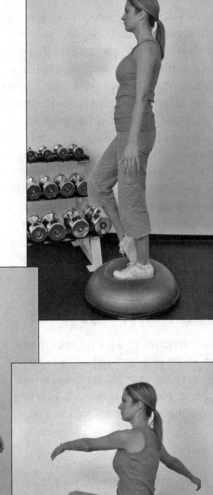

First position.

Second position.

Alternating Lunge Jump

Did you know you can jump higher by leaping off of one foot rather than both feet? It's true, and this exercise lets you practice doing just that. The alternating lunge jump also teaches you to transfer weight from side to side while pumping your arms to produce more power, which can improve your performance in all kinds of sporting activities. Getting your arms involved also engages your abs, although the primary target of this exercise is your lower body. Your glutes, quads, and hamstrings will be working even harder than they do during a regular lunge because you can lower down deeper using the BOSU. That's another thing that helps you jump higher. So go ahead and jump!

Real-Life Activities It Helps You Do

This exercise prepares you for highly athletic movements, including catching a home run as it's flying over the outfield wall, dunking a basketball, jump serving a volleyball, running uphill, or running up the stairs two at a time.

Starting Point

1. Start in a partial lunge with your legs slightly bent with your left foot just shy of the top of the BOSU and the ball of your right foot about 2 feet behind the BOSU. Let your arms hang down at your sides, and keep your torso erect throughout the exercise.

Movement

2. Lunge down as if you were going to kneel on the ground, but don't let your right knee touch the ground. As you lunge, swing your right arm forward and your left arm back in a more exaggerated way than you would when walking normally.

3. Without stopping at the bottom of your lunge, push off your feet to jump as high as you can. In mid-air, swap your arms and legs as if you were running so your right foot and left arm come forward and your left foot and right arm go back.

4. As you land, plant your right foot directly on top of the BOSU and the ball of your left foot on the ground about 2 feet behind the BOSU. Without a rest, immediately go back down into a lunge. Continue alternating sides until you've done 20 to 30 repetitions.

Tips and Precautions

Don't stop or rest in the lunge position or when you land. By making the exercise one fluid motion, you increase the potential to stretch and load your lower body muscles, which provides more power for the jump, and helps you land more gently.

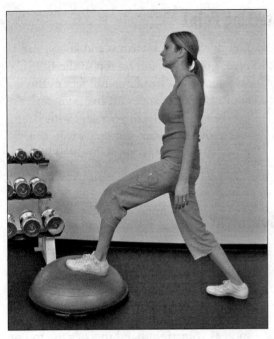

Starting/ending position.

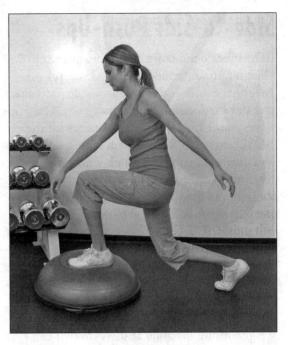

First position.

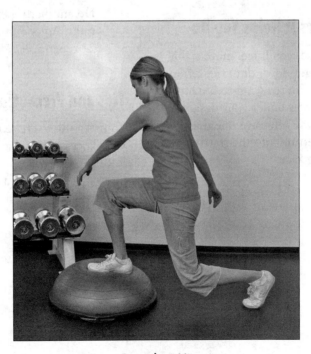

Second position.

Side-to-Side Push-Ups

Remember bend down, walk forward from Chapter 16's intermediate BOSU exercises? Like that exercise, these side-to-side push-ups transfer the focus to your upper body. Only this time, your hands will be in contact with the BOSU, so you'll feel the twitching, shaking, and quivering course through your fingers, forearms, upper arms, shoulders, and chest. That shows that the smaller stabilizing muscles in your upper body are working against the instability of the BOSU. You'll also need to engage the larger muscles in your arms, shoulders, and chest to provide the strength for the push-ups. When you combine all that with the side-to-side movement, you also turn on your ab muscles. There isn't a single traditional weight-lifting machine at the gym that can get all those muscles working at the same time like this exercise does.

Real-Life Activities It Helps You Do

Thanks to this exercise, you'll feel more stable anytime you need to get down onto the ground on all fours, whether you're trying to untangle all those wires and cables under your desk, taking your position on the offensive line during a football game, or getting into the starting position for a running race.

Starting Point

1. Get down on your hands and knees, and place your left hand on top of the BOSU and your right hand about 2 feet to the right. Lift your knees off the floor so you're on the balls of your feet with your feet about shoulder-width apart. In this push-up position, your body should form a relatively straight line.

Movement

2. As smoothly as you can, lower yourself into a push-up, keeping your body straight like a wooden plank. As you rise back up, move your right hand and leg over in unison to meet your left hand and leg. As soon as your right hand touches the top of the BOSU, walk your left hand and foot about 2 feet to the left of the BOSU.

3. Do another repetition moving from left to right. A good goal for this exercise is 20 to 24 repetitions.

Tips and Precautions

To make this exercise easier, do the push-ups on your knees rather than your feet or forego the lowering-down portion of the push-up and simply walk your hands and feet from side to side while maintaining the push-up position.

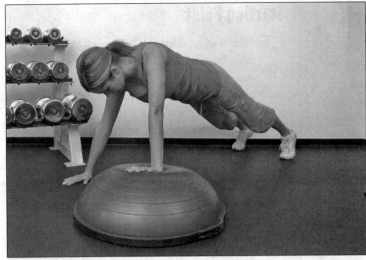

Starting/ending position.

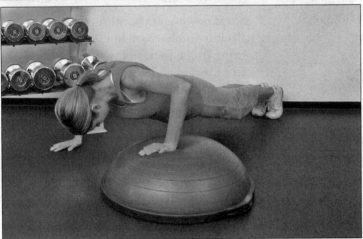

First position.

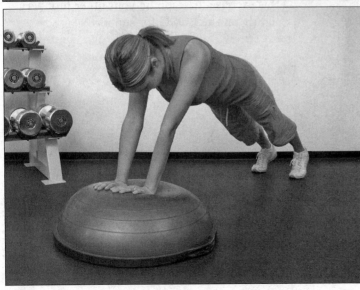

Second position.

One-Leg Squat with Reach

It's time to take your balancing act to new heights. By now, you're very familiar with the one-leg stand, and you're probably getting really good at it. Nice work! That now-familiar move won't feel so comfortable anymore when you try it on the BOSU. When you also throw in a squat and a reach, you're almost guaranteed to lose your balance.

It may take you several attempts before you can perform this exercise without flailing around or having to step off the BOSU. With practice, you'll strengthen the larger muscles in your lower body and train those all-important stabilizing muscles so you can begin smoothing out any herky-jerky motions.

Real-Life Activities It Helps You Do

This exercise helps you feel stable on one leg so you can kick a ball with your other leg or kick up your leg during a dance move. When you tee off in golf, you need stability and balance as your weight shifts from your back foot to your front foot or else your drive will hook or slice.

Starting Point

1. Stand in a one-leg stand with your left foot balancing on top of the BOSU and your right foot as high off the dome as is comfortable. Depending on your balance, your right foot may end up barely off the dome, lifted higher with your right shin parallel to the ground, or anywhere in between. Relax your arms down at your sides, and stand up tall with your torso erect.

Movement

2. Squat down as if you were going to sit in a chair as you let your right leg and left arm swing to the back and you reach your right arm forward and across your body so it ends up near your left knee.

3. Come back to your one-leg stand, and repeat 10 to 15 times before shifting to the other side.

Tips and Precautions

If you simply can't keep your balance during this exercise, try tapping your other foot very lightly on the BOSU for support.

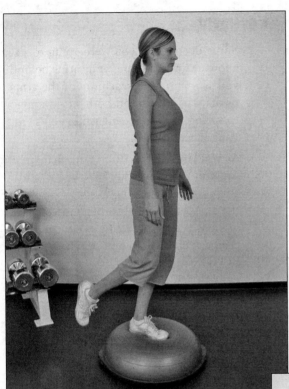

Starting/ending position.

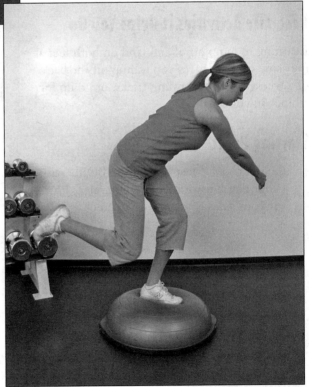

Midpoint position.

Jump and Stick It

Like an Olympic gymnast, you have to stick the landing on this heart-pumping exercise to get all its functional benefits. This advanced movement involves leaping off both feet equally from the ground and landing softly on both feet at the same time on the BOSU.

Most people think this sounds easy, but it takes a combination of power and strength in addition to a healthy dose of confidence. If you get nervous about your ability to perform this exercise, you're likely to lead off with one leg or land on one side first, which can bounce you off the BOSU. Try to imagine you're an athlete whose body moves quickly but whose brain is calm and in the zone. By staying relaxed and confident, you'll increase your chances of sticking the landing and earning a perfect 10 from me, your functional training coach.

Real-Life Activities It Helps You Do

Learning to jump off of and land on both feet at the same time prepares you to hop off the back of a truck, do skateboarding tricks, or go up for a block in volleyball.

Starting Point

1. Stand about 2 feet behind the BOSU with your feet hip-width apart, your arms down at your sides, and your torso erect.

Movement

2. Squat deeply as if you were going to sit in a low chair, and swing your arms behind you as if you were reaching for the arms of that chair. Push off both feet evenly to spring up into the air while you swing your arms forward.

3. As you land on the BOSU, immediately squat by bending your hips, knees, and ankles to cushion your landing, similar to the way the shock absorbers on your car prevent you from feeling every rut in the road as you drive. Then step back off the BOSU with either leg.

4. When you can do 10 to 15 repetitions without stopping, you'll know you've reached the highest echelon of functional fitness.

Tips and Precautions

Although you can perform most of the BOSU exercises in this book barefoot, this one may place a bit too much stress on tender arches. Keep your shoes on while you jump and stick it.

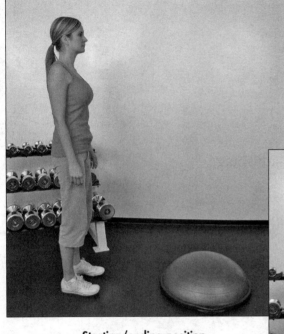

Starting/ending position.

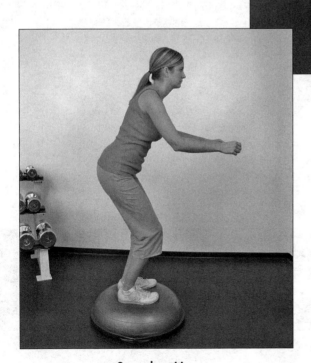

First position.

Second position.

In This Chapter

- ◆ Using momentum to your advantage
- ◆ Coordinating your movements
- ◆ Slowing down the kettlebell
- ◆ Putting it all together

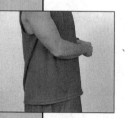
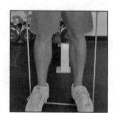
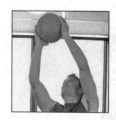
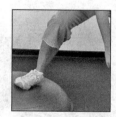
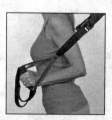
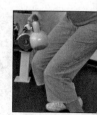

Chapter 23

Advanced Kettlebell Exercises

"Don't use momentum." That's the mantra at most gyms, where personal trainers routinely advise you to keep your movements controlled as you lift weights. That's not the idea behind functional training, though. In real life, momentum is a good thing. It helps you swing a golf club, hand off a heavy sandbag, or hoist a toddler onto your shoulders. That's why I've designed the whole-body exercises in this chapter to incorporate momentum to help you lift and swing the kettlebells.

To use momentum with these advanced exercises, you draw on everything you've learned throughout this book. For example, you have to coordinate and time complex movements so you can avoid smacking yourself with the kettlebells. In addition, you have to slow down your movements, or momentum will make the kettlebells go soaring across the room. Oops!

When you've conquered the exercises in this chapter, you'll know you've reached your goal of functional fitness. Kudos! Remember, though, that your journey to functional fitness doesn't end here. In fact, it never ends. Throughout your life, keep finding new ways to move and challenge your body to keep you moving better and feeling great, regardless of your age.

Transverse Back Squat with Snatch

Momentum is at work in this exercise to help you create the power you need to raise that kettlebell overhead. To gain that momentum, you use your inner thighs and all your core muscles to rotate around your hips. Like a corkscrew winding and unwinding, your body will turn one way and then the other to build energy. With your whole body at work, it will be easier to lift that kettlebell. Making movements easier—isn't that the goal of functional training?

Real-Life Activities It Helps You Do

You'll notice improvement when performing everyday tasks, such as getting out of a car or getting up out of a chair at your desk or at the dining table. You can also expect a better backswing in golf or backhand in tennis.

Starting Point

1. Hold the kettlebells down by your sides with your palms facing your thighs and with your feet hip-width apart.

Movement

2. Lift your right foot off the ground, rotate your body to the right, and place your right foot on the ground about 2 feet behind where it was, the way you would get out of a swivel chair. Your left foot should still be facing forward; your right foot should be facing to the right. As soon as your right foot lands on the ground, squat with your knees pointing outward, similar to a ballet dancer's plié.

3. As you squat, swing the right kettlebell over your right shoulder, keeping your arm straight.

4. Return to the starting position, and rotate to the left while swinging the left kettlebell overhead to complete 1 repetition. Alternate from side to side 12 to 15 times.

Tips and Precautions

On your first attempts, you may want to eliminate the squat and just get the feel for rotating from side to side. To make this exercise even more demanding, do 12 to 15 repetitions on one side first and then the other rather than alternating.

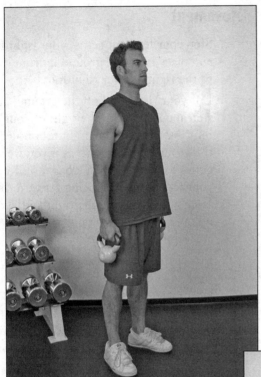

Starting/ending position.

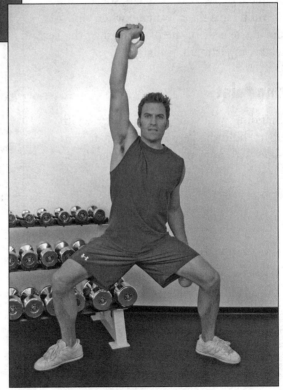

Midpoint position.

Crossover Shuffle and Snatch

Baseball outfielders, soccer players, and tennis players know that if you're chasing down a ball, you have to stop before you can actually catch, kick, or hit the ball. Then you typically have to run in the opposite direction to throw the ball or get back into position on the field or court.

That's the concept behind this exercise. It uses the muscles on one side of your body to create power and strength and then makes you change directions and create that same force on the other side. This helps make both sides of your body equally strong and coordinated, yet another key to better movement.

Real-Life Activities It Helps You Do

In addition to improving your performance in sporting activities like baseball, soccer, and tennis, you'll have the advantage when shuffling down the aisle of the plane to snag the last overhead compartment available.

Starting Point

1. Standing with your feet shoulder-width apart, hold the kettlebells down at your sides with your palms facing your legs.

Movement

2. Step your left foot across your right foot, and place it on the ground in front of and to the right of your right foot.

3. Lift your right foot off the ground, and step about 2 feet to the right of your left foot. As soon as your right foot touches the ground, squat down as if you were going to perch against a barstool. Keep your feet and knees facing forward. In the same motion, swing the right kettlebell up over your right shoulder, keeping your arm straight.

4. Lower the kettlebell as you bring your right foot across your left, and step your left foot to the side as you raise the kettlebell in your left hand over your left shoulder. Now, you've completed 1 repetition. Shoot for a total of 10 to 12 repetitions.

Tips and Precautions

I've designed this exercise so you're moving your leg out of the kettlebell's way as it comes down so you won't hit yourself with it. If you mess up your timing or get confused about which direction you're heading, you might end up with a bruised leg. To avoid hitting yourself, take it slow at first until you get into a nice side-to-side rhythm.

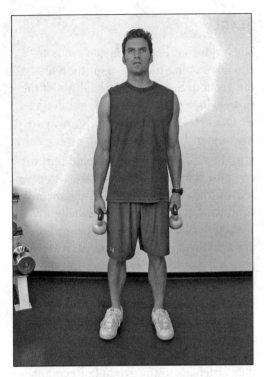

Starting/ending position.

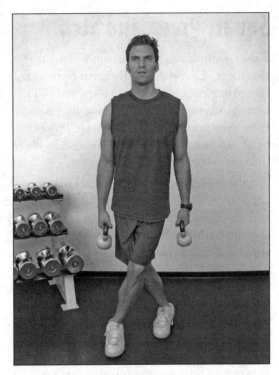

First position.

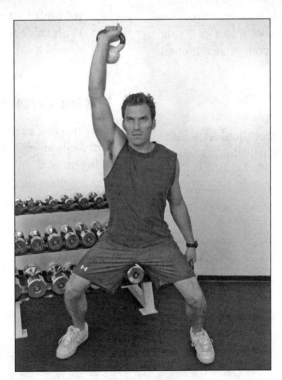

Second position.

Squat, Press, and Step

I always think about Superman when I teach this move. Everybody knows that Superman flies faster than a speeding bullet, but did you ever notice that he has to hit the brakes to land? If he didn't, he would be crash-landing every time and injuring himself. The same holds true for you.

In this exercise, you use momentum to propel you forward—okay, maybe not quite as fast as a speeding bullet—but then you have to slow down, or you'll fall off balance. With practice, this move gives you the best of both worlds—power and finesse. When you possess this superfunctional combo of skills, you'll feel like a superhero.

Real-Life Activities It Helps You Do

Power and finesse give you what you need to lift a heavy object off the floor and pass it to someone up high on a ladder or on a truck bed, pick up a basketball and shoot a half-court shot, push a mugger away from you, or swing open heavy double doors.

Starting Point

1. Standing with your feet shoulder-width apart, hold the kettlebells down at your sides with your palms facing your legs.

Movement

2. Squat down as low as you can go, as if you were going to sit on a cushion on the ground. Squat deep enough to let the kettlebells touch the ground, but don't let them rest on the ground. It's okay to round your back as you squat.

3. Use the muscles in your legs and butt to come back to standing, and take a step forward with your right foot. Simultaneously, bend your elbows so the kettlebells are at shoulder height with your palms facing away from you and without pause, press the kettlebells overhead. In the same motion, raise up onto your toes as you step forward.

4. As soon as your right foot touches the ground, step forward with your left foot so they're parallel, squat down, and lower the kettlebells to the ground. To complete your first repetition, step forward with your left foot and lift the kettlebells high. With this exercise, 10 to 12 repetitions should be about right.

Tips and Precautions

Ease into this exercise by starting with the kettlebells at your shoulders with your palms facing away from you rather than lowering and tapping them on the floor.

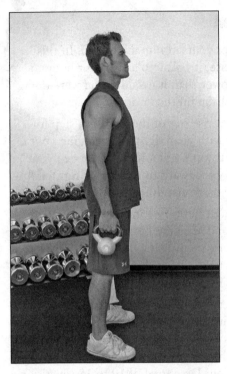

Starting/ending position.

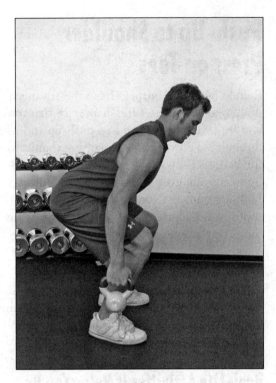

First position.

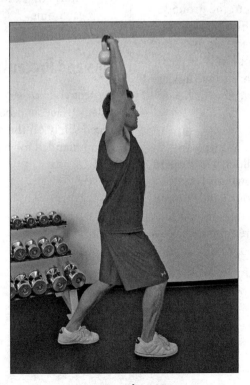

Second position.

Push-Up to Shoulder Press on Toes

Remember those burpees from the advanced body weight exercises in Chapter 18 that took you from standing down to a push-up and back up again? This move is similar, but thanks to the kettlebells, you can go lower in the push-up to activate even more upper body muscles. Holding onto the kettlebells in the push-up position is also great for wrist strength, something that's tough to achieve with other exercises.

One thing you did in the burpees that I absolutely do not recommend for this one is jumping your legs forward and back. With the kettlebells, it's safer for your wrists if you walk one leg up and back at a time. Safety first!

Real-Life Activities It Helps You Do

Anytime you have to get down to the ground quickly, you'll be grateful for this move—when you go camping and have to sleep on the ground, when you play with your kids or pets on the ground, surfing, or even hitting the deck when a foul ball is hurtling toward your head.

Starting Point

1. Place the kettlebells shoulder-width apart on the ground and get down on your hands and knees. Place your hands on the kettlebells, and lift your knees so you're in a push-up position. Tighten the muscles in your torso to help keep your body rigid.

Movement

2. Lower yourself into a push-up. In this exercise, it's okay to allow your body to dip lower than it would if you were doing a push-up on the floor.

3. As you rise out of the push-up, step forward with your right leg, bringing your knee toward your chest. Then step your left foot forward to meet your right and come up to standing.

4. Without hesitating, press up onto your toes and raise the kettlebells overhead by bending your elbows so your palms face away from you at shoulder height and then pressing them up.

5. Lower the kettlebells to the ground by bending at your hips and knees and rounding your back. Step your right foot back and then your left to return to the starting position. Do a total of 10 to 15 repetitions, alternating the leg that steps forward first each time.

Tips and Precautions

Protect your wrists and only do this exercise on a flat surface, and be sure the kettlebells are balanced safely on the ground. This exercise is not recommended for uneven surfaces.

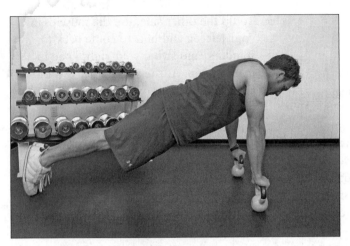

Starting/ending position.

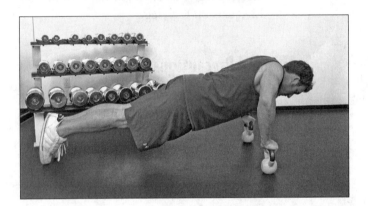

First position.

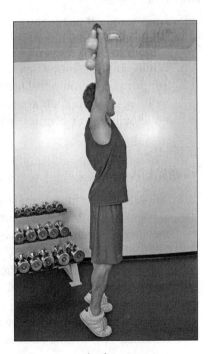

Third position.

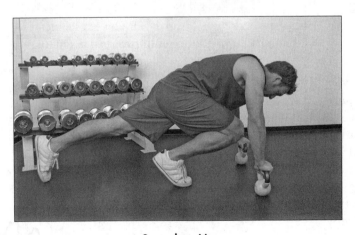

Second position.

Single-Leg Squat to Side Step Press

This exercise has it all—balancing on one leg, strengthening the lower body, rotating the trunk, bending down low, reaching up high, and lifting the kettlebell. That's a lot for one exercise! With so many components, this move can be a bit confusing, which also creates lots of work for your nervous system and your brain. Now that's what I call a whole-body exercise!

Real-Life Activities It Helps You Do

Ice skaters, roller bladders, and downhill runners who have to load up one leg and then transfer weight to the other leg will notice an improvement in performance thanks to this exercise. Even if you're just racing down the stairs at home or at the office, you'll find it's more of a breeze.

Starting Point

1. While standing, raise your left knee in front of you so you're balancing on your right leg. Hold the left kettlebell over your left shoulder with your left arm straight.

Movement

2. Lower your left foot to the ground as you step forward slightly and squat down into your left hip and knee. Lift your right foot off the ground, and let your right leg shift behind you. Let your back round as you reach the right kettlebell across to the left of your left foot, tapping it lightly on the ground. As you squat, lower the left kettlebell to your side and reach it slightly behind you to help you maintain balance. This completes 1 repetition.

3. To do the other side, use the muscles in your left leg and butt to come back to standing, and swing your right knee in front of you. At the same time, swing the right kettlebell up over your right shoulder, keeping your arm straight.

4. Step on your right foot, and bring the kettlebell back down to your right side. Squat on your right leg while shifting your left leg behind you and reaching the left kettlebell across to the outside of your right foot. Now, you've done your second repetition. Ideally, you should move fluidly through this exercise, raising one arm and then the other until you've done 10 to 12 squats on each leg.

Tips and Precautions

Because this exercise is a bit of a brain teaser, you might want to practice it without the kettlebells at first to avoid getting any bumps or bruises. After you get the movement down, add the kettlebells.

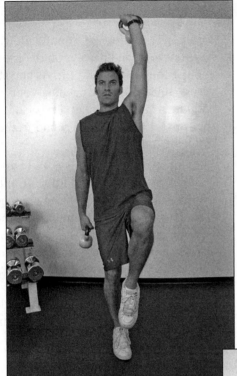

Starting/ending position.

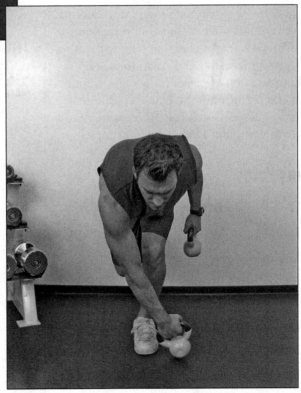

Midpoint position.

Walking Crossover Touch to Snatch

"Awkward" is how most of my clients describe this move, and that's why it's such a great exercise for functional training. In real life, it's when you get twisted into awkward positions that you tend to get injured. With this exercise, you train your body how to react to those clumsy movements without straining yourself.

Specifically, this exercise strengthens your upper and lower body while increasing flexibility in your hips. The result? Better protection for your knees, ankles, and hips and increased confidence that uncomfortable movements won't hurt you.

Real-Life Activities It Helps You Do

This exercise is a big hit with skiers who have to maneuver around while strapped into ski boots that don't move. It also comes in handy if you're in a crowd and have to bend down to pick up something and don't want to hit anyone around you. Of course, anyone who plays recreational or professional sports will benefit from training the body to withstand awkward contortions.

Starting Point

1. Stand with your feet shoulder-width apart, and hold the kettlebells at your sides with your palms facing your legs.

Movement

2. Step your right foot in front of and across your left foot, and place it on the ground about 1 foot to the left of it. As you step across, squat down by bending your hips and knees and rounding your back. Tap the left kettlebell to the ground to the inside of your right foot.

3. Use the muscles in your legs and butt to come up to standing, and lift your left foot off the ground so you're balancing on your right foot. At the same time, swing the left kettlebell over your left shoulder with your arm straight. Now, step your left leg over your right and try it on the other side to complete your first repetition. When you can do 10 to 12 repetitions of this awkward exercise, you'll know you've achieved functional fitness.

Tips and Precautions

On the crossover step, the farther forward you step, the easier it is; the more you step directly across your other foot, the more challenging it is. If you're unsure about this move, start by stepping farther forward and gradually shift to stepping directly across.

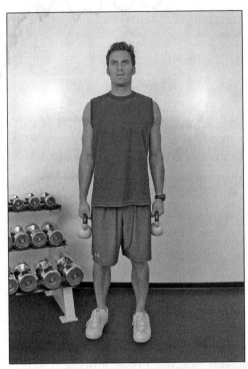

Starting/ending position.

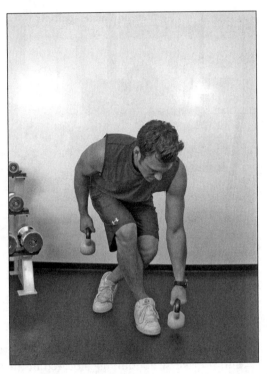

First position.

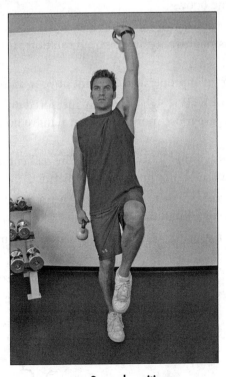

Second position.

Glossary

abdominals A group of four muscles—the internal and external obliques, rectus abdominis, and transverse abdominis—located in the torso that coordinates movement of your upper and lower body.

anterior The front side of the body.

biceps A muscle located on the front of the upper arm that rotates the forearm and flexes the elbow. It also slows down straightening and internal rotation of the forearm, like when you throw a ball.

body alignment The proper or improper arrangement of your muscular and skeletal system.

body weight How much your body weighs, typically measured on a scale. In functional training, body weight exercises are those movements that require no equipment other than the weight of your own body.

BOSU A functional training tool that looks like a stability ball cut in half and attached to a firm platform. The BOSU is a useful tool for improving balance.

cardiovascular exercise An activity that increases your heart rate for a period of time, often recommended to be at least 20 to 30 minutes.

core The muscles in your torso that coordinate movement between your pelvis, rib cage, and spine.

core conditioning A type of exercise program that targets the torso muscles.

erector spinae The muscles and tendons in the lower back that help keep your spine erect and slow down your spine as you bend forward.

endorphins Hormones secreted during strenuous exercises that have an analgesic effect.

extension   The action of moving a part of the body from a bent position to a straight position, such as when you straighten your arm.

external oblique   An abdominal muscle involved in rotation of the torso, bending the chest downward, stabilizing the spine, and bending to the side.

fascia   A three-dimensional web of tissue that holds together all your muscles, ligaments, tendons, and other body parts.

flexion   The act of bending a limb or joint, such as bending the knees and hips when sitting down.

foam roller   A long, foam cylinder used to loosen tight muscles in preparation for a functional training workout.

frontal   A plane of motion in which movement goes from side to side.

functional training   A type of exercise program that focuses on movement that mimics the way you move in everyday life with the goal of helping you move better.

glutes   The three muscles located in the butt.

gluteus maximus   The largest of the glute muscles, its primary task is extension of the hip and to slow down flexion of the hip, like when you sit. It is the most superficial of the glutes and gives the butt its shape.

gluteus medius   A glute muscle located below the gluteus maximus involved in rotation of the hip and leg.

gluteus minimus   The smallest and deepest of the glute muscles that helps with hip and leg rotation.

gravity   A force of nature that pulls your body down to the ground at all times. It provides resistance that your body has to work against while exercising.

hamstrings   A group of three muscles on the back of the thigh that flex the knee and extend the hip and also slow down extension of the knee and flexion of the hip.

heart rate   The number of times your heart beats per minute.

hip extension   A movement in which your hip is straightened rather than being bent, such as when you push your hips forward to stand up straight.

hip flexion   A movement in which the hip is bent. For example, if you are sitting while you read this book, your hip is in flexion.

hip flexor   A group of muscles in the hip that act to pull the knee upward, such as in a walking or running motion. The hip flexors also slow down your leg as it goes behind you when you walk.

internal oblique   One of the four abdominal muscles, it helps rotate the trunk.

kettlebell   A functional training tool that looks like a small cannonball with a flat bottom and a handle. In functional training, kettlebells are used to build strength.

kinesthetic   Relating to the sensation of movement in the muscles or the body as a whole.

kinetic   Anything that produces or is related to motion.

latissimus dorsi   A muscle in the midback that provides movement to the arm and spine.

ligaments   Connective tissues that attach bones to other bones.

lunge   A basic exercise in which you step forward with one foot and lower yourself forward to an object or down toward the ground by bending at the hip, knees, and ankles.

maximum heart rate   According to the American Heart Association, your maximum heart rate is 220 minus your age. For example, if you're 40 years old, your maximum heart rate would be 220 – 40 = 180.

medicine ball   A weighted ball made of rubber or leather used to build strength.

muscles   Tissues within the body that contract to produce movement. You have more than 600 muscles in your body.

myofascial   Tissues that include the muscles (*myo*) and connective tissues (*fascia*).

pelvic tilt   A basic exercise in which you tilt the hips under to flatten or straighten the lower back. This example is a posterior pelvic tilt.

planes of motion   The three directions the body can move: forward and backward, side to side, and rotation.

posterior   The back side of the body.

posture   The position in which you hold your body at any time as you perform any movement.

press   An exercise in which you push an object away from you, such as a kettlebell, by bending your elbows and then pressing your arms overhead.

quadriceps   A group of four muscles located in the front of the thigh that straightens the knee and slows down bending of the knee.

rectus abdominis   The biggest of the four abdominal muscles, it helps round the lower back and slows down straightening of the spine. It is also responsible for the appearance of "six-pack" abs.

repetitions   The number of times you perform an exercise.

resistance   Any force that impedes or slows your movement, such as gravity, body weight, or functional training tools.

resistance bands   A functional training tool consisting of long, rubber band–like tubes with handles on the ends used to provide resistance.

rest   The time between each exercise or each set of repetitions, during which you may remain still, walk, or perform some other activity.

rotation   The act of moving the body in the transverse plane, usually by twisting the torso or a limb.

sagittal   A plane of motion in which you move forward and backward.

sets   A group of repetitions for a particular exercise. In functional training, you may be asked to do 1, 2, or 3 sets of an exercise.

snatch   A basic kettlebell exercise in which you lift the kettlebell overhead while keeping your arm straight.

squat   A basic exercise that involves bending at your hips, knees, and ankles to lower your butt toward the ground as if you were going to sit in a chair.

stability ball   A large, inflatable plastic ball commonly used for fitness training but not specifically for functional training. Also called a Swiss ball or an exercise ball.

stabilizers   Muscles whose primary task is to help stabilize and balance the body or a body part.

strength   In functional training, strength is measured by your ability to support your body weight or lift heavy objects.

tendons   Connective tissues that attach muscles to bones.

transverse   A plane of motion in which the body rotates in any direction.

triceps   A muscle located on the back of the upper arm that straightens the arm and slows down bending of the arm.

TRX   A functional training tool consisting of a lightweight, portable suspension-training device.

vertebrae   The bones that make up the spine.

yoga   A type of exercise that may involve static stretching.

B

Sample Workout Plans

To help you get started with functional training, we've included some sample workout plans. The first two workouts include a series of exercises designed to help you minimize any body alignment problems. When your body alignment is in good shape, you can move on to the other sample workouts.

The beginner, intermediate, and advanced sample workouts are designed to target your entire body and improve your strength, balance, and coordination. They involve a variety of functional training tools to keep you on your toes and keep your workout fun and fresh. Use these workouts as a jumping-off point for your functional training program.

Get Your Body Working Correctly

Before you get started with any type of workout program, be sure your body is correctly aligned and up for the task. Take the time to perform the assessments detailed earlier in the book to ensure you're aware of your body's strengths and weaknesses. For example, if you know your shoulders are rounded, it's a great idea to perform some basic exercises to help strengthen your upper back to help make your spine more erect and pull back your shoulders. You can do these types of exercises every day as part of your workout or at a different time to help improve your alignment.

The sample exercises I've chosen for the rounded shoulder workout are from a couple beginner exercise sections that address specific alignment issues. When you progress to the actual workout, you'll be performing exercises that address the whole body.

Sample Workout for Rounded Shoulders

First, start with foam roller exercises to loosen up:

1. Foam roller upper back (Chapter 5): 2 or 3 minutes.

Next, beginner body weight moves:

2. Lying wave good-bye (Chapter 6): 2 sets, hold for 30 to 60 seconds.
3. Lying straight arm raise (Chapter 6): 2 sets, hold for 30 to 60 seconds.

Next, beginner TRX:

4. Trunk rotations (TRX; Chapter 9): 2 sets of 8 to 10 reps.
5. Squat row (TRX; Chapter 9): 2 sets of 10 to 12 reps.

Sample Workout for Arched Lower Back

If you discover that your lower back is arched too much, it's a good idea to perform a selection of exercises that addresses this imbalance. Do each exercise in the order listed as little as three times per week or as often as every day.

First, start with foam roller exercises to loosen up:

1. Foam roller glutes (Chapter 5): 1 or 2 minutes each leg.
2. Foam roller side of thigh (Chapter 5): 1 or 2 minutes each leg.
3. Foam roller front of thigh (Chapter 5): 1 or 2 minutes each leg.

Next, beginner body weight moves:

4. Pelvic tilt (Chapter 6): 2 sets of 10 to 15 reps.

Next, beginner TRX:

5. Tri-planar hip flexor (with TRX; Chapter 9): 2 sets of 6 to 8 reps.
6. Rotating hip and back (with TRX; Chapter 9): 2 sets of 6 to 8 reps.

Follow with beginner medicine ball exercises:

7. Bend down, reach up (with medicine ball; Chapter 8): 2 sets of 8 to 10 reps.

Beginner Workouts

After you've addressed some of your imbalances, you can begin a basic functional workout. Remember, be sure you can do all the beginner body weight exercises listed in Chapter 6 before you move on to incorporate exercises that use different pieces of equipment. Choose exercises that work your lower and upper body and get you moving in as many directions as possible. Rest between exercises as you need to.

Remember: always do the foam roller and dynamic warm-up before any workout (see Chapter 5).

Beginner Workout Sample 1

1. Standing rotations (resistance bands; Chapter 7): 1 set, 10 to 12 reps each side.
2. One-leg stand with row (resistance bands; Chapter 7): 1 set, 10 to 15 reps each side.
3. Partial squat with high-low rotation (medicine ball; Chapter 8): 1 set, 10 to 15 reps each side.
4. Side step with partial squat (BOSU; Chapter 10): 1 set, 12 reps each side.
5. Side step with bend (TRX; Chapter 9): 1 set, 10 to 12 reps each side.
6. Partial squat with front-back arm swings (kettlebell; Chapter 11): 1 set, 10 to 15 reps each side.

Beginner Workout Sample 2

1. Band shuffle (resistance bands; Chapter 7): 1 set, 10 steps to each side.

2. Standing alternating high pulls (resistance bands; Chapter 7): 1 set, 10 reps each side.

3. Rotations with side step (medicine ball; Chapter 8): 1 set, 10 to 15 reps each side.

4. Hip flexor with partial lunge (TRX; Chapter 9): 1 set, 8 to 10 reps each side.

5. Squat row (TRX; Chapter 9): 1 set, 10 to 15 reps.

6. Side step two-arm opposite swing (kettle-bell; Chapter 11): 1 set, 10 to 15 reps.

Intermediate Workouts

As you gain confidence in your abilities and your body is prepared for further action, you're ready to move on to an intermediate-level workout. Choose exercises that get you moving in all three planes of motion and reaching up and down. The rest period between exercises should be shorter than when doing a beginner workout.

Remember: always do the foam roller and dynamic warm-up before any workout (refer to Chapter 5).

Intermediate Workout Sample 1

1. Partial lunge with crossover reach (body weight; Chapter 6): 1 or 2 sets, 8 to 12 reps each side.

2. Partial side squat with lateral reach (body weight; Chapter 6): 1 or 2 sets, 8 to 12 reps each side.

3. Forward crawl (body weight; Chapter 12): 1 or 2 sets, crawl for 30 yards, or about 15 steps.

4. Lunge with rotation (body weight; Chapter 12): 1 or 2 sets, 8 to 12 reps each side.

5. Single-leg squat with row (resistance bands; Chapter 13): 1 or 2 sets, 8 to 12 reps each side.

6. Reverse lunge to shoulder press (medicine ball; Chapter 14): 1 or 2 sets, 10 to 12 reps each side.

7. Lateral lunge with opposite rotation (medicine ball; Chapter 14): 1 or 2 sets, 8 to 10 reps each side.

8. Isolated I with squat (TRX; Chapter 15): 1 or 2 sets, 10 to 12 reps.

9. Side-to-side jump (BOSU; Chapter 16): 1 or 2 sets, 20 to 30 reps.

10. Partial side squat to one-arm snatch (kettlebell; Chapter 17): 1 or 2 sets, 10 to 15 reps.

Intermediate Workout Sample 2

1. Side-to-side squat with overhead press (body weight; Chapter 12).

2. Back lunge with overhead reach (body weight; Chapter 12).

3. Single-leg squat with reach (body weight; Chapter 12): 1 or 2 sets, 10 to 12 reps each side.

4. Lunge to hip stretch (body weight; Chapter 12): 1 or 2 sets, 6 to 10 reps each side.

5. Lunge row (resistance bands; Chapter 13): 1 or 2 sets, 8 to 12 reps each side.

6. Transverse step with rear fly (resistance bands; Chapter 13): 1 or 2 sets, 10 to 12 reps each side.

7. Side squat with floor touch (medicine ball; Chapter 14): 1 or 2 sets, 8 to 10 reps each side.

8. Alternating crossover step (TRX; Chapter 15): 1 or 2 sets, 10 to 15 reps.

9. Side squat (TRX; Chapter 15): 1 or 2 sets, 10 to 15 reps each side.

10. Lunge with open side reach (BOSU; Chapter 16): 1 or 2 sets, 10 to 15 reps each side.

Advanced Workouts

When you feel confident to advance to this level, it's time to really test yourself. Move in all three planes of motion; reach up and down; add jumping; increase the weight; and rest for shorter periods, if at all, between sets of exercise. Add jumping rope, running up hill, or jumping jacks between sets to keep your heart rate up. For the advanced workouts, do 1 set of each exercise, and depending on your time and fitness level, either end your workout or repeat the entire workout 1 or 2 more times.

Remember: always do the foam roller and dynamic warm-up before any workout (refer to Chapter 5).

Advanced Workout Sample 1

1. Forward crawl (body weight; Chapter 12): crawl for 30 yards, or about 15 steps.

2. Lunge with rotation (body weight; Chapter 12): 10 to 15 reps each side.

3. Lunge to hip stretch (body weight; Chapter 12): 10 to 15 reps each side.

 Fit Fact

You can perform a superset by doing one set of exercise and then going straight into the next exercise with no rest.

4. One-leg stand to side squat with rotations (resistance bands: Chapter 13): 8 to 12 reps each side.

5. One-leg wood chops (resistance bands: Chapter 13): 8 to 12 reps each side.

6. Rest for 30 seconds to 1 minute.

7. One-leg reverse rotational lunge (body weight: Chapter 18): 10 to 12 reps each side.

8. Burpees with push-up (body weight: Chapter 18): 10 to 15 reps.

9. Rest for 30 seconds to 1 minute.

10. Backward crawl (body weight: Chapter 18): crawl 20 to 30 yards, or about 10 to 15 steps.

11. Rotational push-ups (body weight; Chapter 18): 10 to 16 reps.

12. Rest for 30 seconds to 1 minute.

13. Stork stance with shoulder flexion (resistance bands; Chapter 19): 8 to 12 reps each side.

14. Multiplanar lunge (medicine ball; Chapter 20): 10 to 15 reps each side.

15. Rest for 30 seconds to 1 minute.

16. Sprinter's start (TRX; Chapter 21): 12 to 15 reps each side.

17. Rotating power jump (TRX; Chapter 21): 20 to 30 reps.

18. Rest for 30 seconds to 1 minute.

19. Reverse lunge to hop up (BOSU; Chapter 22): 10 to 15 reps each side.

20. Side-to-side push-ups (BOSU; Chapter 22): 20 to 24 reps.

21. Rest for 30 seconds to 1 minute.

Advanced Workout Sample 2

1. Forward lunge with rotation (medicine ball; Chapter 14).

2. Side squat with floor touch (medicine ball; Chapter 14).

3. Lateral lunge with opposite rotation (medicine ball; Chapter 14).

4. One-leg side squat with reach (body weight; Chapter 18): 6 to 10 reps each side.

5. One-leg ice skater with one-arm chest fly (resistance bands; Chapter 19): 8 to 12 reps each side.

6. Single-leg squat to high pull (resistance bands; Chapter 19): 8 to 12 reps each side.

7. Side-to-side jumps with opposite reach (medicine ball; Chapter 20): 10 to 15 reps.

8. Jump rope for 1 minute.

9. Suspended lunge jump (TRX; Chapter 21): 10 to 15 reps each side.

10. Seesaw to pike (TRX; Chapter 21): 15 to 20 reps.

11. Suspended hip twist (TRX; Chapter 21): 6 reps.

12. Jump and stick it (BOSU; Chapter 22): 10 to 15 reps.

13. Run uphill for 1 minute.

14. Transverse back step with snatch (kettlebell; Chapter 23): 12 to 15 reps each side.

15. Squat, press, and step (kettlebell; Chapter 23): 10 to 12 reps.

16. Single-leg squat to side step press (kettlebell; Chapter 23): 10 to 12 reps each side.

17. Walking crossover touch to snatch (kettlebell; Chapter 23): 10 to 12 reps.

18. Do jumping jacks for 1 minute.

Sample Training Log

Using a training log is an excellent way to keep track of your functional progress. By recording the type, intensity, duration, and purpose of every training session you do, you can become aware of your improvements and begin to understand your individual movement needs and accomplishments.

As your functional capabilities improve, it's easy to forget how difficult activities may have been in the early stages, so don't overlook this important opportunity to document your incredible journey from Couch Potato to James Bond functional superhero.

Training Log

Date: Monday 3/2

What I Did Today	Sets/Reps	Activities Between Sets
Intermediate 1 Workout		
Warm-Up:		
Foam roller glutes and quads	2 minutes total	No rest
Leg swings (forward and back and side to side)	2 minutes total	No rest
Partial lunge with crossover reach	2 minutes	No rest
Partial side squat with lateral reach	2 minutes	No rest
Exercises:		
Forward crawl	30 yards, or about 15 steps	Rest 90 seconds
Lunge with rotation	12 reps × 2 sets	Rest 90 seconds
Single leg squat with row	12 reps × 2 sets	Rest 90 seconds
Reverse lunge to shoulder press	12 reps × 2 sets	Rest 90 seconds
Lateral lunge with opposite rotation	12 reps × 2 sets	Rest 90 seconds
Isolated I with squat	12 reps × 2 sets	Rest 90 seconds
Side-to-side jump	20 reps × 2 sets	Rest 90 seconds
Partial side squat to one-arm snatch	12 reps × 2 sets	Rest 90 seconds

Total Workout Time:

45 minutes

Comments:

Felt good and loose after the warm-up, but the crawling was more tiring than I thought! Made it through the whole workout though, and afterward, felt surprisingly limber and ready for anything. Off to chug some water and reflect on a job well done.

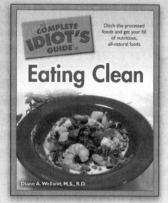
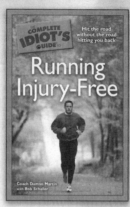
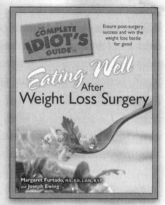
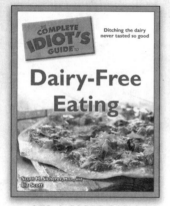
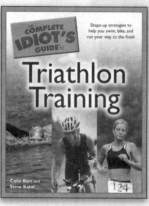
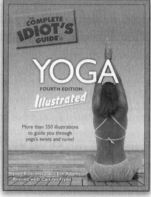
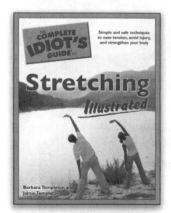
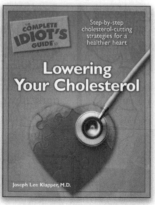
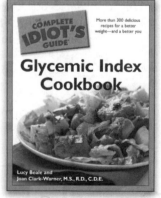

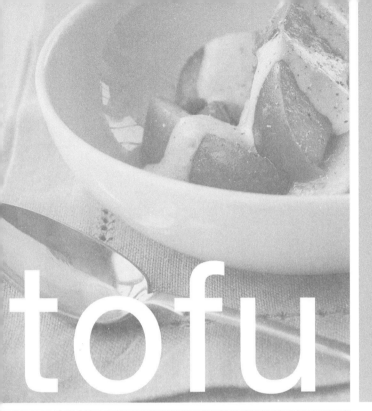

tofu 1-2-3

by Maribeth Abrams

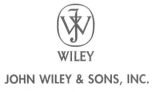

WILEY

JOHN WILEY & SONS, INC.

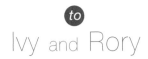

to

Ivy and Rory

Copyright © 2006 by Maribeth Abrams. All rights reserved
Photography © 2006 by Joseph De Leo

Published by John Wiley & Sons, Inc., Hoboken, New Jersey
Published simultaneously in Canada

For general information about our other products and services, please contact our Customer Care Department within the United States at (800) 762-2974, outside the United States at (317) 572-3993 or fax (317) 572-4002.

Wiley also publishes its books in a variety of electronic formats. Some content that appears in print may not be available in electronic books. For more information about Wiley products, visit our web site at www.wiley.com.

Library of Congress Cataloging-in-Publication Data:
Abrams, Maribeth.
   Tofu 1-2-3 / Maribeth Abrams.
       p. cm.
   Includes bibliographical references and index.
   ISBN-13: 978-0-471-74809-0 (pbk.)
   ISBN-10: 0-471-74809-9 (pbk.)
   1. Cookery (Tofu) 2. Tofu. I. Title.

   TX814.5.T63A27 2005
   641.6'5655--dc22
                                    2005023409

Printed in the United States of America

10 9 8 7 6 5 4 3 2 1

contents

acknowledgments

I would like to thank my family for supporting me in all that I do: Ivy and Rory, Ellen and Martin Abrams, Ilyse, Stephen, Reed, Rachel and Harrison Wells, and my beloved Peter Trivelas.

I would also like to thank the wonderful staff at Vitasoy USA for so generously providing me with an abundance of Nasoya tofu to use for recipe development, and for their support in my teaching of natural foods cooking.

I am grateful to friend and colleague Diane Wagemann for her culinary creativity and her early contact with Wiley Publishing that led to this body of recipes.

And thank you to those who tested recipes from a reader's perspective: Kristin Bourbeau, Kathleen Bowen, Kristin Bowen, Heidi Colescott-Aleman, Kathy Cuomo, Heather Davis, Amy Diezemann, Carol Frieberg Reese, Suzie Keeney, Aimee Kuelling, Jill Lambert, Wendy Lobel, Cassie Magzaman, Robin Meloy Goldsby, Janel Ricci, Elaine Schechter, Barbara Traverso, Claudia Trivelas, Helen Trivelas, Jonathan Trivelas, Peter Alexander Trivelas, Jackie Troccki, Mary Webster, and Robin Webster. I appreciate the seriousness with which you viewed this task.

I thank Garden of Light Natural Foods in Glastonbury, CT, for handling logistical details; Mark Bailin for legal consultation; Michael Greger, MD, for his contribution to the health section; Aaron Schechter, David Kidd, and Brian and Sharon Graff for their ongoing support and encouragement; and Justin Schwartz at John Wiley & Sons for his vision of this cookbook.

preface: taking the mystery out of the big white blob

I love to cook and am happy to say that I've been blessed with many opportunities to integrate my passion for preparing whole, natural foods into my livelihood. One such instance occurred in the mid-1990s when I started working for the North American Vegetarian Society as the managing editor of its publication *Vegetarian Voice*.

My job with NAVS includes testing recipes and reviewing cholesterol-free, natural foods cookbooks, duties that provide me with an abundance of first-hand experience with foods typically considered unfamiliar in our culture.

Soon after joining NAVS, people in my community started to bring me their questions on natural foods cooking. I quickly noticed a trend: a surprisingly high percentage of people want to add tofu to their diets but have absolutely no idea how to go about doing it. That's when I started teaching tofu cooking classes that continue today, with an emphasis on easy recipes for the home cook.

Since that time, I collaborated with colleagues Diane Wagemann and Peter Trivelas to produce *Tofu 1-2-3,* a tofu cooking video/DVD with special guest Olympian Carl Lewis. This is the companion cookbook.

Interestingly, even though cholesterol-free cooking is totally vegetarian by definition (see "Tofu: It's Not Just for Vegetarians," page ix), I have found that most of the people who attend my cooking classes and view the *Tofu 1-2-3* video do, in fact, still eat meat. When asked about this, I always say, "Well, as everyone who enjoys a good plate of spaghetti marinara with garlic bread knows, you don't have to be vegetarian to eat like one!"

I invite you to delight in the versatility of tofu with these recipes. I encourage you to roll up your sleeves and engage in the mashing, slicing, dicing, baking, broiling, blending, and crumbling of tofu. Touch it. Taste it. Experiment with it in ways you never dreamed, such as in Beer-Battered Coconut Tofu (page 28), Chocolate Chip Cookie Bars (page 192), and Manicotti Florentine (page 44).

And may it be known that each and every recipe here in *Tofu 1-2-3* has been double-tested by a member of my Tofu Testing Team to ensure that even novices handling "the big white blob" for the first time will be pleased with the outcome. Now it's your turn. Let your taste-buds discover why so many people embrace tofu as the basis of easy, scrumptious meals.

preface

tofu: it's not just for vegetarians

Tofu contains all nine essential amino acids found in animal protein, but it has no cholesterol and much less saturated fat. Tofu comes from soybeans, and research shows that consuming at least 25 grams of soy protein in place of animal protein lowers blood cholesterol levels by 5 to 10 percent. This research is so strong that the U.S. Food & Drug Administration now makes the official claim that "Diets low in saturated fat and cholesterol that include 25 grams of soy protein per day may reduce the risk of heart disease." One serving of tofu contains 10 grams of soy protein.

Cholesterol is a necessary component in human cell membranes and we make all the cholesterol we need, just like we make all of the blood that we need. Nonhuman animals make all the cholesterol they need too, and we consume that cholesterol when we eat meat, dairy, and eggs. Saturated animal fat raises your LDL "bad" cholesterol, the number one dietary risk factor for heart disease, the number one killer of both men and women in our culture.

Tofu, on the other hand, comes from soybeans, a plant. Cholesterol is made in the liver, and unlike animals, plants don't have livers. To capitalize on the fact that tofu is cholesterol-free and to support the FDA recommendation to increase our consumption of soy protein while minimizing our cholesterol intake, all of the other ingredients used in this book are cholesterol-free as well.

Some studies show that a component in soybeans called *isoflavones* may decrease the negative symptoms associated with menopause such as hot flashes, night sweats, insomnia, vaginal dryness, and headaches. With 24.74 milligrams of isoflavones per 100 grams (about half a cup), tofu is one of the richest sources of isoflavones in the supermarket. (For comparison, 100 grams of beef contain 1.14 milligrams; 100 grams of peanuts contain 0.26 milligrams.)[1]

Researchers looking at breast cancer, prostate cancer, and gastrointestinal cancer (like colon cancer) have found highly significant reductions in cancer risk among consumers of soy products. This evidence is so strong that there is now another health claim before the FDA, and we may soon see labels saying that soy products protect against certain kinds of cancer as well.

"Between the heart benefits and the fact that soy may help prevent osteoporosis and even certain cancers, it is no wonder that soy is considered a superfood," says Michael Greger, MD, physician, author, and internationally recognized speaker.

For detailed information on the health benefits of tofu, I encourage you to read *The Simple Soybean and Your Health,* by Mark Messina and Virginia Messina (Avery Publishing Group).

[1] Source: USDA-Iowa State University Database on the Isoflavone Content of Foods

tofu: it's not just for vegetarians

everything you need to know about cooking with tofu but didn't know who to ask

I am convinced that there is only one reason why many people in our culture consider tofu to be unfamiliar or "weird," and it has absolutely nothing to do with its taste, texture, or appearance. Rather, it's because our parents didn't prepare tofu for us when we were children.

Just think about it. Imagine having absolutely no knowledge of the existence of raw ground beef. That means having never come in visual or direct contact with it, never seeing it in your refrigerator, never shaping a meatball with your hands, never cooking a hamburger on the grill, never seeing anyone else handle or prepare it in any way or form. Now, consider encountering raw ground beef for the first time as an adult. How would you view it? Probably the way many people look at tofu—with skepticism!

But now that tofu is touted as healthful and desirable by the medical and health communities, many people once cautious about tofu are now interested in integrating this versatile and nutritious food into their and their families' meals.

Before we begin, determine your Tofu Habit Quotient by checking all that apply:

a *I saw tofu in the store and wanted to buy it but chose not to because I didn't know what to do with it.*

b *I bought tofu but didn't know what to do with it so I threw it away after a few weeks.*

c *I bought tofu and tried to prepare it but the meal didn't come out right so I threw it away and went out for pizza.*

d *Any combination of A, B, and C*

e *I have successfully cooked with tofu but am in need of easy, creative recipes that my friends and family will love.*

If you checked A, B, C, D, or E, then everything you need to know is right here at your fingertips.

What Is Tofu?

Soft, white, and resembling a block of cheese, tofu is made from soybeans that have been soaked, ground, and boiled. The resulting liquid is drained to remove pulp, and a natural coagulent such as calcium sulfate is added to make it firm. There are two main kinds of tofu—regular and silken. Both come in varying densities and are used in different ways.

Regular Tofu

Also known as water-packed tofu, regular tofu is packaged in water and kept refrigerated at all times, even before the package has been opened. Regular tofu is available in three densities (extra-firm, firm, and soft) and each is good for a particular style of cooking. Keep in mind, however, that there is no standard from brand to brand. In other words, one brand's extra-firm may be softer than another brand's firm. Experimenting with different brands is one way to determine how soft or firm regular tofu can be.

In general, extra-firm or firm (regular) tofu is good for sautéing, stir-frying, and pan-frying because it is sturdy enough to maintain its shape while cooking. On the other hand, soft (regular) tofu works better in creamy recipes that call for pureeing or blending such as cheesecake and thick, rich dips.

All packages of regular tofu sold in retail stores do not weigh the same, but they are usually about 1 pound. Also, the type of packaging may vary from brand to brand, but you will most often find regular tofu sealed in plastic rectangular tubs. Alternatively, some regular tofu is sold in clear, vacuum-packed plastic. Always check the expiration date before purchase.

everything you need to know about cooking with tofu

What to Do about the Water

As mentioned, regular tofu comes immersed in water. This water needs to be drained off before use, and the easiest way to do so is to hold the tub of tofu over a sink and to cut a slit or two at the edge of the top of the package, avoiding cutting into the tofu. Tilt the slit-open tofu package to drain the water directly into the sink, slice or peel off the rest of the top, transfer the block of tofu into your hand, and gently rinse it under cool, running water. Finally, pat the tofu dry with a clean dishtowel and voilà! You are ready to prepare something delicious.

Silken Tofu

Silken tofu is available in the same three densities as regular tofu (extra-firm, firm, and soft) but is entirely different. First of all, it is most often sold in 12-ounce cardboard boxes. This packaging is aseptic (sterilized in the package), so the tofu does not have to be refrigerated until after the box has been opened. Sometimes, silken tofu is sold in packaging similar to regular tofu. Make sure to check the "use-by" date before purchase.

As its name implies, silken tofu is as smooth as, well, silk. It's extremely soft and creamy, ideal for such foods as puddings, sauces, cream pies, and smoothies.

While the variation between the densities of silken tofu are not as great as those between regular tofu, there are still some guidelines to help select the best kind: the sturdier the creamy dish, the denser the silken tofu needs to be. For example, pumpkin pie is creamy but must be sturdy enough to maintain its shape once cut into individual portions, so extra-firm silken tofu would be the best choice. On the other hand, soft silken tofu is ideal for puddings and cream sauces.

Tofu Storage

A recipe might not call for an entire package of tofu. To store unused tofu (regular or silken), put it in a storage container, cover it with cold water, seal it tightly, and refrigerate for up to three or four days, changing the water daily. If the part about changing the water every day sounds like a chore, then you are a lot like me. And that's why I offer an easy, tasty alternative: make a smoothie right on the spot with the unused tofu.

The Impromptu Smoothie

There are more than fourteen smoothie recipes in this cookbook and all call for any density of silken tofu. But I'll let you in on a little secret: smoothies can also taste great with regular tofu. You may have to increase the amount of liquid, however, so the smoothie isn't too thick. As you would expect, you may want to increase the liquid more if using firm or extra-firm (regular) tofu and less if using soft (regular) tofu.

Fortunately, making delicious smoothies is a lot like making spaghetti sauce in that using the proper ingredients is oftentimes more important than conforming to exact measurements. So keep a bag or two of frozen berries tucked away in your freezer for those times you need to use up some unused tofu.

In many instances, doubling a recipe is another way to avoid having to store unused tofu.

Pressing Tofu for Added Firmness

Sometimes it's nice to bite into a dense, succulent piece of tofu—especially tofu that has been grilled, pan-fried, baked, or broiled. In those instances (as mentioned earlier), "regular" firm or extra-firm tofu yields the best results. But you can alter this kind of tofu to further increase its density and firmness, and to improve its overall texture. In fact, many recipes contained here embrace this easy and beneficial procedure, called "pressing."

To press tofu, wrap a rinsed and drained block of regular tofu in a clean dishtowel and place it on a plate. Cover it with a heavy cutting board, and lay a book or two on top. (The cookbook *Professional Vegetarian Cooking* by Ken Bergeron works for me!)

everything you need to know about cooking with tofu

Allow the tofu to "press" in this manner for 10 to 20 minutes. Remove the book(s) and cutting board, gently open the dishtowel (it will be water-soaked), and you will find that the tofu has significantly increased in density. Now it's even more suited for grilling, frying, baking, broiling, or other methods of cooking that optimally yield a very dense texture.

Freezing (and Defrosting) Tofu to Make It Chewy

If frozen blocks of tofu conjure up images of edible igloos, then consider the fact that there is actually a very practical reason to freeze (and then defrost) tofu—it changes its texture. More specifically, the act of freezing and then defrosting tofu makes it very chewy, perfect for use in recipes such as Garden Vegetable Chili with Kale and Black Beans (page 114) and Sloppy Joes (page 153).

It's easy to freeze tofu; you can simply transfer the container from grocery bag to freezer. However, it is important to keep two things in mind when doing so: defrosting and pressing.

Defrosting

Optimally, tofu is defrosted in the refrigerator overnight or one day in advance. However, when time is limited, frozen tofu can be removed from its package, placed in a glass bowl, and microwaved on the defrost setting for about 10 minutes. It is normal for frozen tofu that has been defrosted to be slightly yellow in color.

Pressing (Frozen) Tofu

In order for defrosted frozen tofu to reach its full chewy potential, it should be pressed to remove excess water. (See "Pressing Tofu for Added Firmness," page xiv.) Pressing can take place before or after it has been frozen and defrosted. I prefer to press in advance and to store the pressed tofu in a sealed freezer-proof bag or container in the freezer until I need it for a recipe. However, it is sometimes more convenient to transfer the tofu directly from grocery bag to freezer, and to do the pressing after it has fully defrosted at a later date.

In any case, defrosted tofu that has also been pressed is a magnificent way to manipulate its texture. On the other hand, be aware that if you freeze tofu simply as a way to extend its shelf-life, you will be somewhat limited in the kinds of recipes you can use it for once it has been defrosted.

everything you need to know about cooking with tofu

glossary of ingredients

There once was a time, very long ago, that I skipped recipes that called for ingredients I had never used before. Miso? Flip that page! Nutritional yeast flakes and tahini? Yikes! But I overcame that fear by simply giving these unfamiliar yet readily available ingredients a try.

Here's what I discovered: the act of scooping out a teaspoon of miso or tahini requires the exact same motion as scooping out a teaspoon of peanut butter (no mystery there!), and in terms of flavor, I found a whole world of fabulously flavored and health-supporting foods. The vast majority of recipes here in *Tofu 1-2-3* use ingredients typically found in mainstream kitchens. But you will discover a few new items too, so use the following glossary if you would like more information on something listed that is unfamiliar.

Agave Nectar

A liquid sweetener made from the extract of wild agave. Has about 1.4 times the sweetening power of white sugar. Will keep for at least one year, does not require refrigeration, and will not crystallize so it remains pourable even when cold. Available in both light and amber varieties; light is neutral in flavor.

Almond Butter

Made from ground almonds, a spreadable nut butter used in desserts, sauces, dressings, or as a topping for breads. Stir upon opening because oil separation occurs. Will last for about three months if kept sealed and refrigerated after each use.

XVii

Arrowroot

A starch that is used as a thickener, derived from the root of a tropical plant. Has a more neutral flavor than cornstarch and can be used in place of it ounce for ounce. Found in the bulk spices section in natural food stores.

Cashew Butter

A rich-flavored spread made from ground cashews. Used for flavor and texture in dairy-free cheeses, cheese sauces and cream sauces, soups, dips, and as a topping for bread. Stir upon opening because of oil separation. Will last for about three months if kept sealed and refrigerated after each use.

Dairy-Free Chocolate Chips

Found in the baking section and in the bulk bin area at natural food stores, and in the natural foods section of large grocery stores. Can be used in place of milk chocolate chips, and may be labeled "vegan chocolate chips." Regular dark chocolate chips are usually dairy-free too.

Dairy-Free Cream Cheese

There are several brands of soy-based, dairy-free cream cheese, oftentimes available in different flavors. Good for use in baking and as a spread for crackers and toast, dairy-free cream cheese can be found in the refrigerated section of natural food stores and in the natural foods section at large grocery stores. Check label to avoid hydrogenated fat (see Soy Margarine, below).

Dairy-Free Parmesan Cheese

Some brands of rice- and soy-based Parmesan cheese contain casein, a milk product, so check labels to ensure that it is dairy-free. Sold in natural food stores and in the natural foods section of large grocery stores.

Dairy-Free Sour Cream

Can be used in place of dairy sour cream in baked goods, dips, and of course on baked potatoes. Sold in the refrigerated section of natural food stores and in the natural foods section of large grocery stores. Check the label to avoid hydrogenated fat (see Soy Margarine, below).

Dulse Flakes

A sea vegetable available in dried, flake form, delicious sprinkled into soups, salads, stews, pastas, and sauces, adding a bit of "ocean flavor" to fish-free recipes. Find in the sea vegetable section (such as nori, for making sushi) of natural food stores, or in specialty stores. Like other sea

glossary of ingredients

vegetables, dulse flakes are rich in minerals and trace elements including calcium, magnesium, iron, potassium, iodine, manganese, and chromium, and provide vitamins, fiber, enzymes, and high-quality protein.

Eggless Mayonnaise

There are several brands of eggless mayonnaise based on ingredients such as tofu and oil, and all vary significantly in flavor. Most are sold on the shelf, but at least one brand is sold refrigerated. Large supermarkets typically carry at least one brand of eggless mayonnaise in their natural foods section, but natural food stores usually have at least two or three from which to choose. Experiment with different brands to discover the one you like best.

Flax Seeds

A rich source of omega-3 fatty acids, flax seeds can be blended with water or other liquid to become a thick egg substitute perfect for baking and for use in battering. Look for flax seeds in the baking or bulk bin section at natural food stores, or in the natural foods section of large grocery stores. Store in a tightly sealed jar and keep refrigerated.

Miso

Fermented soybean paste that comes in several varieties ranging from light to dark. Sold in the refrigerated section of natural food stores, miso can last for a year or more if stored in the refrigerator. Use in miso soup and for flavoring in gravies, sauces, and dressings.

Nori

A dried, dark green sea vegetable sold in paper-thin sheets, most often used to wrap sushi or rice balls. Find in the Asian section of large grocery stores, and in the sea vegetable section of natural food stores and specialty stores. See Dulse Flakes (above) for general nutrition information.

Nutritional Yeast Flakes

A dried, inactive yeast, nutritional yeast flakes impart a cheesy, nutty flavor and are a rich source of B vitamins. Excellent in dairy-free cheese sauces, soups, scrambled tofu, and gravies, and sprinkled on cooked vegetables, stews, and chili. Find in the bulk bin section in natural food stores. If kept tightly sealed in a jar in a cupboard, will last about a year.

Pure Maple Syrup

More than just a pancake and French toast topper, pure maple syrup is an ideal liquid sweetener in savory and sweet dishes. Artificially flavored and colored syrups are not a replacement for pure maple syrup when cooking and baking.

Rice Milk

Like other dairy-free milks, rice milk can be substituted ounce for ounce for dairy milk when baking or making smoothies, sauces, etc., and in cereal and hot beverages. Many brands of rice milk have flavors such as plain, vanilla, chocolate, and carob, and have varieties enriched with vitamins and calcium. Look for rice milk in both refrigerated and non-refrigerated sections of natural food stores and supermarkets.

Soy Margarine (Non-Hydrogenated)

Can be used in place of butter or hydrogenated margarine. Sold in plastic tubs in the refrigerated section of natural food stores and the natural foods section of large grocery stores. Look for labels that say "non-hydrogenated," "no trans-fats," or "no trans-fatty acids."

Tahini

A smooth spread made from ground-up sesame seeds, tahini (also known as sesame paste) adds rich flavor and creaminess to dips, sauces, spreads, and stews. Although it has a strong, nutty flavor, it's also delicious spread on toast. Tahini is rich in essential fatty acids, is sold in both jars and cans, and can be found with other seed- or nut-butters in natural food stores or in the natural foods section of large grocery stores. Stir until smooth upon opening.

Tamari

Tamari is a flavorful liquid brewed from whole soybeans. Similar to soy sauce except that it is wheat-free and has a more delicate taste. Soy sauce and tamari may be used interchangeably but you might make a permanent switch to tamari after experiencing its flavor.

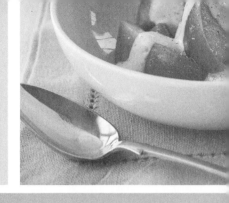

breakfast:
delectable ways
to start the day

1

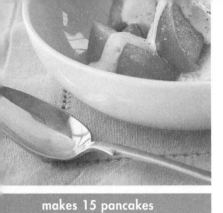

banana–chocolate chip pancakes

Tofu and fresh banana give the all-time favorite breakfast a nutritious boost.

dry ingredients

2$\frac{1}{2}$ cups whole wheat flour

2 teaspoons baking powder

$\frac{1}{2}$ teaspoon baking soda

$\frac{1}{2}$ teaspoon cinnamon

$\frac{1}{8}$ teaspoon ground nutmeg

Pinch salt

liquid ingredients

2$\frac{1}{4}$ cups water or rice milk

1 whole banana

$\frac{1}{3}$ cup soft tofu

$\frac{1}{4}$ cup vegetable oil

$\frac{1}{4}$ cup pure maple syrup

1 teaspoon vanilla extract

$\frac{1}{2}$ cup dairy-free chocolate chips or carob chips

1   Combine the dry ingredients in a large mixing bowl and stir with a wire whisk. Combine the liquid ingredients in a blender and process until smooth. Pour the

2

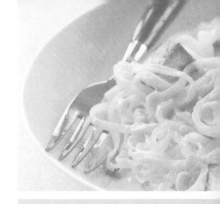

liquid ingredients into the dry ingredients and stir until combined. (Do not over-mix.) Stir in the chocolate chips.

2 Mist a nonstick skillet with nonstick cooking oil spray and set over medium-high heat. Drop the batter into the skillet using a $1/3$-cup measuring cup. Cook both sides until golden brown. Cook until small bubbles appear on top, about 2 minutes. Flip the pancake and cook until the bottom is golden brown, about 2 minutes. Remove from pan, repeat with remaining batter, and serve with pure maple syrup.

per pancake: 0mg cholesterol • 152 calories • 5g fat • 23g carbohydrate • 3g protein

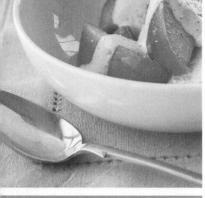

pumpkin pancakes

You don't have to wait until autumn to make pancakes with the quintessential orange squash. After all, pumpkin is high in powerful vitamins known as antioxidants, and is readily available in cans year-round.

dry ingredients

$2^1/_2$ cups whole wheat flour

1 tablespoon baking powder

$^1/_2$ teaspoon baking soda

$^1/_2$ teaspoon cinnamon

$^1/_4$ teaspoon ground ginger

$^1/_4$ teaspoon ground nutmeg

Pinch salt

liquid ingredients

$2^1/_4$ cups water

$^1/_2$ cup pumpkin puree

$^1/_3$ cup soft silken tofu

$^1/_4$ cup vegetable oil

$^1/_4$ cup pure maple syrup

1 Combine the dry ingredients in a large mixing bowl and stir with a wire whisk. Combine the liquid ingredients in a blender and process until smooth. Pour

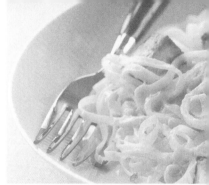

the liquid ingredients into the dry ingredients and stir until combined. (Do not overmix.)

2 Mist a nonstick skillet with nonstick cooking oil spray and set over medium heat. Drop the batter into the skillet using a $\frac{1}{3}$-cup measuring cup. Cook until small bubbles appear on top, about 2 minutes. Flip the pancake and cook until the bottom is golden, about 2 minutes. Remove from pan, repeat with remaining batter, and serve with pure maple syrup.

per pancake: 0mg cholesterol • 124 calories • 4g fat • 19g carbohydrate • 3g protein

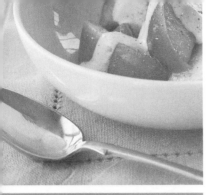

makes 12 pancakes

blueberry-buckwheat pancakes

After one heavenly taste of this easy recipe, you'll be bidding your instant buckwheat pancake mix goodbye.

dry ingredients

1 cup buckwheat flour

1 cup unbleached all-purpose flour

1 tablespoon baking powder

liquid ingredients

2¹/₄ cups water or rice milk

¹/₃ cup soft silken tofu

2 tablespoons pure maple syrup

1 cup blueberries (fresh or frozen/defrosted)

1   Combine the dry ingredients in a large mixing bowl and stir with a wire whisk. Combine the liquid ingredients in a blender and process until smooth. Pour the liquid ingredients into the dry ingredients and stir until combined. (Do not over-mix.) Stir in the blueberries.

2   Mist a nonstick skillet with nonstick cooking oil spray and set over medium heat. Drop the batter into the skillet using a ¹/₃-cup measuring cup. Cook until small bubbles appear on top, about 2 minutes. Flip the pancake and cook until the bottom is golden brown, about 2 minutes. Remove from pan, repeat with remaining batter, and serve with pure maple syrup.

per pancake: 0mg cholesterol • 101 calories • 1g fat • 24g carbohydrate • 2g protein

coconut french toast

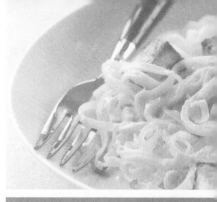

Thick, rich coconut milk is an ideal alternative to eggs when it comes to making perfect, cholesterol-free French toast.

$^1/_2$ cup soft silken tofu

2 tablespoons pure maple syrup

2 tablespoons apple juice or rice milk

1 teaspoon vanilla extract

1 (14-ounce) can coconut milk

15 slices whole grain bread

1. Combine the tofu, pure maple syrup, apple juice, and vanilla extract in a blender and process until smooth. Transfer to a shallow baking dish and whisk in the coconut milk.

2. Mist a large nonstick skillet with nonstick cooking oil spray and set over medium heat. Dip each piece of bread into the coconut mixture, scrape off most of the excess using the back of a spoon, place in the hot pan, and fry each side until brown, about 7 minutes per side. Remove from heat, repeat with the remaining bread, and serve with pure maple syrup.

per slice: 0mg cholesterol • 166 calories • 7g fat • 21g carbohydrate • 4g protein

breakfast: delectable ways to start the day

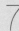

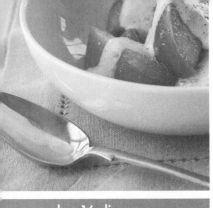

cashew french toast

When it comes to preparing spectacular brunch fare or when loading children up with ultimate nutrition before they head off to school, this recipe works absolute wonders.

1 cup raw, unsalted cashews

2 tablespoons flax seeds

3 cups water or rice milk

$^2/_3$ cup raisins

$^1/_2$ cup soft silken tofu

$^1/_4$ cup nutritional yeast flakes (optional)

1 teaspoon cinnamon

16 slices whole grain bread

1   Combine the cashews and flax seeds in a blender with $1^1/_2$ cups of the water. Blend for 2 minutes or until completely smooth. Add the raisins and remaining water and blend until completely smooth. Add the tofu, nutritional yeast flakes (if using), and cinnamon and blend until completely smooth. Transfer the mixture to a shallow baking dish.

2   Mist a nonstick skillet with nonstick cooking oil spray, and set over medium heat. Dip each piece of bread into the cashew mixture, scrape off most of the excess using the back of a spoon, and fry each side until brown, about 7 minutes per side. Remove from heat, repeat with the remaining bread, and serve with pure maple syrup.

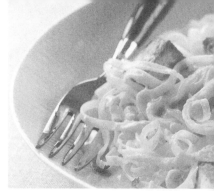

note Carefully monitor the heat while frying the French Toast, because if the skillet gets too hot, it will burn even if not yet cooked on the inside. Start with medium heat or a tiny bit above, and reduce the heat while cooking if necessary.

per slice: 0mg cholesterol • 192 calories • 6g fat • 28g carbohydrate • 8g protein

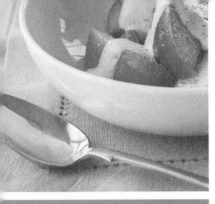

sunday morning scramble

Nutritional yeast flakes might sound overly healthy and devoid of flavor, but they actually add a phenomenal cheeselike flavor when used as a seasoning. Here, they join oven-browned potatoes and sautéed vegetables to make scrambled tofu hearty enough to carry you through an active weekend day. Serve with toast and meatless breakfast links for a healthy version of the full American breakfast, or wrap in warm tortillas with extra salsa for breakfast burritos.

1 medium potato, peeled and cut into $1/2$-inch cubes

2 tablespoons olive oil

1 onion, chopped

1 red bell pepper, chopped

3 ounces mushrooms, sliced (about $2/3$ cup)

1 pound firm tofu, rinsed and patted dry

$1/3$ cup salsa (your choice, preferably chunky)

3 tablespoons nutritional yeast flakes

$1/4$ teaspoon freshly ground black pepper

1 Put the potato cubes into a pot of boiling water, and boil for 2 minutes. Drain the potatoes and return to the dry pot. Drizzle with 1 tablespoon of the olive oil and stir to coat. Mist a baking sheet with nonstick cooking oil spray. Spread the potatoes on the baking sheet in a single layer and place under the broiler for 5 minutes or until golden brown. Remove from the heat and set aside.

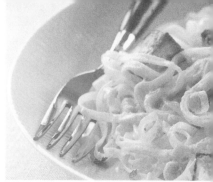

2 Put the remaining tablespoon of olive oil in a large nonstick skillet and set over medium-high heat. Add the onion and cook, stirring, until softened, about 3 minutes. Add the red bell pepper and mushrooms and cook, stirring, for 5 minutes. Crumble the tofu into the pan and cook, stirring, for 2 minutes. Stir in the salsa, nutritional yeast flakes, pepper, and reserved potatoes. Cook until heated through and serve immediately while hot.

per serving: 0mg cholesterol • 202 calories • 12g fat • 11g carbohydrate • 14g protein

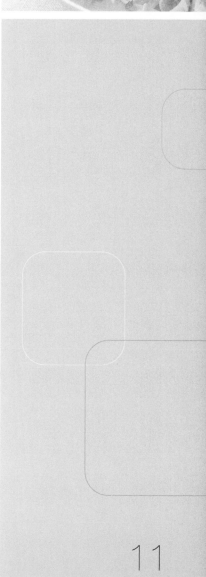

breakfast: delectable ways to start the day

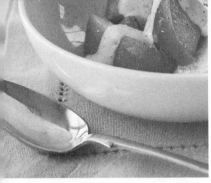

hot apples with cashew cream

Steaming, cinnamon-spiked apples pair lusciously with rich, cashew cream. Use Fuji apples for optimal taste and texture.

$1/_2$ pound soft tofu

3 tablespoons cashew butter

3 tablespoons pure maple syrup

1 teaspoon vanilla extract

2 tablespoons water

4 dates, pitted and chopped

4 whole cloves

4 sweet, red apples, cored and cut into medium wedges

$1/_2$ teaspoon cinnamon

$1/_8$ teaspoon ground nutmeg, plus extra for garnish

1 Put the tofu in a food processor and blend for 2 minutes or until completely smooth and free of graininess, stopping at least once to scrape down the sides of the bowl. Add the cashew butter, maple syrup, and vanilla and blend until smooth. Set aside.

2 Combine the water, dates, and cloves in a small, heavy-bottomed pot. Bring to a boil, cover, reduce the heat, and simmer for 3 minutes. Stir in the apples, cinnamon, and nutmeg and simmer, covered, for 5 minutes or until the apples are soft. Remove from the heat and discard the cloves.

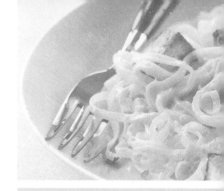

3   Spoon the apples into small dessert bowls and top with the cashew cream. Garnish with a pinch of nutmeg if desired.

per serving: 0mg cholesterol • 272 calories • 9g fat • 43g carbohydrate • 7g protein

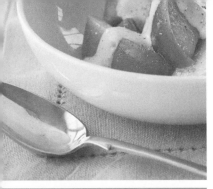

corn muffins

Making muffins first thing in the morning isn't really a big deal. As a matter of fact, it takes just minutes to prepare batter and spoon it into muffin cups. Then, while the yummy baked goods are in the oven, you can relax or get morning chores done and then be rewarded with the splendid taste and aroma of fresh, baked muffins. (Don't forget the fruit spread!)

dry ingredients

1¼ cups yellow cornmeal

¾ cup unbleached all-purpose flour

2 teaspoons baking powder

1 teaspoon salt

½ teaspoon baking soda

liquid ingredients

1¼ cups apple juice

¼ cup soft silken tofu

5 tablespoons pure maple syrup

3 tablespoons vegetable oil

1   Preheat oven to 350°F. Mist 12 muffin cups with nonstick cooking oil spray and set aside.

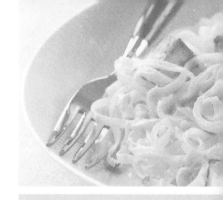

2   Combine the dry ingredients in a large mixing bowl and stir with a wire whisk. Combine the liquid ingredients in a blender and process until smooth. Pour the liquid ingredients into the dry ingredients and mix until combined. (Do not over-mix.)

3   Spoon the batter into the prepared muffin cups. Bake for 15 minutes or until a toothpick inserted into a muffin comes out dry. Remove from the heat and let cool for 10 minutes before releasing the muffins. Serve with fruit spread.

per muffin: 0mg cholesterol • 148 calories • 4g fat • 25g carbohydrate • 2g protein

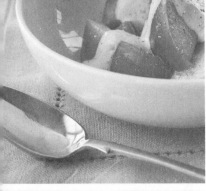

peanut butter and jelly muffins

Kids consider these a special morning treat, but Peanut Butter and Jelly Muffins work equally well as an anytime snack, or as a stand-in for the classic sandwich for lunch.

dry ingredients

2 cups unbleached all-purpose flour

1 tablespoon baking powder

$^1/_2$ teaspoon salt

liquid ingredients

1 cup pure maple syrup

$^2/_3$ cup soft silken tofu

$^1/_2$ cup natural peanut butter (smooth)

3 tablespoons dairy-free milk

1 teaspoon vanilla extract

2 tablespoons fruit spread (grape, strawberry, or blueberry recommended)

1   Preheat oven to 350°F. Mist 12 muffin cups with nonstick cooking oil spray and set aside.

2   Sift the dry ingredients into a large mixing bowl and set aside. Combine the liquid ingredients (not including the fruit spread) in a blender and process until smooth. Pour the liquid ingredients into the dry ingredients and stir until blended. (Do not overmix.)

16

tofu 1-2-3

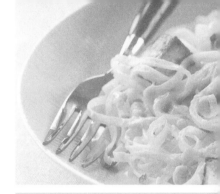

3 Put about ¹/₄ cup of batter into each muffin cup. Top each with ¹/₂ heaping teaspoon fruit spread. Cover with remaining batter and bake for 20 minutes or until
a toothpick inserted into the center of a muffin comes out dry. Remove from heat,
let cool for 10 minutes, and gently release the muffins. Serve warm or at room
temperature.

per muffin: 0mg cholesterol • 231 calories, 6g fat • 39g carbohydrate • 5g protein

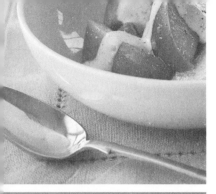

blueberry muffins

Yet another example of how easy it is to replace eggs with silken tofu when preparing classic baked goods.

dry ingredients

2 cups unbleached all-purpose flour

1 tablespoon baking powder

$^1/_2$ teaspoon salt

liquid ingredients

1 cup pure maple syrup

$^2/_3$ cup soft silken tofu

$^1/_3$ cup vegetable oil

1 teaspoon vanilla extract

$^1/_2$ cup blueberries (fresh or frozen/defrosted)

1   Preheat oven to 350°F. Mist 12 muffin cups with nonstick cooking spray oil.

2   Sift the dry ingredients into a large bowl. Combine the liquid ingredients in a blender and process until smooth. Pour the liquid ingredients into the dry ingredients and stir just enough to combine; do not overmix. Stir in the blueberries.

3   Spoon the batter into the prepared muffin cups and bake for 20 minutes or until a toothpick inserted into the middle of a muffin comes out dry. Let cool for 10 minutes before releasing the muffins from the cups.

per muffin: 0mg cholesterol • 212 calories • 6g fat • 34g carbohydrate • 3g protein

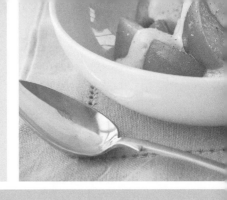

2 appetizers and
other finger-lickin'
party pleasers

19

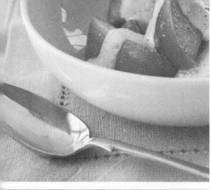

hot fiesta dip

Spinach and salsa lend flavor to this festive dip, best served piping hot with corn chips on the side.

¹/₂ pound soft tofu

1 cup dairy-free sour cream

1 tablespoon freshly squeezed lemon juice

1 tablespoon olive oil

1 onion, chopped

1 (10-ounce) package frozen chopped spinach, defrosted and drained

1 cup chunky salsa (your choice)

¹/₃ cup sliced black olives (optional)

1 tablespoon nutritional yeast flakes (optional)

1   Preheat oven to 375°F. Mist an 8 × 8-inch baking dish with nonstick cooking oil spray.

2   Combine the tofu, dairy-free sour cream, and lemon juice in a food processor and blend until smooth. Set aside.

3   Heat the oil in a skillet over medium-high heat. Add the onion and cook, stirring, until softened, about 5 minutes. Add the spinach and cook, stirring, until all of the water from the spinach has evaporated, about 5 minutes more. Remove from the heat and stir in the salsa, reserved tofu mixture, olives, and nutritional yeast flakes, if using.

4. Transfer to the prepared baking dish and bake, uncovered, for 20 minutes or until bubbly. Remove from the heat, let cool for 5 minutes, and serve with corn chips.

per tablespoon: 0mg cholesterol • 17 calories • 1g fat • 1g carbohydrate • 1g protein

appetizers and other finger-lickin' party pleasers

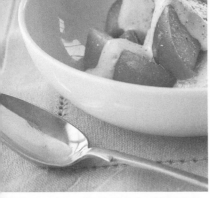

hot-n-cheesy layer dip

When it comes to making delectably cheesy dishes based on tofu rather than dairy, nutritional yeast flakes step in as the superstar of flavor. Just imagine hot, bubbly bean dip blanketed with melty cheese sauce and cold, crunchy lettuce. Bring on the margaritas!

1 (16-ounce) can vegetarian refried beans

$1/2$ cup salsa (your choice)

$1/2$ cup silken tofu

1 (4.5-ounce) can chopped green chiles

2 tablespoons nutritional yeast flakes

5 teaspoons freshly squeezed lemon juice

1 tablespoon sweet white miso

$1/4$ teaspoon onion granules

$1/8$ teaspoon salt

1 cup shredded lettuce

$1/4$ cup sliced jalapeño peppers (optional)

1 Preheat oven to 375°F.

2 Combine the vegetarian refried beans and salsa in an 8 × 8-inch baking pan. Stir together and spread over the bottom of the pan. Combine the remaining ingredients except the lettuce and jalapeño peppers in a blender and process until smooth. Drizzle over the beans.

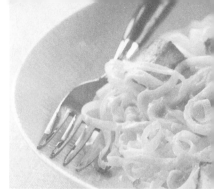

3 Bake for 20 minutes or until the beans are hot and bubbly. Remove from the oven, top with lettuce and jalapeños (if using), and serve with corn chips for dipping.

per serving: 0mg cholesterol • 114 calories • 2g fat • 15g carbohydrate • 8g protein

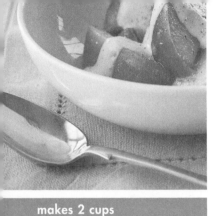

hot artichoke dip

For total party success, serve this awesome dip with crusty bread rounds.

1 pound soft tofu

1/4 cup dairy-free Parmesan cheese

1 garlic clove, minced

1 tablespoon freshly squeezed lemon juice

1 tablespoon fresh basil or 1 teaspoon dried

1 teaspoon arrowroot powder or cornstarch

1/2 teaspoon salt

2 (6-ounce) jars marinated artichoke hearts

Paprika for garnish

1 Preheat oven to 350°F. Mist an 8 × 8-inch baking dish with nonstick cooking oil spray. Set aside.

2 Combine all of the ingredients except one of the jars of the marinated artichoke hearts and the paprika in a food processor and blend until smooth. Add the second jar of artichoke hearts and pulse a few times until the second jar of artichokes is coarsely chopped. The dip should be somewhat chunky.

3 Transfer to the prepared baking dish, dust lightly with paprika, and bake, uncovered, for 20 minutes. Remove from the heat and serve with crackers or crusty bread rounds.

per tablespoon: 0mg cholesterol • 39 calories • 3g fat • 1g carbohydrate • 1g protein

tofu 1-2-3

chile con queso

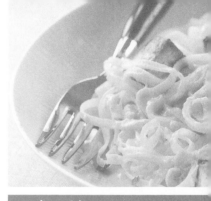

For a zippy nacho dip free of dairy and cholesterol, look no further than Chile Con Queso made with silken tofu, nutritional yeast flakes, and miso—three ingredients that when blended together taste a lot like, well, cheese! Serve with multicolored corn chips for a festive flair.

¹/₂ cup silken tofu

1¹/₂ tablespoons nutritional yeast flakes

¹/₂ tablespoon sweet white miso

³/₄ teaspoon freshly squeezed lemon juice

¹/₄ teaspoon onion granules

¹/₈ teaspoon salt

¹/₂ cup tomato salsa (your choice)

1 (4.5-ounce) can chopped green chiles

Combine the tofu, nutritional yeast flakes, miso, lemon juice, onion granules, and salt in a food processor or blender and process until smooth. Transfer to a medium saucepan and stir in the salsa and green chiles. Heat over low heat until warm, then transfer to a serving bowl and serve with corn chips for dipping.

per tablespoon: 0mg cholesterol • 12 calories • .6g fat • 1g carbohydrate • 1g protein

appetizers and other finger-lickin' party pleasers

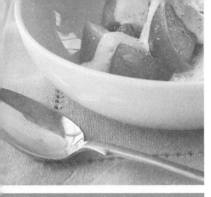

spinach dip in a bread crust

One of the best ways to introduce tofu to a skeptic is with this fanciful dip because the taste and texture are downright delectable.

1 cup eggless mayonnaise

$1/2$ pound soft tofu, rinsed and patted dry

1 tablespoon freshly squeezed lemon juice

$1/2$ teaspoon salt

1 (10-ounce) package frozen spinach, defrosted and drained well

5 scallions, chopped (both green and white parts)

3 tablespoons fresh parsley

3 tablespoons fresh dill or 1 tablespoon dried

Half of an 8-ounce can of water chestnuts, coarsely chopped (optional)

1 round loaf of rye or other crusty bread

1 Combine the eggless mayonnaise, tofu, lemon juice, and salt in a food processor, and blend until completely smooth. Add the spinach, scallions, parsley, and dill. Pulse several times in the food processor until mixed but not totally smooth. Transfer to a storage container and stir in the water chestnuts, if using. Cover and refrigerate for at least 1 hour before preparing the bread.

2 Cut the top quarter off the bread. Form a "bowl" by hollowing out the bread using your fingers or a spoon, leaving about 1 inch of crust all the way around. Place the bread bowl on a large serving dish. Cube the sliced-off top and the bread that

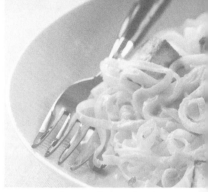

was scooped out of the loaf. (The cubes should be approximately 1 × 1 inch.) Arrange the cubes around the bread bowl for dipping. Fill the bread bowl with the spinach dip and serve.

per serving: 0mg cholesterol • 42 calories • 3g fat • 2g carbohydrate • 1g protein

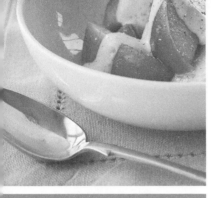

beer-battered coconut tofu
with apricot-dijon dipping sauce

Tofu replaces shrimp in this indulgent treat for the adventurous cook.

2 tablespoons warm water

1 tablespoon flax seeds

$1^1/_2$ teaspoons baking powder

$^2/_3$ cup beer

$^1/_3$ cup unbleached all-purpose flour

$2^1/_2$ cups unsweetened coconut flakes

1 pound firm or extra-firm tofu, pressed (see page xiv)

Vegetable oil for frying

Apricot-Dijon Dipping Sauce (recipe follows), for serving

1 Combine the water and flax seeds in a blender and process until emulsified. Transfer the mixture to a medium bowl. Whisk in the baking powder and stir in the beer.

2 Put the flour in a medium, flat-bottomed baking dish. Put the coconut flakes in a separate flat-bottomed baking dish. Cover a baking sheet with parchment paper and set aside.

3 Slice the tofu widthwise into $^1/_2$-inch slices; you will have about 8 or 9 rectangles. Now, cut each rectangle in half widthwise so that you have 16 or 18 squares. One by one, dredge each tofu square in the flour, then in the beer mixture, then

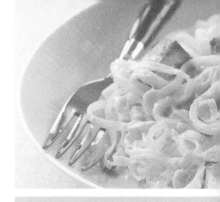

lay in the shredded coconut. Gently flip over the tofu in the shredded coconut in order to coat each side. Set the coated tofu pieces on the parchment paper until all are complete.

4 Pour ¼-inch layer of oil into a large skillet over high heat. Fry each piece of tofu for 3 minutes on each side or until brown and crispy. Remove from the pan and let drain on a wire rack. Serve immediately with Apricot-Dijon Dipping Sauce.

per piece: 0mg cholesterol • 133 calories • 10g fat • 8g carbohydrate • 3g protein

apricot-dijon dipping sauce

makes about ¹/₂ cup

¹/₂ cup apricot fruit spread

1 tablespoon rice vinegar

1¹/₂ teaspoons Dijon mustard

¹/₈ teaspoon ground ginger

Combine all of the ingredients in a small bowl and stir.

per ¹/₂ tablespoon: 0mg cholesterol • 20 calories • 0g fat • 5g carbohydrate • 0g protein

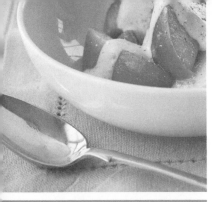

wish sticks with tartar sauce

Children go crazy over these crunchy, delicious, finger-lickin' sticks—and so will you.

1 cup cornmeal

1 pound extra-firm tofu, rinsed and patted dry

Vegetable oil for frying (about $^1/_4$ cup depending on the size of the pan)

Tartar Sauce (recipe follows), for serving

1   Put the cornmeal into a shallow baking dish, spread it evenly over the bottom, and set aside.

2   Slice the block of tofu lengthwise into 5 equal rectangles. Then, slice each rectangle lengthwise into 3 equal "sticks" (15 sticks total). Lay the tofu sticks on top of the cornmeal. Gently shake the baking dish until all sides of each tofu stick are coated, using your fingers to gently coat them if necessary. You may have to do this in more than one batch depending on the size of the dish.

3   Pour a thin layer of oil into a large, nonstick skillet, and heat over medium-high heat. When a bead of water dropped into the oil sizzles, the oil is ready for frying. Carefully lay the tofu sticks into the oil, and fry all four sides of each stick for 3 to 4 minutes each until crispy all over, using tongs or a fork to flip the tofu. (This will take about 12 to 15 minutes.) You may have to cook the tofu sticks in more than one batch depending on the size of your pan, although one whole batch will fit into most large, home-kitchen pans.

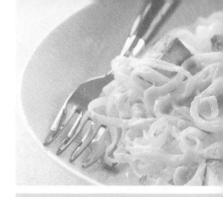

4 When done, remove the tofu sticks and place on a wire rack for 5 minutes to drain. Serve immediately with Tartar Sauce.

per stick: 0mg cholesterol • 88 calories • 5g fat • 7g carbohydrate • 3g protein

tartar sauce

makes about ¹/₃ cup

¹/₃ cup eggless mayonnaise

1–2 tablespoons relish

¹/₂ teaspoon onion granules

Combine all of the ingredients in a small bowl and mix well.

per teaspoon: 0mg cholesterol • 15 calories • 1g fat • 1g carbohydrate • 0g protein

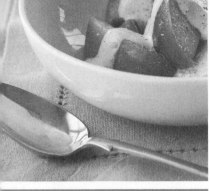

stuffed mushrooms
with sun-dried tomato pesto

Consider making a double batch, because these stuffed mushrooms disappear fast when presented to munchie-loving party guests.

2 (10-ounce) packages white mushrooms

1 tablespoon olive oil

1 garlic clove, minced

$^1/_2$ cup silken tofu, crumbled

$^1/_2$ cup pine nuts

$^1/_3$ cup packed fresh basil leaves

1 (6.5-ounce) jar sun-dried tomatoes packed in oil

Salt and freshly ground black pepper, to taste

1 Preheat oven to 350°F. Mist a baking sheet with nonstick cooking oil spray and set aside.

2 Separate the mushroom caps from the stems. Reserve the caps and trim and chop the stems. Heat the oil in a skillet over medium-high heat. Cook the garlic and mushroom stems, stirring, until soft, about 5 minutes. Remove from the heat and set aside.

3 Combine the tofu, pine nuts, and basil in a food processor and blend until combined. Add the sautéed mushroom stems and sun-dried tomatoes (including their oil) and pulse several times until a thick paste has formed. Some pieces of tomato should remain intact. Season to taste with salt and pepper.

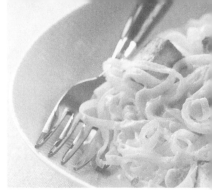

4 Fill each mushroom cap with about 1 tablespoon of stuffing. Arrange the stuffed mushrooms on the baking sheet and bake for 30 to 40 minutes, or until the mushrooms are soft and their tops are brown. Let cool for 5 minutes, transfer to a serving platter, and serve.

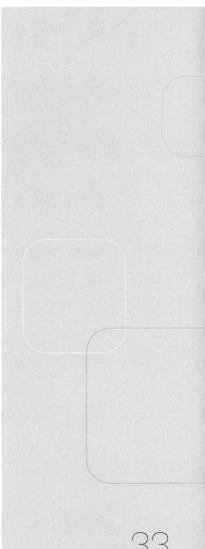

note Make sure that your oil-packed sun-dried tomatoes do not contain vinegar. Fortunately, most brands do not. However, it is important to check the label because vinegar will ruin the recipe.

per mushroom: 0mg cholesterol • 34 calories • 2g fat • 2g carbohydrate • 1g protein

appetizers and other finger-lickin' party pleasers

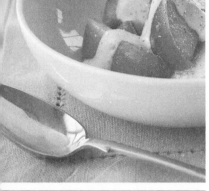

teriyaki tofu with peanut dipping sauce

To showcase this Asian-flavored broiler-crisped tofu, serve with a knife on a cutting board with a small bowl of Peanut Dipping Sauce on the side.

$1/2$ cup tamari or soy sauce

1 tablespoon rice vinegar

1 tablespoon pure maple syrup

1 teaspoon toasted sesame oil

$1/4$ teaspoon ground ginger

$1/4$ teaspoon garlic granules

1 pound firm or extra-firm tofu, rinsed and pressed (see page xiv)

Peanut Dipping Sauce (recipe follows), for serving

1   Combine all the ingredients except the tofu and Peanut Dipping Sauce in a medium bowl and whisk together until emulsified. Pour into a loaf pan or small baking dish of similar size.

2   Cut the tofu widthwise in half into 2 blocks. Put the 2 pieces of tofu in the marinade and let them sit, covered and refrigerated, for at least 15 minutes; flip to marinate the other three sides for at least 15 minutes per side. (This step can be done overnight for optimal flavor, and if the tofu sits for several hours, it is only necessary to marinate the tops and bottoms.)

34

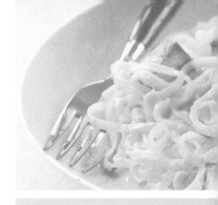

3 Mist a baking sheet with nonstick cooking oil spray. Lay the marinated tofu on the baking sheet, and cook under the broiler for about 5 minutes per side or until all four sides are crispy brown. Remove from the heat and serve on a cutting board with a knife and small bowl of Peanut Dipping Sauce.

per serving: 0mg cholesterol • 64 calories • 3g fat • 6g carbohydrate • 6g protein

peanut dipping sauce

makes about $^1/_2$ cup

3 tablespoons natural peanut butter (smooth)

3 tablespoons pure maple syrup

4 teaspoons tamari or soy sauce

$^3/_4$ teaspoon rice vinegar

Combine all of the ingredients in a small bowl and whisk until emulsified.

per teaspoon: 0mg cholesterol • 18 calories • 1g fat • 2g carbohydrate • .5g protein

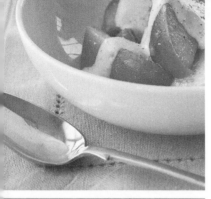

nori rolls with teriyaki tofu and fresh pea shoots

Few appetizers compare in presentation to an artful platter of nori rolls made with a beautiful array of fillings.

1$^1/_2$ cups short-grain white rice

1$^3/_4$ cups water

1$^1/_2$ tablespoons rice vinegar

1 tablespoon sugar

$^3/_4$ teaspoon salt

4 sheets nori

Several pieces pickled ginger (see Note)

$^1/_2$ recipe of Teriyaki Tofu (page 34), cut into thin strips

Handful fresh pea shoots or watercress

Tamari and wasabi mustard (optional), for serving

1 Wash the rice and let it dry in a strainer for 1 hour. Put the rice and water in a small, heavy-bottomed saucepan, and bring it to a boil. Cover, reduce the heat, and simmer for 15 minutes. Remove from heat and let stand, covered, for 10 minutes.

2 Combine the vinegar, sugar, and salt in a small saucepan and set over medium heat. Simmer until the salt and sweetener are dissolved, 2 to 3 minutes.

3 Transfer the cooked rice into a large, non-metal bowl. Pour the vinegar mixture over the surface of the rice. Using a wooden spoon or rubber spatula, mix the

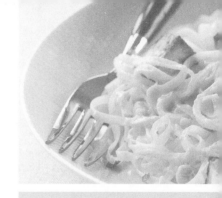

vinegar into the rice using up and down cutting motions (rather than circular stirring motions). Fan the rice with a magazine, thin book, or hand-held fan for 1 minute. (This gives it a shiny look.)

4. Place a sushi-rolling mat in front of you on a flat surface, and cover it with a sheet of nori with the shiny side face-down. Spread a thin layer of rice on the nori, leaving a 1-inch gap at the top. Lay several strips of pickled ginger over the rice in a horizontal line about 1 inch from the bottom of the nori (the end closest to you). Cover the pickled ginger with several strips of Teriyaki Tofu. Next, lay pea shoots over the tofu.

5. Starting with the end closest to you, gently roll the mat and the nori sheet over the filling. Press down firmly, and continue rolling until you reach the end of the space at the end of the nori. Dab a bit of water across the top of the nori, and continue rolling to the end. Press down to seal. Using a very sharp knife with a touch of water on its blade, cut the nori roll in half. Then, cut each of the halves two more times to make a total of 6 pieces.

6. Repeat with the remaining 3 pieces of nori. Arrange the cut nori on a serving platter with a dish of tamari and/or a dollop of wasabi mustard, if desired.

note Look for pickled ginger in natural food stores, Asian grocery stores, and in the Asian section of large grocery stores.

per piece: 0mg cholesterol • 70 calories • 1g fat • 14g carbohydrate • 1g protein

appetizers and other finger-lickin' party pleasers

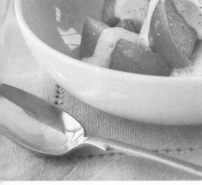

loaded nachos

Whether fully loaded or merely dotted with jalapeños, everyone's favorite group appetizer has now gone guilt-free thanks to cheesy-flavored yet dairy-free nutritional yeast flakes.

1 cup silken tofu

3 tablespoons nutritional yeast flakes

1¹/₂ tablespoons freshly squeezed lemon juice

1 tablespoon sweet white miso

¹/₂ teaspoon onion granules

¹/₄ teaspoon salt

¹/₂ cup tomato salsa (your choice)

1 (4.5-ounce) can chopped green chiles

1 medium bag baked corn chips (about 16 ounces)

additions (your choice)

2 cups warm vegetarian chili (fresh or canned)

2 cups shredded lettuce

1 tomato, chopped

1 ripe Haas avocado, cubed

¹/₂ cup sliced black olives

¹/₂ cup sliced jalapeño peppers

38

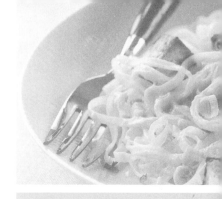

1 Preheat oven to 200°F.

2 Combine the tofu, nutritional yeast flakes, lemon juice, miso, onion granules, and salt in a blender or food processor. Blend until smooth, transfer to a medium saucepan, and stir in the salsa and chiles. Heat gently over low heat to keep warm until the chips are ready.

3 Spread the corn chips on an ungreased baking sheet and put in the oven for 6 minutes or until warm but not toasted. Transfer the chips to a serving platter and drizzle with the warm sauce. Top with your choice of additions in the order in which they appear and serve immediately with plenty of napkins.

per serving: 0mg cholesterol • 294 calories • 7g fat • 51g carbohydrate • 12g protein

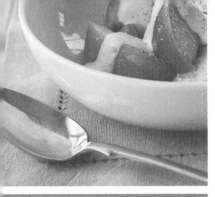

mini fillo cups

Many entrées, stews, and salads become instant appetizers when stuffed into mini fillo shells, easily accessible in the frozen section of large grocery stores. Since these fillo shells are already shaped into tiny edible cups and baked, they need nothing more than a few minutes of defrosting before being filled and served.

1 (2-ounce) package frozen mini fillo shells (about 15 prebaked shells)

1 cup of one of the following fillings:

hot fillings

Garden Vegetable Chili with Kale and Black Beans (page 114)

Cannellini Beans and Roasted Potatoes in Cashew Cream Sauce (page 88)

Kale and Chickpea Chardonnay (page 106)

Mixed Sautéed Mushrooms and White Wine Stroganoff (page 84), omit the farfalle

Hot Artichoke Dip (page 24), unbaked

cold fillings

Chickenless Salad (page 141)

Eggless Salad (page 144)

Spinach Dip (page 26)

Waldorf Salad (page 145)

Ambrosia (page 146)

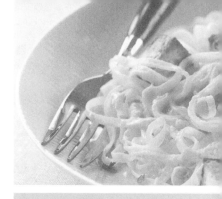

1   If preparing a hot appetizer, preheat oven to 350°F.

2   If preparing a hot appetizer, remove the frozen mini fillo shells from the package, arrange on a baking sheet, and let sit to defrost for 10 minutes. Using a very small spoon, fill the cups with your filling of choice. Bake for about 10 minutes or until filling is hot. Serve immediately.

3   If preparing a cold appetizer, remove the frozen mini fillo shells from package, arrange on a serving platter, and let sit to defrost for 10 to 15 minutes. Using a very small spoon, fill each cup with your cold filling of choice and serve immediately.

note   Mini fillo shells can only hold up to 1 tablespoon of filling per cup. Therefore, when preparing any of these fillings for the cups, chop the ingredients a little bit smaller than the recipes indicate so there won't be any big chunks.

note   If preparing cups with Chili, Cannellini Beans and Roasted Potatoes in Cashew Cream Sauce, Mushroom Stroganoff, or Kale and Chickpea Chardonnay, consider making the filling one day in advance because the texture becomes more suitable to this recipe after the recipes have had a chance to cool completely. The filling can heat up with the shells at serving time. If preparing Hot Artichoke Dip as filling, it does not have to be baked before going into the cups.

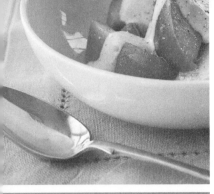

english muffin pizzas

For easy, guilt-free, taste-tempting pizza, reach for silken tofu, nutritional yeast flakes, and miso—three ingredients that lead to delectable dairy-free pizza-topping cheese.

makes 12 mini pizzas

1 cup silken tofu

3 tablespoons nutritional yeast flakes

4 teaspoons freshly squeezed lemon juice

1 tablespoon light miso

3/4 teaspoon onion granules

1/2 teaspoon salt

6 English muffins, sliced in half

1 cup pizza sauce (your choice)

1 tablespoon Italian seasoning

1 Preheat oven to 375°F.

2 Combine the tofu, nutritional yeast flakes, lemon juice, miso, onion granules, and salt in a food processor. Blend until smooth. Lay the English muffin halves face-up on a baking sheet and spread the top of each with pizza sauce. Top each with about 1 tablespoon of the tofu mixture and sprinkle with Italian seasoning.

3 Bake for 8 to 10 minutes or until edges are golden brown. Cool for 5 minutes and serve as is or cut into quarters.

per serving: 0mg cholesterol • 102 calories • 1g fat • 17g carbohydrate • 6g protein

tofu 1-2-3

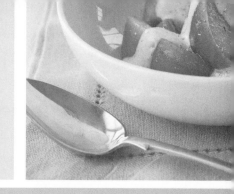

3 enticing entrées

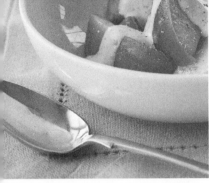

manicotti florentine

serves 4

A blend of tofu, spinach, and parsley makes a fabulous filling for manicotti, yielding only 7 grams of fat and of course absolutely no cholesterol per serving. Compare that to manicotti made with dairy, which contains about 15 grams of fat and 103 milligrams of cholesterol for the same amount! Serve with garlic bread and a crisp, green salad for the healthy update of a traditional Italian meal.

1 pound soft tofu, rinsed and patted dry

3 tablespoons fresh, chopped parsley or 1 tablespoon dried

$1/4$ teaspoon salt

$1/4$ teaspoon freshly ground black pepper

2 (10-ounce) packages frozen chopped spinach, thawed and well drained

1 (8-ounce) package manicotti

1 (26-ounce) jar spaghetti sauce

1 tablespoon dairy-free Parmesan cheese

1 Preheat oven to 350°F.

2 Put the tofu in a large bowl and mash with a fork or potato masher. Add the parsley, salt, and pepper, mashing and stirring until evenly mixed. Make sure the spinach is completely drained of water and stir it into the tofu mixture. Set aside.

3 Cook the manicotti according to the package directions. Drain and gently rinse with cold water until cool enough to handle.

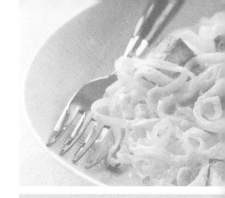

4   Pour a thin layer of spaghetti sauce in the bottom of a 9 × 13-inch baking dish and set aside. Using a small spoon or a pastry bag, stuff the manicotti with the tofu filling and arrange in a single layer over the sauce. Spoon the remaining sauce over manicotti and sprinkle with Parmesan cheese. Cover and bake for 35 minutes or until bubbly. Uncover, bake for 5 minutes, then remove from heat and let stand for 5 minutes before serving.

per serving: 0mg cholesterol • 381 calories • 7g fat • 61g carbohydrate • 22g protein

enticing entrées

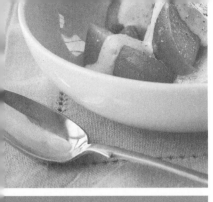

spanakopita

It's not necessary to wait for a special occasion to prepare this classic Greek spinach pie made with a tofu mixture in lieu of feta cheese. It's important to work quickly when using fillo dough, but using olive oil spray rather than the bottled form makes it relatively easy.

Olive oil spray (see Note)

1 pound firm tofu, rinsed and patted dry

2 tablespoons light miso

2 tablespoons freshly squeezed lemon juice

3 tablespoons fresh dill or 1 tablespoon dried

1 tablespoon nutritional yeast flakes (optional)

$1/4$ teaspoon ground nutmeg

2 (10-ounce) packages frozen chopped spinach, defrosted and drained well

4 scallions, chopped (both green and white parts)

12 sheets fillo dough

1 Preheat oven to 350°F. Mist a 9 × 13-inch baking dish with olive oil spray. Set aside.

2 Put the tofu in a large bowl and mash with a fork or potato masher. Add the miso, lemon juice, dill, nutritional yeast flakes (if using), and nutmeg, mashing and stirring until evenly mixed. Make sure the spinach is completely drained of water and stir it into the tofu mixture along with the scallions. Set aside.

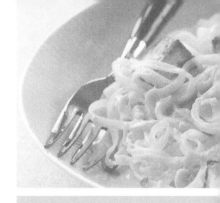

3 Unroll the fillo dough and lay it on a flat, dry surface. Cover the stack with a damp dishtowel to prevent drying. Lay 1 sheet of fillo dough in the prepared baking dish and heavily mist it with olive oil spray. Work quickly and repeat with 5 more sheets of fillo dough, heavily misting each before adding the next sheet. Keep the pile of unused fillo dough sheets covered with the damp towel as much as possible during this process to prevent the fillo dough from tearing.

4 After misting the sixth sheet of fillo dough, cover with the tofu/spinach filling. Top with 6 more sheets of fillo dough, working quickly and misting each with olive oil spray like before. Mist the top sheet, then tuck down its edges against the sides of the pan.

5 Bake for 35 minutes or until golden brown. Serve hot or cold, cut into squares of desired size.

note Using olive oil spray makes it very easy to prepare this dish. However, it does not result in extra-crispy, golden-brown fillo dough the way brushed-on olive oil does. If you prefer, brush olive oil onto the individual fillo sheets instead of misting them with olive oil spray.

per serving: 0mg cholesterol • 282 calories • 10g fat • 34g carbohydrate • 16g protein

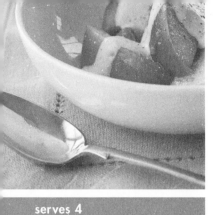

tofu parmesan

A bit of an indulgence, it's the breading that makes these crispy-coated cutlets so scrumptious. Serve with a crisp green salad and spaghetti on the side for an ultra-satisfying meal.

$^1/_2$ cup unbleached all-purpose flour

1 cup warm water

2 tablespoons flax seeds

1 cup bread crumbs

2 tablespoons Italian seasoning

$^3/_4$ teaspoon poultry seasoning

$^1/_2$ cup dairy-free Parmesan cheese

1 pound firm or extra-firm tofu, rinsed and patted dry

Vegetable oil for frying (about $^1/_4$ cup)

$2^1/_2$ cups spaghetti sauce

1   Preheat oven to 350°F. Mist a 9 × 13-inch baking dish with nonstick cooking oil spray. Set aside.

2   Put the flour in a shallow baking dish and set aside.

3   Combine the water and flax seeds in a blender and process until emulsified. Transfer to a small bowl and set aside.

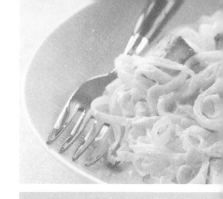

4   Put the bread crumbs in a shallow baking dish and stir in Italian seasoning, poultry seasoning, and $^1/_4$ cup of the Parmesan cheese. Set aside.

5   Cut the tofu widthwise into $^1/_4$-inch slices (you will have about 12 rectangles). Pour a thin layer of oil into a nonstick skillet and heat over medium-high heat. Dip each piece of tofu into the flour, then the flax mixture, and then dredge in the bread crumbs, coating well. Fry for 3 minutes on each side or until brown and crispy. You will need to do this in batches to avoid overcrowding.

6   Lay half of the fried tofu pieces, side by side, in the prepared baking dish. Cover with half of the spaghetti sauce and sprinkle with 2 tablespoons of the Parmesan cheese. Lay the remaining tofu pieces, side by side, over the sauce. Cover with remaining sauce and Parmesan cheese. Bake, uncovered, for 30 minutes or until bubbly. Remove from the heat and serve.

per serving: 0mg cholesterol • 568 calories • 28g fat • 61g carbohydrate • 21g protein

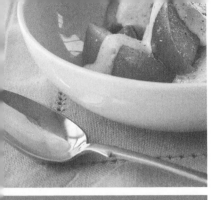

serves 8

shepherd's pie

This hearty casserole is a great dish for the holiday table. You might want to prepare it the day before or at least several hours in advance because its texture gets even better once cooled completely and reheated.

mashed potato topping

4 medium potatoes, peeled and cut into medium chunks

$1/3$–$1/2$ cup plain-flavored dairy-free milk (soy-, rice-, or oat-based)

3 tablespoons olive oil

Salt and freshly ground black pepper, to taste

filling

1 tablespoon vegetable oil

1 large onion, chopped

3 garlic cloves, minced

2 tablespoons all-purpose flour

2 cups vegetable broth

$1/4$ cup sherry cooking wine

1 teaspoon dried basil

1 teaspoon dried parsley

1 teaspoon vegetarian Worcestershire sauce

$1/2$ teaspoon garlic granules

50

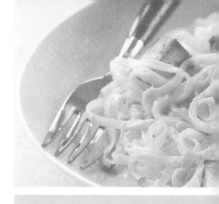

$^1/_2$ teaspoon poultry seasoning

$^1/_2$ teaspoon salt

$^1/_8$ teaspoon freshly ground black pepper

1 pound firm or extra-firm tofu, patted dry and cut into $^1/_2$-inch cubes

1 (16-ounce) package frozen mixed vegetables, defrosted (peas, corn, green beans, and carrots are a good combination)

Salt and freshly ground black pepper, to taste

1 To make the mashed potato topping, cook the potatoes in boiling water until tender, about 15 minutes. Drain them and mash in a medium bowl with the dairy-free milk, olive oil, salt, and pepper. Set aside.

2 Preheat oven to 400°F. Mist a deep-sided 10 × 10-inch casserole dish with non-stick cooking oil spray and set aside.

3 To make the filling, heat the oil in a large skillet over medium-high heat. Add the onion and garlic and cook, stirring, until the onion is soft, about 10 minutes. Sprinkle the flour over the onions and stir to coat. Gradually pour in the vegetable broth, stirring constantly to prevent lumps. Stir in the sherry and simmer, stirring constantly, until thick, about 2 minutes.

4 Stir in the basil, parsley, Worcestershire sauce, garlic granules, poultry seasoning, salt, and pepper. Gently stir in the tofu and defrosted vegetables, and adjust the seasonings to taste.

(continues)

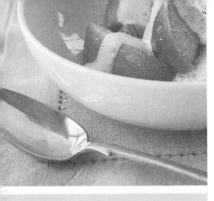

shepherd's pie

(continued)

5 Transfer the tofu/vegetable mixture to the prepared casserole dish. Spoon the mashed potatoes over the top. Smooth out the surface of the mashed potatoes with the back of a spoon. Cover and bake for 30 minutes or until bubbly. Let cool for 15 minutes before serving.

per serving: 0mg cholesterol • 228 calories • 10g fat • 24g carbohydrate • 8g protein

tofu 1-2-3

chili-stuffed peppers

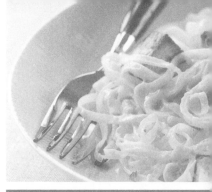

Sure, personal pizzas are great. But when was the last time you gave friends and family the opportunity to reach for their own personal peppers!

makes 12 stuffed peppers

1 recipe Garden Vegetable Chili with Kale and Black Beans (page 114)

12 bell peppers in assorted colors

1 (15-ounce) can tomato sauce

$1/2$ cup nutritional yeast flakes or shredded dairy-free cheddar cheese

1 Preheat oven to 375°F.

2 Prepare the chili and set aside.

3 Cut the top off each bell pepper, removing stems and seeds. Drop the peppers into a large pot of boiling water for 5 minutes, then drain upside down on a wire rack. (You may have to do this in more than one batch depending on the size of the pot.)

4 Stand the peppers up in a shallow baking dish so that they touch and support each other. Spoon the chili into the peppers. Bake for 20 minutes. Remove from oven and spoon tomato sauce over the chili. Sprinkle with the nutritional yeast flakes or shredded dairy-free cheddar cheese. Return to oven and bake for 10 minutes. Remove from heat and serve.

per pepper: 0mg cholesterol • 246 calories • 4g fat • 38g carbohydrate • 18g protein

enticing entrées

53

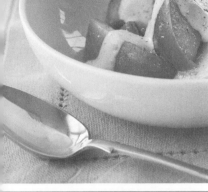

captain tofu

Here, tofu replaces chicken in the dish traditionally referred to as Country Captain, a.k.a. East Indian Curry. It's truly astounding that the simple combination of tomatoes, curry powder, thyme, onion, and green pepper can create such amazing flavor. Best served over white basmati rice.

$1/4$ cup whole wheat flour

2 tablespoons nutritional yeast flakes (optional)

$1/2$ teaspoon salt

$1/8$ teaspoon freshly ground black pepper

1 pound extra-firm tofu, rinsed, pressed, and cut into $1/2$-inch cubes (see page xiv)

3 tablespoons olive oil

1 onion, chopped

1 green bell pepper, chopped

2 garlic cloves, minced

2–3 teaspoons curry powder

$1/2$ teaspoon thyme

1 (28-ounce) can whole tomatoes

1 Preheat oven to 350°F.

2 Combine the flour, nutritional yeast flakes (if using), salt, and pepper in a shallow baking dish and stir with a wire whisk. Place the tofu cubes in the flour mixture and gently shake the baking dish until the tofu is completely coated.

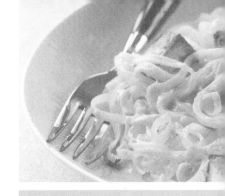

3 Put 2 tablespoons of the olive oil in a large nonstick skillet and heat over medium-high heat. Add the tofu and cook all sides until golden brown, 7 to 10 minutes. Transfer the tofu to a 9 × 11-inch baking dish and set aside. Return the unwashed skillet to the stove.

4 Heat the remaining tablespoon of olive oil in the skillet over medium-high heat. Add the onion, bell pepper, and garlic and cook, stirring, until softened, about 5 minutes. Stir in the curry powder and thyme and cook, stirring, for 1 minute. Add the canned tomatoes and break them apart with a wooden spoon. Bring to a simmer and cook, stirring, for 1 minute. Remove from heat and pour over the tofu.

5 Bake, uncovered, for 35 minutes or until hot and bubbly. Remove from the heat and let cool for 5 minutes before serving.

per serving: 0mg cholesterol • 269 calories • 16g fat • 19g carbohydrate • 16g protein

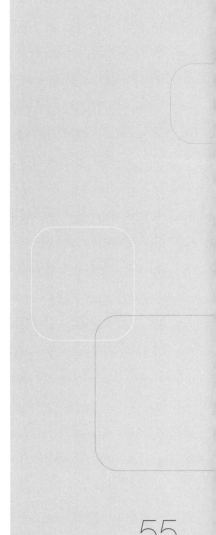

enticing entrées

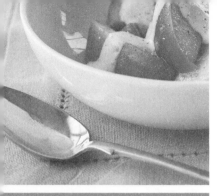

baked penne florentine

Nutritional yeast flakes and miso bring cheesy flavor to this luscious mixture of pasta and spinach topped with bread crumbs and baked to perfection. Warmly suitable for a wintry day.

1 pound penne, boiled for 5 minutes and drained

1 (10-ounce) package frozen spinach, defrosted and drained well

1 (12-ounce) package soft silken tofu (1^1/$_2$ cups)

1 cup water

^{1}/$_4$ cup nutritional yeast flakes

2 tablespoons non-hydrogenated soy margarine

1 tablespoon light miso

1 tablespoon white wine

1 tablespoon freshly squeezed lemon juice

^{1}/$_2$ small onion, coarsely chopped

1 teaspoon mustard powder

^{1}/$_4$ teaspoon paprika

^{1}/$_4$ teaspoon salt

^{1}/$_4$ teaspoon dried basil

Pinch ground nutmeg

1 cup bread crumbs

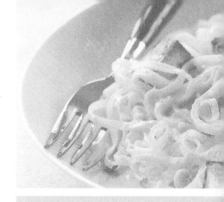

1. Preheat oven to 350°F. Mist a deep casserole dish with nonstick cooking oil spray and set aside.

2. Combine the partially cooked penne and spinach in a large mixing bowl and stir well. Put the remaining ingredients except the bread crumbs in a blender and process until smooth. Pour over the pasta and stir well.

3. Transfer the mixture to the prepared casserole dish and sprinkle the bread crumbs over the top. Bake for 35 minutes or until bubbly. Remove from the oven and let it rest for 10 minutes before serving.

per serving: 0mg cholesterol • 476 calories • 9g fat • 76g carbohydrate • 22g protein

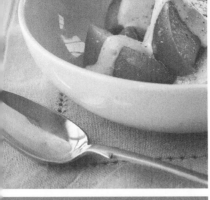

roasted vegetable lasagna

A mélange of colorful vegetables takes center stage in this remarkably "light" lasagna.

2 red bell peppers

1 eggplant, thinly sliced lengthwise

2 zucchini, thinly sliced lengthwise

2 yellow summer squash, thinly sliced lengthwise

Olive oil for drizzling

Salt and freshly ground black pepper, to taste

1 pound firm or extra-firm tofu, rinsed and patted dry

$^1/_3$ cup eggless mayonnaise

1 (10-ounce) package frozen kale, defrosted and drained well

1 tablespoon Italian seasoning

$^1/_2$ teaspoon onion granules

$^1/_8$ teaspoon garlic granules

2 (26-ounce) jars spaghetti sauce

12–15 lasagna noodles, uncooked

1 Preheat the broiler.

2 Put the red bell peppers (whole) on a large baking sheet and place directly under the broiler. Rotate the peppers every few minutes until they are partially blackened all over. Remove from heat and put the peppers in a paper bag. Roll up the

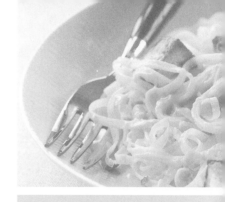

top of the bag, let sit for 10 minutes, and remove the peppers. Core the peppers, remove the seeds, and scrape off the skin. (The skin will come off easily.) Cut the peppers into wide strips and transfer them to a large bowl or pan. Set aside. Do not turn off the broiler.

3   Mist a large baking sheet with nonstick cooking oil spray and lay the slices of eggplant, zucchini, and yellow squash on it. (You may have to do this in more than one batch depending on the size of the baking sheet.) Drizzle with olive oil and sprinkle with salt and pepper. Place under the broiler for 3 to 5 minutes or until soft and light brown. Flip, drizzle with a bit more olive oil, and return to the broiler for 3 to 5 minutes or until light brown. (Watch to avoid burning.) Remove from heat and transfer to the bowl or pan of peppers.

4   Preheat oven to 350°F.

5   Put the tofu in a large bowl and mash with a fork or potato masher. Stir in the eggless mayonnaise, defrosted kale, Italian seasoning, onion granules, and garlic granules. Set aside.

6   Pour half of one of the jars of spaghetti sauce into a 9 × 13-inch baking pan. Lay 3 or 4 of the uncooked lasagna noodles lengthwise over the sauce, and 1 of the noodles horizontally at one of the ends (break to fit if necessary). There will be a lot of space between the noodles but they will expand as they cook.

7   Lay half of the roasted vegetables over the noodles, also covering the spaces between the noodles. Spread the tofu mixture over the vegetables. Cover with

(continues)

enticing entrées

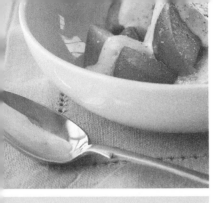

roasted vegetable lasagna

(continued)

the remaining half of the open jar of sauce. Arrange 4 more lasagna noodles in the same manner as the first noodle layer. Cover with remaining vegetables. Pour on half of the second jar of sauce. Arrange the last 4 lasagna noodles over the sauce, and top with remaining sauce.

8   Cover tightly with foil and bake for 55 minutes, removing the cover for the last 10 minutes. Let cool for at least 10 minutes before serving.

note   For optimal texture, prepare one day in advance. (To reheat, cover and cook for about 40 minutes at 350°F.)

note   It's not necessary to use special "no-cook" lasagna noodles for this recipe. Simply cooking the lasagna for the time specified in this recipe will make them nice and soft.

per serving: 0mg cholesterol   •   450 calories   •   16g fat   •   66g carbohydrate   •   14g protein

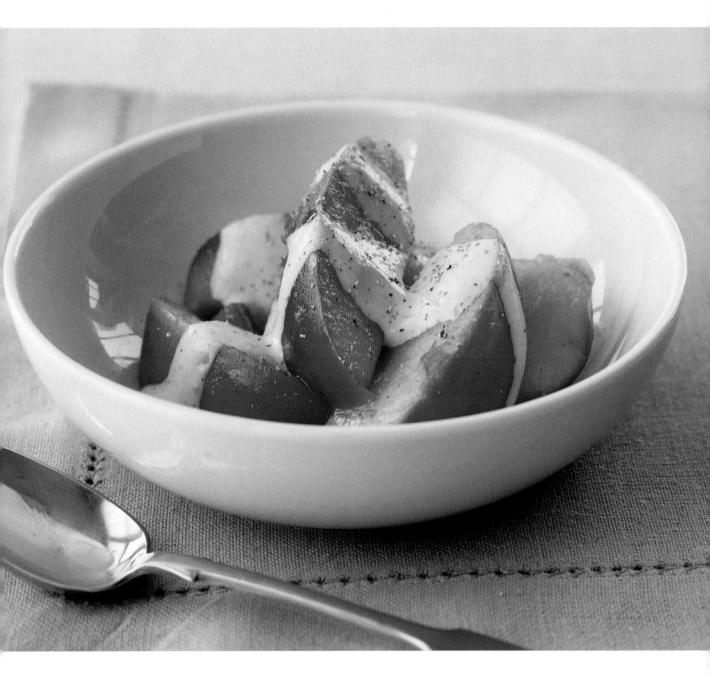

hot apples with cashew cream   *page 12*

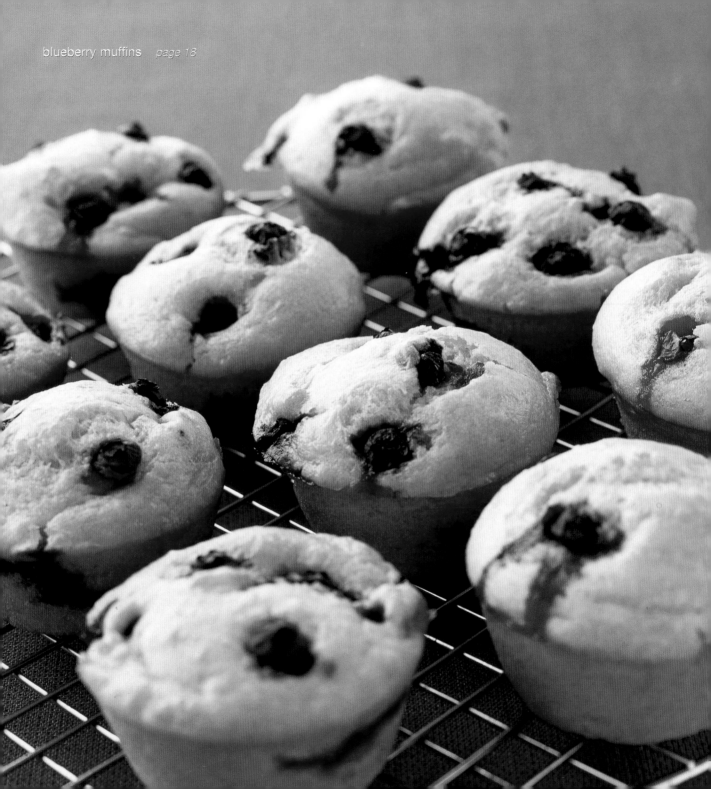

blueberry muffins   page 18

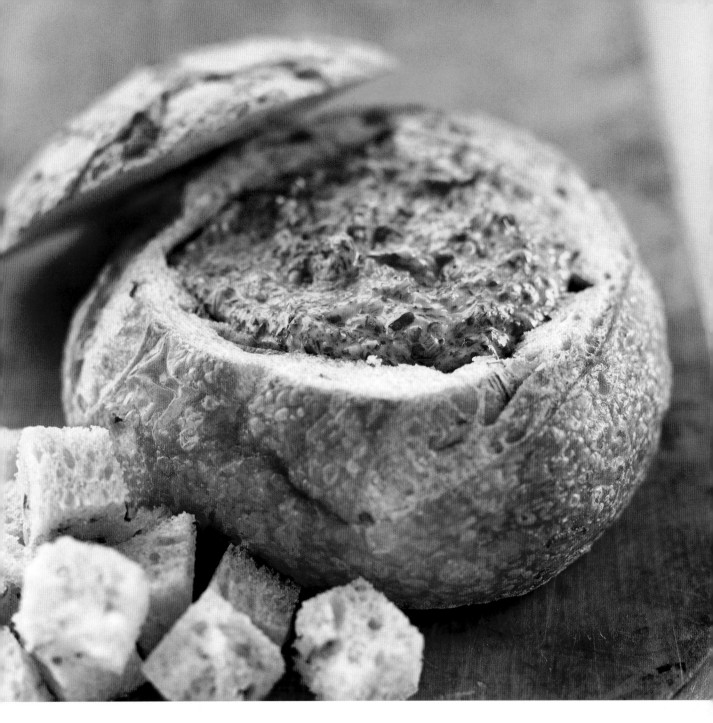

spinach dip in a bread crust   *page 26*

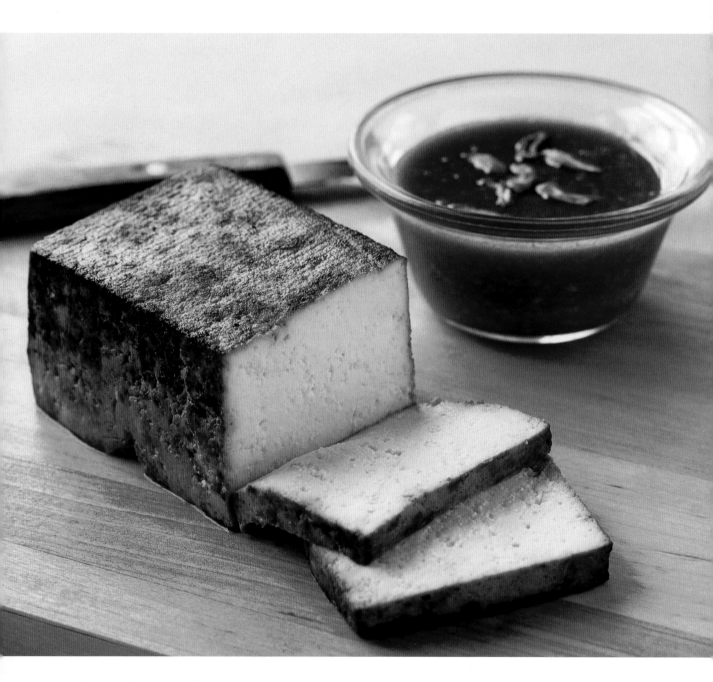

terriyaki tofu with peanut dipping sauce   *page 34*

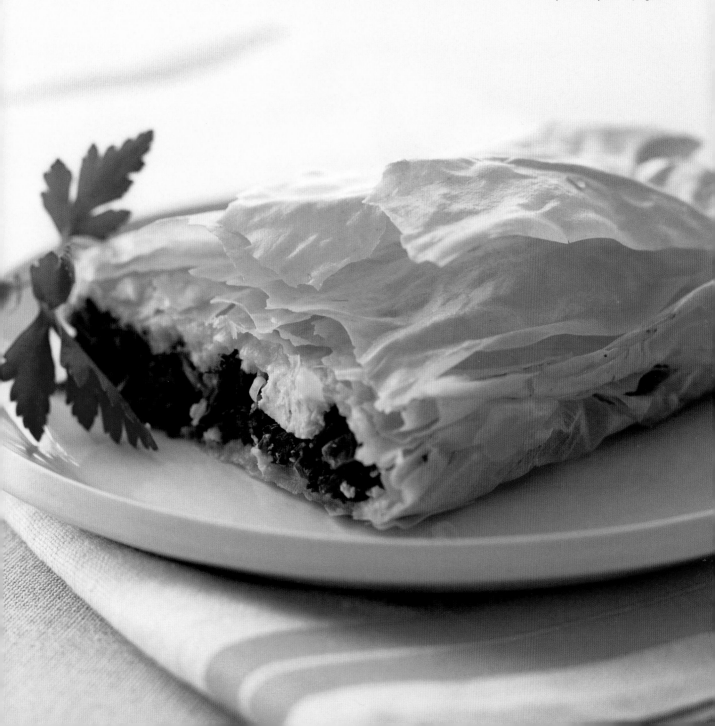

spanakopita *page 46*

spicy peanut noodles *page 66*

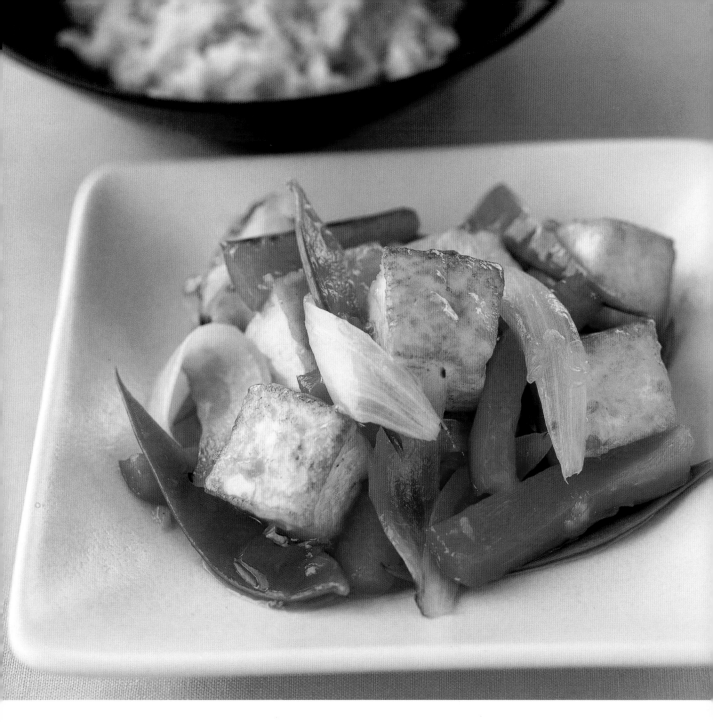

glazed apricot stir fry   *page 74*

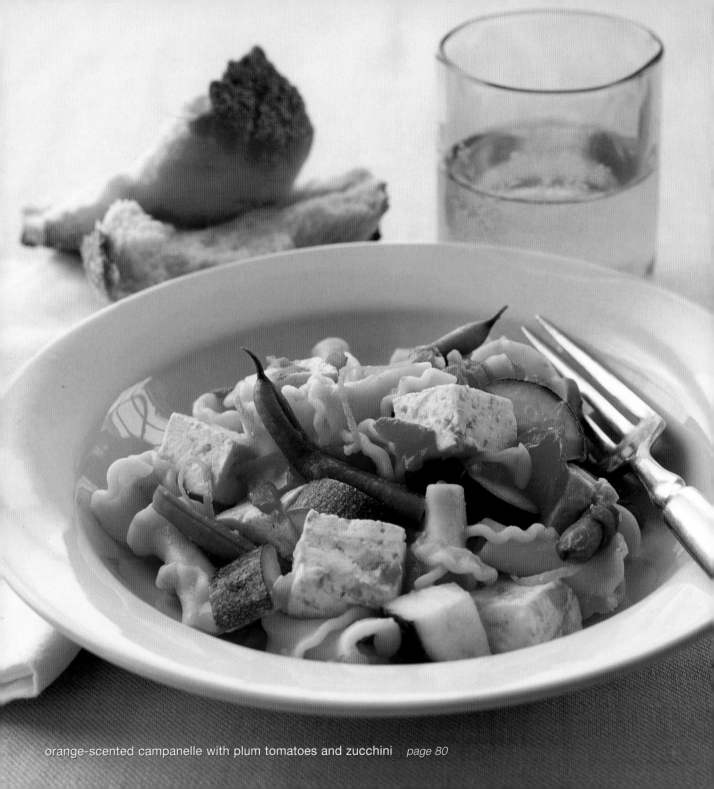

orange-scented campanelle with plum tomatoes and zucchini   *page 80*

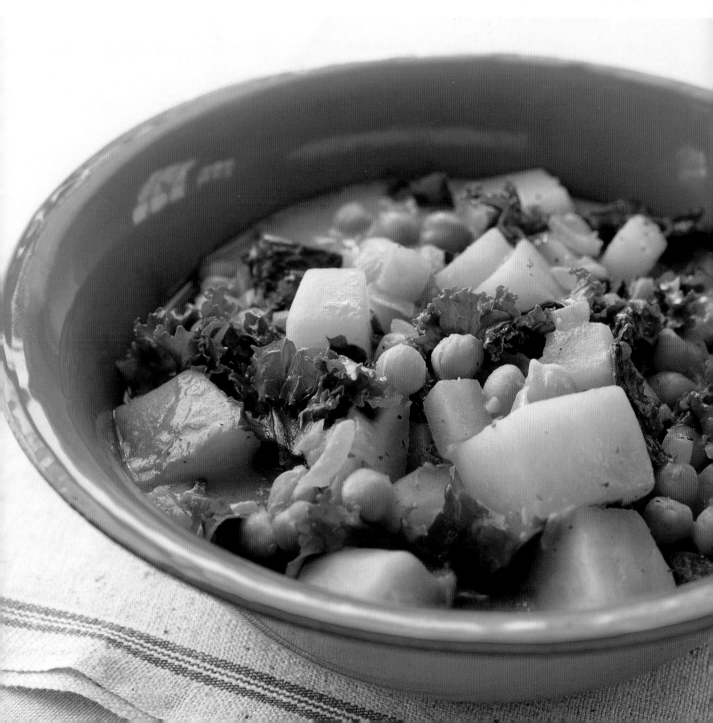

southwestern corn chowder *page 117*

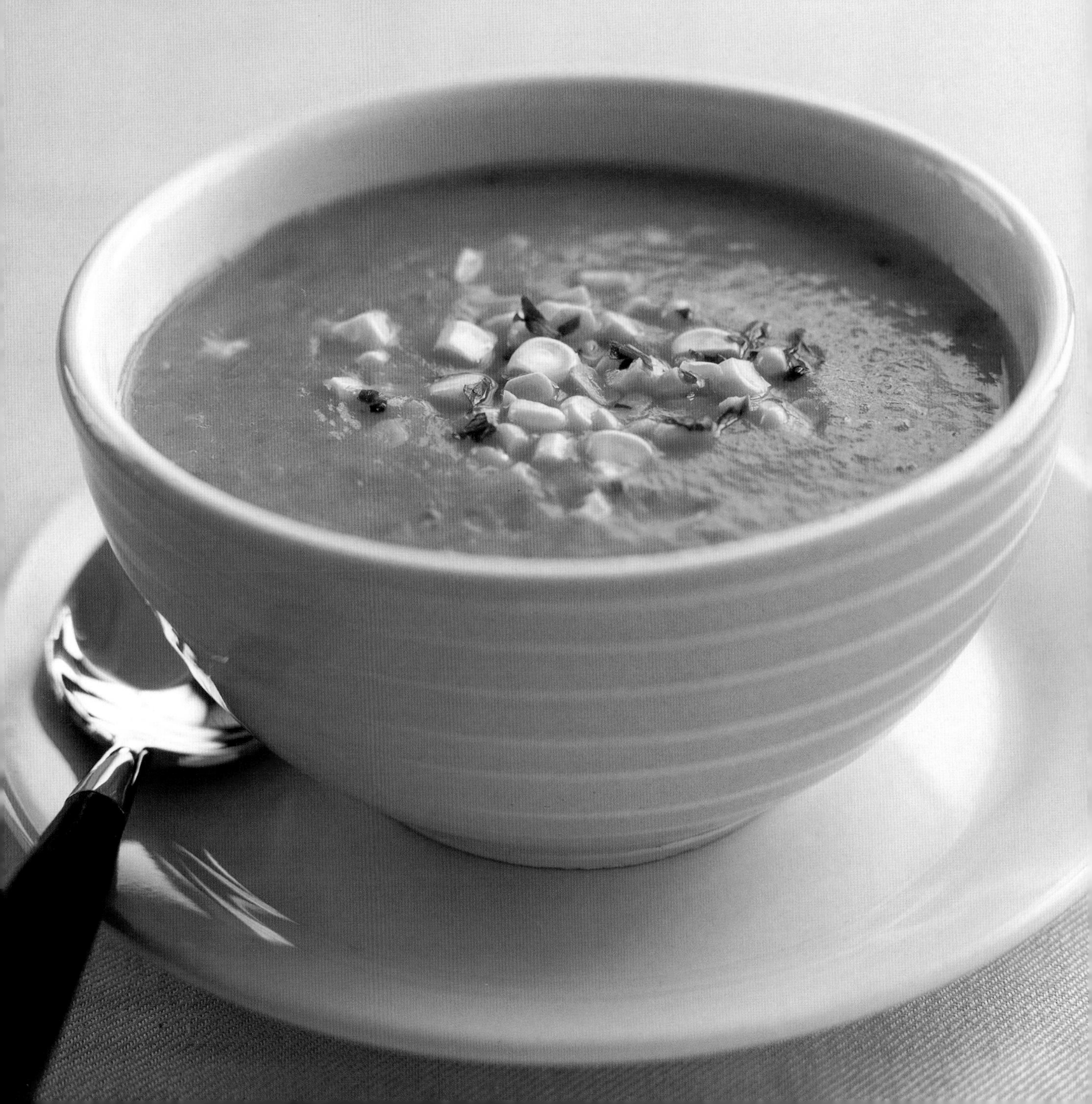

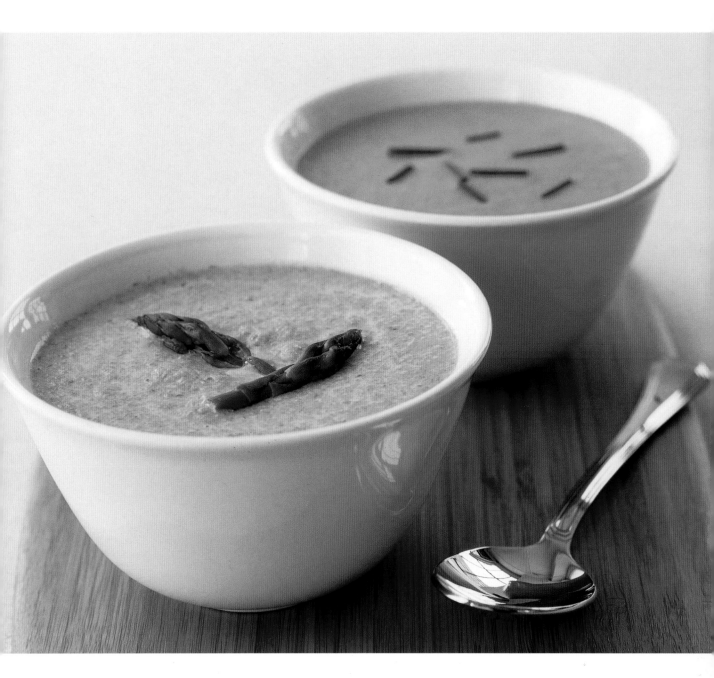

two soups: cream of asparagus (front)   *page 123*   carrot-ginger soup (back)   *page 131*

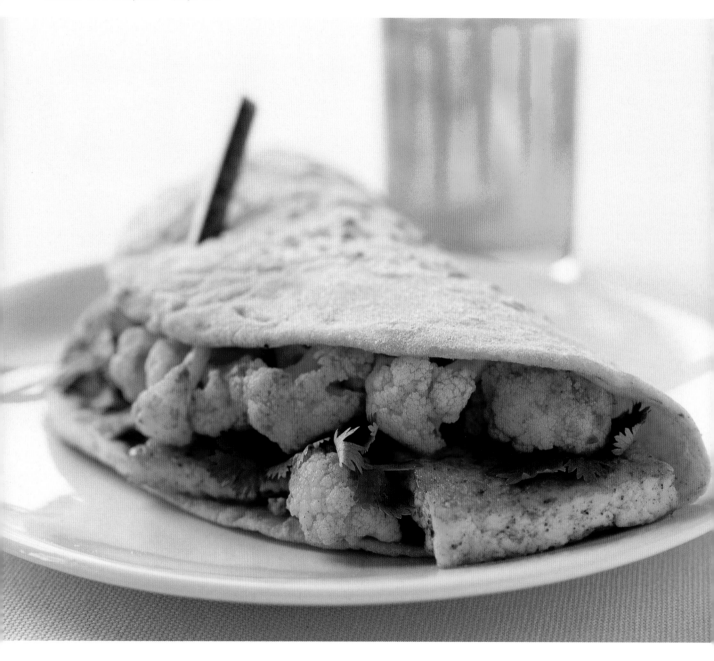

curried tofu chapatis   *page 156*

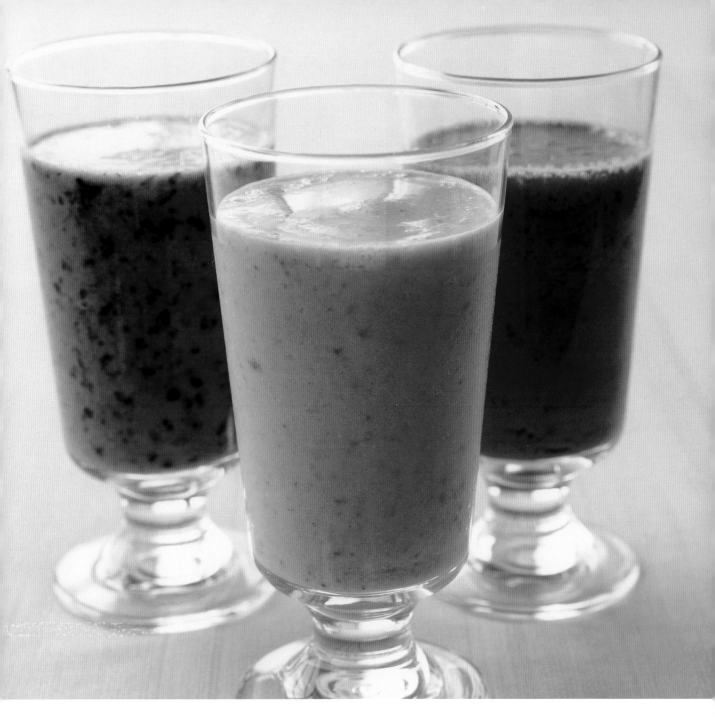

three smoothies: blueberry thrill (left)   *page 166*   strawberry fields (center)   *page 172*
and cherry citrus frost (right)   *page 176*

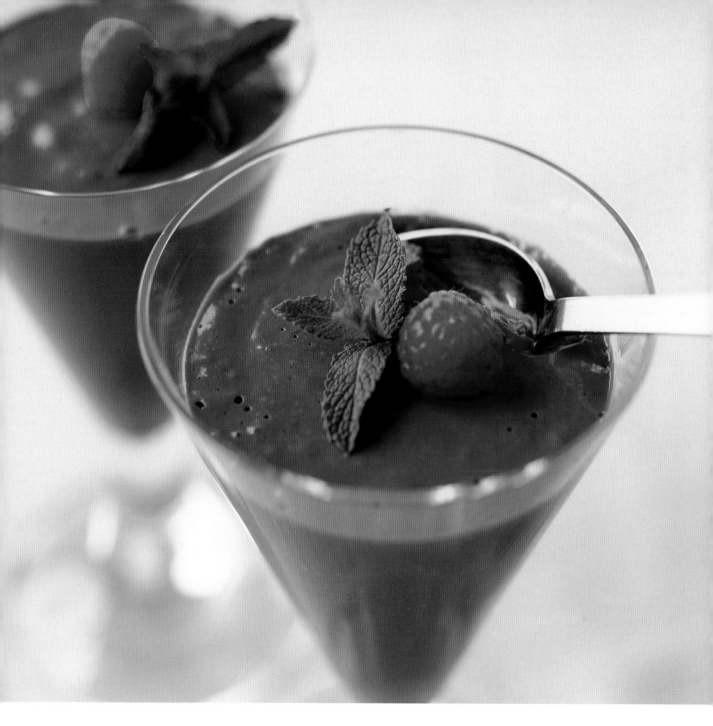

chocolate mousse *page 204*

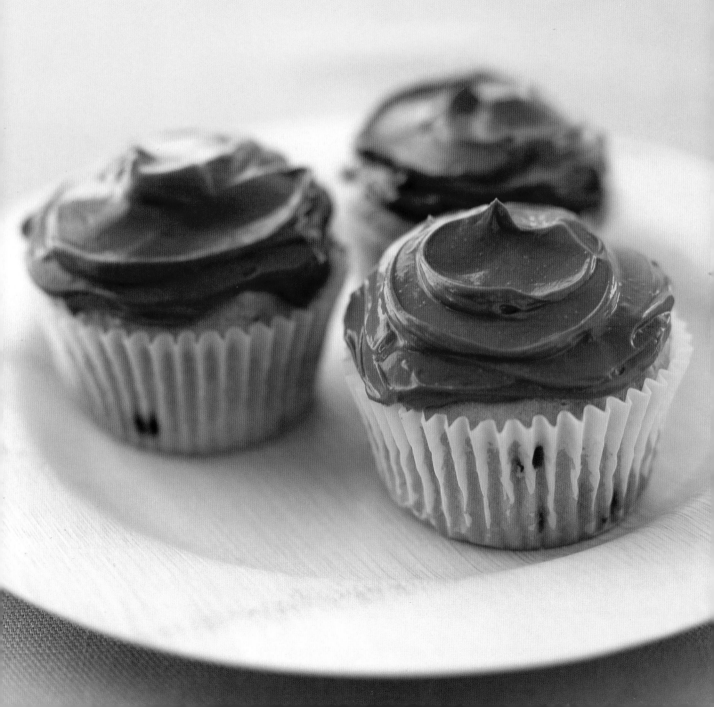
chocolate chip peanut butter cupcakes *page 202*

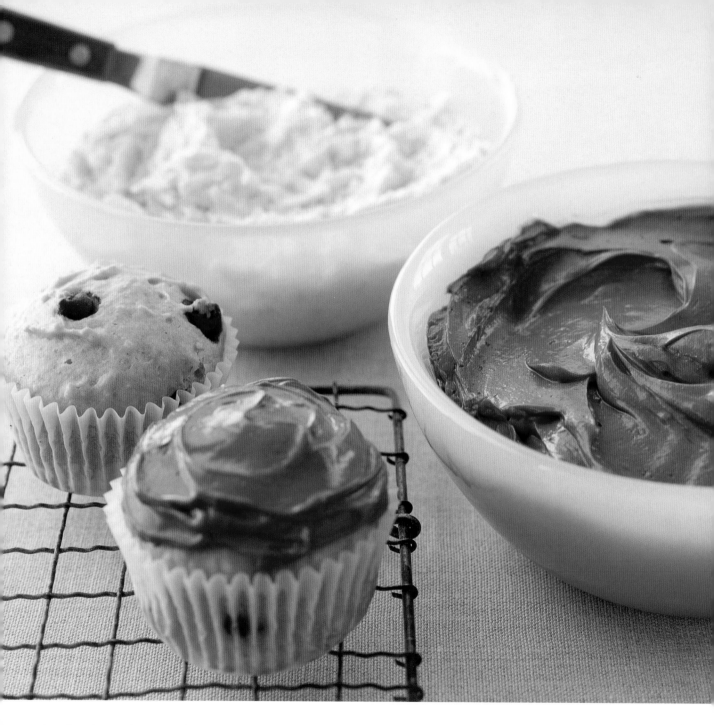

two frostings: chocolate frosting (right)   *page 205*   coconut frosting (left)   *page 206*

stuffed cabbage

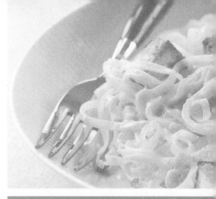

makes about 12 stuffed leaves

If you grew up with Stuffed Cabbage at Grandma's house or on the holiday table, then the smell of cooked cabbage basking in sweet and sour tomato sauce probably brings back fond memories. Here, tofu, vegetables, and brown rice replace the traditional filling of ground beef. Incidentally, Grandma's ground beef–stuffed cabbage contained about 47 milligrams of cholesterol per serving, while this version is of course cholesterol-free.

1 tablespoon olive oil

1 onion, chopped

2 medium carrots, chopped

1 zucchini, chopped

1 pound firm or extra-firm tofu, rinsed, patted dry, and crumbled

1 cup short- or long-grain brown rice

2 cups vegetable broth

2 (28-ounce) cans whole tomatoes

2 (6-ounce) cans tomato paste

1/4 cup sugar

1/4 cup apple cider vinegar

2 tablespoons grated orange zest

1 teaspoon salt

1 head of cabbage, frozen for at least one day, and defrosted (see Note)

(continues)

enticing entrées

61

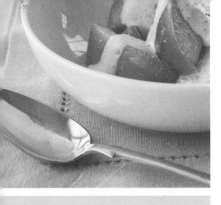

stuffed cabbage

(continued)

1 Heat the olive oil in a large skillet over medium-high heat. Add the onion and carrots and cook, stirring, until soft, about 7 minutes. Add the zucchini and tofu and cook, stirring, until there is no excess liquid in the skillet, 5 to 7 minutes. (Liquid might come out of the tofu as it cooks so make sure to keep cooking until it has all evaporated.) Add the rice and stir to coat. Add the vegetable broth and bring to a boil. Cover, reduce the heat, and simmer for 35 to 45 minutes or until all of the liquid is absorbed. Remove from the heat.

2 Meanwhile, combine the tomatoes, tomato paste, sugar, apple cider vinegar, orange zest, and salt in a large pot. Break apart the tomatoes with a wooden spoon. Bring to a boil, cover, reduce the heat, and simmer for 15 minutes. Remove from heat and set aside.

3 Meanwhile, preheat oven to 350°F.

4 Remove a leaf from the defrosted cabbage and lay it on a flat surface. Place $1/3$ cup of the filling in the center of the leaf. Fold the two sides over the filling. Fold the core end over the two sides and the filling. Roll it up the rest of the way and place it, seam-side down, in a large baking dish. Repeat with the remaining leaves. (There is enough filling for about 12 leaves.) Coarsely chop remaining cabbage and tuck it in the pan around the stuffed cabbage rolls.

5 Pour the tomato sauce over the cabbage rolls. Cover with foil and bake for $1^{1}/_{2}$ hours. Remove the cover and bake for 15 minutes more. Remove from the heat, cool for 15 minutes, and serve.

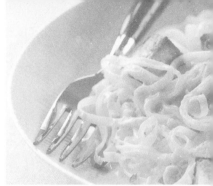

note Making stuffed cabbage is easy when you freeze the whole head of cabbage a few days in advance and let it defrost in the refrigerator the day before you prepare the dish. Once frozen and defrosted, cabbage leaves are soft, pliable, and easy to remove from the cabbage without tearing.

per stuffed cabbage leaf: 0mg cholesterol • 213 calories • 4g fat • 38g carbohydrate • 8g protein

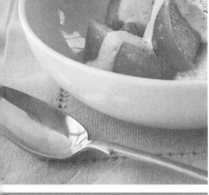

eggplant rollatini

The healthful version of this classic dish is easy yet elegant, using a tofu mixture as a stand-in for ricotta cheese.

1 pound firm or extra-firm tofu, rinsed and patted dry

1 (10-ounce) package defrosted chopped spinach, drained well

2 tablespoons eggless mayonnaise

1 tablespoon Italian seasoning

1 large eggplant, ends removed, sliced thinly lengthwise

Olive oil or olive oil spray

2 cups spaghetti sauce

1 Preheat broiler.

2 Put the tofu in a medium bowl and mash with a fork or potato masher. Stir in the spinach, eggless mayonnaise, and Italian seasoning. Set aside.

3 Mist a baking sheet with nonstick cooking oil spray. Lay the eggplant slices on top, and spray or drizzle them with olive oil. Place under the broiler for 3 to 5 minutes or until brown. Flip the eggplant, spray or drizzle with olive oil, and cook for another 3 to 5 minutes until brown, watching carefully to avoid burning. Remove from heat and let cool.

4 Reduce the oven temperature to 350°F. Spray an 8 × 8-inch baking dish or shallow casserole dish of a similar size with nonstick cooking oil spray and set aside.

tofu 1-2-3

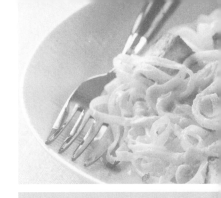

5 Top each slice of eggplant with a $1/4$-inch layer of the tofu mixture. Gently roll up the slices, starting with the large ends. Place the rolled eggplant slices in the prepared baking dish, seam-side down. The rolled eggplant slices should be nestled close to each other.

6 Pour the spaghetti sauce over the eggplant and bake for 35 minutes or until bubbly. Remove from heat and let cool for 5 minutes before serving.

per serving: 0mg cholesterol • 304 calories • 16g fat • 30g carbohydrate • 13g protein

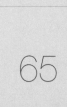

enticing entrées

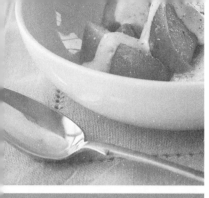

spicy peanut noodles

Sure, the sauce and noodles are great. But it's the manner in which the tofu is prepared that is most valuable to home chefs everywhere. After making this recipe, you may find yourself preparing the crispy tofu by itself and tossing it with nearly any kind of sauce under the sun.

4 tablespoons tamari or soy sauce

$1/2$ teaspoon ground ginger

1 pound firm or extra-firm tofu, rinsed, patted dry, and cut into $1/2$-inch cubes

$1/3$ cup natural peanut butter (crunchy)

3 tablespoons pure maple syrup

2 tablespoons rice vinegar

1 tablespoon water

1 tablespoon sesame seeds

1 garlic clove, minced

$1/2$–1 teaspoon chili paste

1 pound fettuccine, wide rice noodles, or other pasta

2 scallions, thinly sliced (both green and white parts)

1 Preheat broiler.

2 Stir together 1 tablespoon of the tamari and ginger in a medium bowl. Add the cubed tofu and stir gently to coat. Mist a baking sheet with nonstick cooking oil

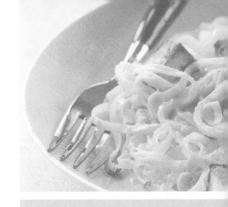

spray. Spread the tofu on the baking sheet in a single layer. Place under a broiler for 5 minutes. Flip the tofu and broil for 5 minutes or until light brown and crispy. Set aside.

3   In a medium bowl, whisk together the remaining 3 tablespoons tamari with the peanut butter, maple syrup, rice vinegar, water, sesame seeds, garlic, and chili paste and set aside.

4   Cook the noodles according to the package directions. Rinse and drain the noodles, transfer to a large bowl, and toss with the peanut sauce. Serve the noodles topped with the tofu cubes and scallions.

per serving: 0mg cholesterol • 401 calories • 11g fat • 59g carbohydrate • 17g protein

enticing entrées

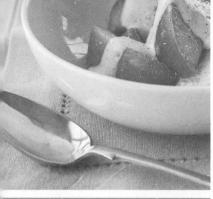

thai-style tofu
with butternut squash

If you've yet to experience butternut squash cooked in Thai sauce, then you're in for a real treat. Here, it is prepared with everyday spices, coconut milk, and of course tofu to form a visually dazzling and utterly scrumptious dish.

2 tablespoons peanut oil

6 scallions, chopped (both green and white parts)

2 garlic cloves, minced

1 tablespoon curry powder

1 teaspoon chili powder

1 teaspoon ground ginger

1 teaspoon sugar

3 tablespoons tamari or soy sauce

1 pound firm or extra-firm tofu, rinsed and cut into $1/2$-inch cubes

1 (15-ounce) can coconut milk

1 cup vegetable broth

1 butternut squash, peeled and cut into $3/4$-inch cubes

1 red bell pepper, cut into 1-inch squares

1 cup broccoli florets

$1/3$ cup chopped fresh basil

tofu 1-2-3

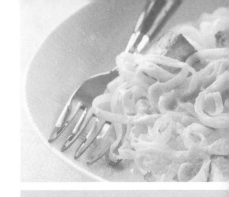

1   Heat the oil in a large, heavy-bottomed pot over medium-high heat. Add the scallions and garlic and cook, stirring, for 3 minutes. Stir in the curry powder, chili powder, ground ginger, and sugar. Add the tamari and stir. Add the tofu cubes, toss gently in the spice mixture to coat, and cook for 10 minutes, stirring occasionally. Stir in the coconut milk, broth, and squash. Bring to a boil, cover, reduce the heat, and simmer, stirring occasionally, for 15 minutes.

2   Add the red bell pepper and broccoli and continue to simmer, covered, until the vegetables are tender, 10 to 15 minutes. Add the basil and simmer for 3 minutes. Remove from the heat and serve.

per serving: 0mg cholesterol • 358 calories • 26g fat • 26g carbohydrate • 11g protein

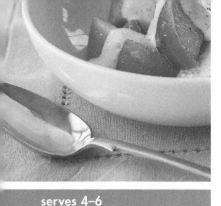

sweet and sour tofu

This is best served over brown rice and eaten with chopsticks for a complete sensory feast.

1 (20-ounce) can pineapple chunks packed in juice

1 tablespoon peanut oil or olive oil

7 ounces green beans, cut into 1-inch lengths (about $1^1/_2$ cups)

1 red bell pepper, cut into 1-inch strips

5 ounces mushrooms, sliced (about $1^1/_2$ cups)

1 teaspoon minced fresh ginger

1 pound firm or extra-firm tofu, rinsed, pressed, and cut into $^3/_4$-inch cubes
  (see page xiv)

1 cup vegetable broth

$^1/_3$ cup pure maple syrup

$^1/_3$ cup rice vinegar

3 tablespoons tamari or soy sauce

2 tablespoons arrowroot or cornstarch

1   Strain the pineapple chunks from their juice (reserving both) and set aside.

2   Heat the oil in a wok or large skillet over medium-high heat. Add the green beans and red bell pepper and cook, stirring, for 3 minutes. Add the mushrooms and ginger and cook, stirring, for 2 minutes. Add the tofu and cook, stirring, for 3 minutes.

tofu 1-2-3

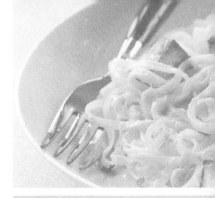

Add the drained pineapple chunks, $1/2$ cup of the pineapple juice, $1/2$ cup of the vegetable broth, the pure maple syrup, rice vinegar, and tamari. Bring to a boil.

3 In a small bowl, mix the arrowroot into remaining $1/2$ cup of vegetable broth and add to the boiling mixture. Reduce the heat and simmer for 1 to 2 minutes, stirring constantly, until the sauce has thickened. Season to taste and serve.

per serving: 0mg cholesterol • 288 calories • 8g fat • 47g carbohydrate • 11g protein

enticing entrées

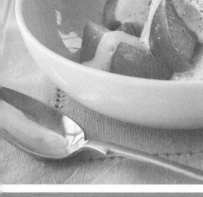

szechuan tofu

Hot, spicy sauce and crisp-tender broccoli join tofu in this all-time favorite stir-fry.

1 tablespoon peanut oil or vegetable oil

1 onion, cut into chunks

1 green bell pepper, cut into 2-inch strips

1 red bell pepper, cut into 2-inch strips

1 cup broccoli florets cut into bite-size pieces

3 tablespoons sherry cooking wine

3 tablespoons toasted sesame oil

$^3/_4$ teaspoon–2 tablespoons hot sauce, depending on desired spiciness

2 tablespoons pure maple syrup

2 teaspoons minced fresh ginger or 1 teaspoon ground

$^1/_4$ teaspoon cayenne pepper

$^1/_4$ teaspoon red pepper flakes

1 pound firm or extra-firm tofu, rinsed, patted dry, and cut into $^3/_4$-inch cubes

$1^1/_2$ tablespoons water

2 teaspoons arrowroot or cornstarch

1 tablespoon sesame seeds

3 cups hot, cooked rice

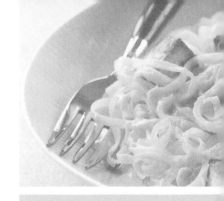

1 Heat the oil in a wok or large nonstick skillet over medium-high heat. Add the onion and cook, stirring, for 2 minutes. Add the bell peppers and broccoli and cook, stirring, for 5 minutes more.

2 In a small bowl, whisk together the sherry, sesame oil, hot sauce, maple syrup, ginger, cayenne, and red pepper flakes. Pour over the cooked vegetables and stir to coat. Gently fold in the tofu cubes and simmer for 5 minutes.

3 In a small bowl, mix together the water and arrowroot and stir into the tofu and vegetables. Simmer for 2 minutes, stirring constantly, until the mixture thickens and becomes bubbly. Stir in the sesame seeds. Remove from the heat and serve over the hot rice.

per serving: 0mg cholesterol • 399 calories • 11g fat • 63g carbohydrate • 10g protein

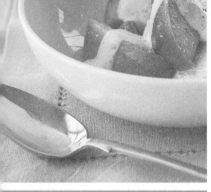

glazed apricot stir-fry

Pretty colors and delicate sweetness highlight this Chinese-style dish.

1 tablespoon peanut oil or vegetable oil

1 onion, cut into wedges

1 red bell pepper, cut into 2-inch strips

4 ounces pea pods, cut on the diagonal (about 1 cup)

$^1/_2$ cup apricot fruit spread

$^1/_2$ teaspoon onion granules

2 tablespoons vegetable oil

2 teaspoons fresh ginger or 1 teaspoon ground

1 teaspoon tamari or soy sauce

1 pound firm or extra-firm tofu, rinsed, patted dry, and cut into $^3/_4$-inch cubes

2 tablespoons apple juice

2 teaspoons arrowroot or cornstarch

3 cups hot, cooked rice

1   Heat the oil in a wok or large nonstick skillet over medium-high heat. Add the onion and cook, stirring, for 3 minutes. Add the red bell pepper and cook, stirring, for 2 minutes. Add the pea pods and cook, stirring, for 2 minutes.

74

tofu 1-2-3

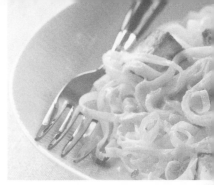

2   In a medium bowl, combine the fruit spread, onion granules, vegetable oil, ginger, and tamari. Add to the vegetables and stir to coat. Gently fold in the tofu cubes and simmer for 5 minutes.

3   In a small bowl, mix together the apple juice and arrowroot. Pour over the tofu/vegetables and simmer for 2 minutes, stirring constantly until bubbly and thickened. Remove from the heat and serve over the hot rice.

per serving: 0mg cholesterol • 471 calories • 11g fat • 82g carbohydrate • 12g protein

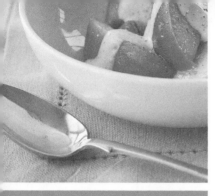

vegetable fried rice

Fried rice often takes on the role of side dish. But here, tofu, vegetables, and brown rice make this Chinese dish stand front and center as the main event.

2 cups water

1 cup uncooked brown rice

2 tablespoons peanut oil, olive oil, or vegetable oil

1 pound firm or extra-firm tofu, rinsed, patted dry, and cut into tiny $1/8$-inch cubes

2 garlic cloves, minced

1 teaspoon minced ginger

1 red bell pepper, chopped

4 ounces snow peas, trimmed and halved diagonally (about 1 cup)

3 ounces white mushrooms, thinly sliced (about 1 cup)

3 scallions, chopped (both green and white parts)

2 tablespoons tamari or soy sauce

$1/2$–1 tablespoon pure maple syrup

1 teaspoon toasted sesame oil

1 Add the water to a heavy-bottomed pot and bring to a boil. Stir in the rice and return to a boil. Cover, reduce the heat, and simmer until the rice is tender, 30 to 40 minutes. Remove from the heat.

tofu 1-2-3

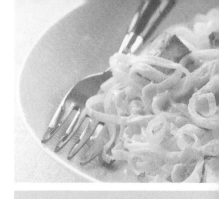

2   Meanwhile, heat 1 tablespoon of the peanut oil in a wok or large, nonstick skillet over medium-high heat. Add the tofu and cook, stirring frequently, until the tofu is very dry, 6 to 8 minutes. Drain off any excess water that the tofu may release while cooking. Remove the tofu from the wok and set aside.

3   Heat the remaining tablespoon of peanut oil in the wok. Add the garlic and ginger, stir for a minute, then add the red bell pepper, snow peas, and mushrooms, and cook, stirring, until the vegetables are crisp-tender, about 5 minutes.

4   Add the cooked rice, scallions, tamari, maple syrup, sesame oil, and reserved tofu. Stir gently but thoroughly and cook until heated through. Serve immediately.

per serving: 0mg cholesterol • 296 calories • 11g fat • 37g carbohydrate • 12g protein

enticing entrées

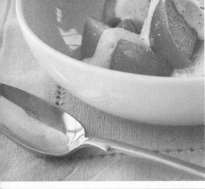

thai rice noodles
with tofu and mixed vegetables

It doesn't take a lot of work to create restaurant-quality flavor with just three ingredients—coconut milk, rice noodles, and curry paste—all conveniently available in most large grocery stores.

1 (13.5-ounce) can coconut milk

1 cup vegetable broth

2 teaspoons–1 tablespoon curry paste

1 (6-ounce) can bamboo shoots, drained

1 zucchini, cut into 1¹/₂-inch strips

1 red bell pepper, cut into 1¹/₂-inch strips

6 ounces Thai rice noodles

1 pound firm or extra-firm tofu, rinsed, pressed, and cut into ¹/₂-inch cubes
(see page xiv)

Handful fresh basil, chopped

1 In a large saucepan, mix together the coconut milk, vegetable broth, and curry paste and bring to a boil. Add the bamboo shoots, zucchini, red bell pepper, and rice noodles. Return to a boil, reduce the heat, and simmer, stirring occasionally, for 8 minutes.

2 Stir in the tofu and basil and simmer for 5 minutes or until vegetables and noodles are tender. Remove from the heat and serve.

per serving: 0mg cholesterol • 337 calories • 19g fat • 32g carbohydrate • 13g protein

tofu 1-2-3

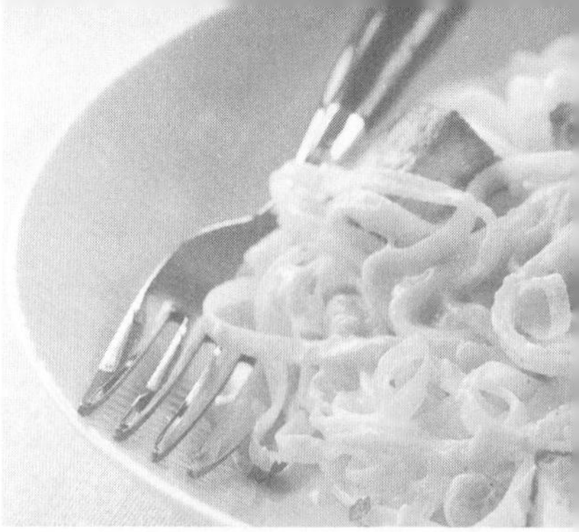

creste di galli in butternut crème

Creste di galli is a short, tubular pasta with a ruffle along the length of the outside curve. Here, it is tossed with a dairy-free butternut "cheese" sauce containing nutritional yeast flakes, an ingredient that imparts a cheesy flavor for creamy, cholesterol-free dishes. Any small shape pasta can be used in place of the creste di galli.

1 medium butternut squash, peeled and cut into 2-inch cubes (discard the seeds)

$1/2$ cup silken tofu

$1/4$ cup light miso

$1/4$ cup nutritional yeast flakes

3 tablespoons hot water

1 tablespoon tamari or soy sauce

1–2 teaspoons Dijon mustard

1 pound creste di galli or other shape pasta, cooked according to the package directions

1 Put 1 to 2 inches of water in a large saucepan with a steamer basket and bring to a gentle boil. Place the butternut squash in the steamer basket, cover, and steam until the squash is tender, about 12 minutes.

2 Put the steamed squash into a food processor with the tofu, miso, nutritional yeast flakes, hot water, tamari, and mustard. Blend until smooth and creamy. Season to taste, pour over the hot, cooked pasta, and toss to coat. Serve immediately.

per serving: 0mg cholesterol • 393 calories • 3g fat • 74g carbohydrate • 18g protein

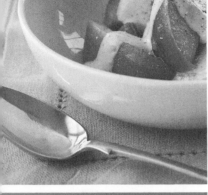

orange-scented campanelle
with plum tomatoes and zucchini

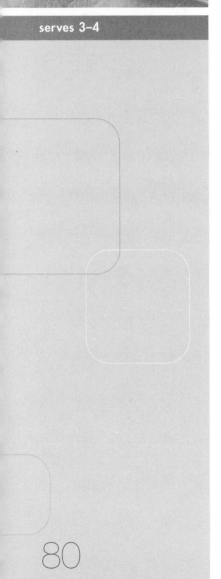

Orange plays an important yet subtle role in the fantastic flavors of this scrumptious dish.

1 tablespoon olive oil

5 plum tomatoes, chopped

1 medium zucchini, chopped (about 1 cup)

3 garlic cloves

1½ teaspoons Italian seasoning

¼ teaspoon salt

⅛ teaspoon freshly ground black pepper

1 (8-ounce) package frozen green beans, defrosted and cut into bite-size lengths

½ cup orange juice

½ pound firm or extra-firm tofu, rinsed, pressed, and cut into ½-inch dice
(see page xiv)

1 tablespoon balsamic vinegar

2–3 teaspoons grated orange zest

1 teaspoon pure maple syrup

6 ounces campanelle, radiatore, or other shape pasta, cooked according to package
directions

1 Heat the olive oil in a large, heavy-bottomed pot or skillet over medium-high heat.
Add the plum tomatoes, zucchini, garlic, Italian seasoning, salt, and pepper.
Bring to a simmer, cover, and cook, stirring occasionally, for about 10 minutes.

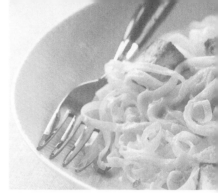

2 Stir in the green beans, orange juice, tofu, balsamic vinegar, orange zest, and maple syrup and bring to a boil. Cover, reduce the heat, and simmer for 20 minutes, stirring in the cooked pasta during the last 5 minutes. Remove from the heat, adjust the seasonings to taste, and serve.

per serving: 0mg cholesterol • 303 calories • 7g fat • 49g carbohydrate • 12g protein

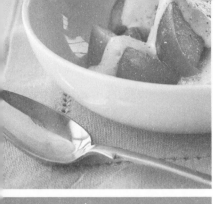

fettuccine with sun-dried tomato crème

Perhaps the simplest way to transform silken tofu into outstanding pasta sauce is to blend it with sun-dried tomatoes. Serve with roasted asparagus spears and a green salad for a simple yet elegant meal.

1 (6.5-ounce) jar sun-dried tomatoes packed in oil (see Note)

1 (12-ounce) package soft silken tofu (1$\frac{1}{2}$ cups)

1 tablespoon water

2 teaspoons freshly squeezed lemon juice

1 teaspoon dried basil

$\frac{3}{4}$ teaspoon salt

$\frac{1}{8}$ teaspoon freshly ground black pepper

1 pound fettuccine, cooked according to the package directions

1 Strain the sun-dried tomatoes, reserving both oil and tomatoes. Put the tomatoes and 1 tablespoon of the reserved oil in a food processor with the tofu, water, lemon juice, basil, salt, and pepper. Blend for 1 to 2 minutes, stopping at least once to scrape down the sides. Set the mixture aside and store the remaining oil for future use.

2 Transfer the hot, cooked fettuccine to a large mixing bowl. Pour the sauce over the pasta and stir to coat. Serve immediately.

note Make sure that your oil-packed sun-dried tomatoes do not contain vinegar. Fortunately, most brands do not. However, it is important to check the label because vinegar will ruin the recipe.

per serving: 0mg cholesterol • 385 calories • 7g fat • 64g carbohydrate • 15g protein

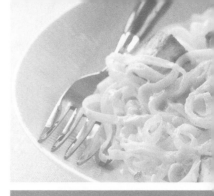

chef rory macaroni

Named for my son Rory, this trio of pasta, tomato sauce, and dairy-free cheese sauce tastes similar to (but a lot better than!) canned "O-shaped" spaghetti that many children find appealing. Use fun pasta shapes like wagon wheels, letters, or numbers when treating the little ones in your life. By the way, if you've never used nutritional yeast flakes before, you will be pleased with the cheesy flavor they impart—not to mention the fact that they're loaded with B vitamins.

1¹/₂ cups tomato sauce

1 pound pasta (elbows, spirals, or wagon wheels), cooked according to the package directions and returned to the empty pot

1 (12-ounce) package soft silken tofu (1¹/₂ cups)

5 tablespoons nutritional yeast flakes

2 tablespoons sweet white miso

4 teaspoons freshly squeezed lemon juice

¹/₂ teaspoon salt

¹/₄ teaspoon onion granules

1 Add the tomato sauce to the pot with the hot, cooked pasta, stir well, and heat gently to keep warm.

2 In a blender, combine the tofu, nutritional yeast flakes, miso, lemon juice, salt, and onion granules and process until smooth. Pour over the pasta and stir well to coat. Heat gently to the desired temperature and serve.

per serving: 0mg cholesterol • 346 calories • 3g fat • 64g carbohydrate • 14g protein

enticing entrées

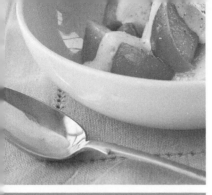

farfalle with mixed sautéed mushrooms and white wine stroganoff

Shiitake and oyster mushrooms lend exotic taste and texture to this light brown, creamy sauce—a perfect match for farfalle (a.k.a. bow-tie) pasta.

1 pound farfalle, cooked according to the package directions

1$\frac{1}{3}$ cups vegetable broth

$\frac{2}{3}$ cup soft silken tofu

5 tablespoons white wine or sherry

1 tablespoon tamari or soy sauce

2 teaspoons nutritional yeast flakes (optional)

$\frac{1}{2}$ teaspoon paprika

$\frac{1}{2}$ teaspoon salt

$\frac{1}{4}$ teaspoon garlic granules

$\frac{1}{4}$ teaspoon freshly ground black pepper

1 tablespoon olive oil

2 pounds assorted mushrooms, cleaned and sliced (about 4 cups)

Grated dairy-free Parmesan cheese (optional)

1   While the pasta is cooking, put the broth in a blender with the tofu, 4 tablespoons of the wine or sherry, the tamari, nutritional yeast flakes (if using), paprika, salt, garlic granules, and pepper. Process until smooth and set aside.

84   tofu 1-2-3

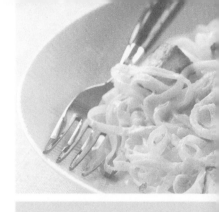

2 Heat the oil in a large skillet over medium-high heat. Add the mushrooms and cook, stirring, for 5 minutes. Stir in the remaining tablespoon of white wine or sherry and cook, stirring, for 3 minutes more.

3 Stir the tofu sauce into the mushrooms and bring to a boil. Cover, reduce the heat, and simmer, stirring occasionally, for 5 minutes. Season to taste with salt, pepper, white wine or sherry, and Parmesan cheese, if using. Serve over the hot, cooked farfalle.

per serving: 0mg cholesterol • 403 calories • 5g fat • 70g carbohydrate • 16g protein

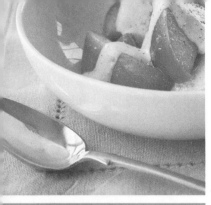

family favorite shells with tomato sauce and cottage cheese

I have sampled this dairy-free dish out to hundreds of people at food events and can attest to the fact that everybody loves it, every time. (And it's an especially good way to serve tofu to kids.)

1½ cups tomato sauce

1 pound small shell pasta, cooked according to the package directions and returned to the empty pot

1 pound firm tofu

⅓ cup eggless mayonnaise

1 tablespoon Italian seasoning (optional)

1   Add the tomato sauce to the hot, cooked pasta, stir well, and heat gently to keep warm.

2   Put the tofu in a large bowl and mash with a fork or potato masher. Stir in the eggless mayonnaise and Italian seasoning, if using. Add the tofu mixture to the pasta. Heat gently to the desired temperature, season to taste, and serve.

per serving: 0mg cholesterol • 348 calories • 7g fat • 63g carbohydrate • 16g protein

pesto fusilli
with sun-dried tomatoes

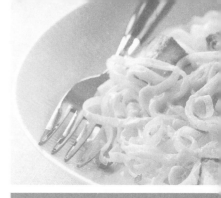

Fusilli is a pasta that looks like twisted spaghetti and is excellent coated with pesto. Here, the addition of sun-dried tomatoes adds a burst of flavor to the classic mixture, and tofu makes it even creamier. If you can't find fusilli, rigatoni works equally well.

1 cup chopped or whole sun-dried tomatoes packed in oil (see Note)

$1/2$ cup pine nuts

$1/3$ cup packed fresh basil

$1/2$ cup silken tofu, crumbled

1 pound fusilli, cooked according to package directions

$1/4$ cup sliced kalamata olives (optional)

1. Strain the sun-dried tomatoes, reserving both the tomatoes and the oil. If necessary, add extra olive oil to the liquid to make $1/4$ cup of oil. If the tomatoes are whole, cut them in half.

2. Combine the pine nuts and basil in a food processor and blend until combined. Add the reserved $1/4$ cup of oil and blend until it forms a paste. Add the silken tofu and blend.

3. Toss the cooked pasta with the pesto and gently stir in the reserved sun-dried tomatoes. Garnish with olives if using.

note Make sure that your oil-packed sun-dried tomatoes do not contain vinegar. Fortunately, most brands do not. However, it is important to check the label because vinegar will ruin the recipe.

per serving: 0mg cholesterol • 385 calories • 9g fat • 62g carbohydrate • 14g protein

enticing entrées

87

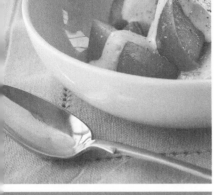

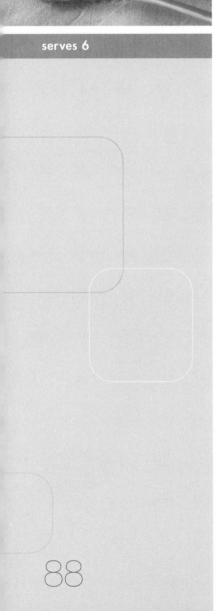

cannellini beans and roasted potatoes in cashew cream sauce

For comfort food with sophistication, this creamy mixture of potatoes and white beans delivers. Serve with a green vegetable, or better yet, two!

3 medium potatoes, peeled and cut into $1/2$-inch cubes

1 tablespoon olive oil

$1/4$ teaspoon salt

$1/8$ teaspoon freshly ground black pepper

1 (15.5-ounce) can cannellini beans, rinsed and drained

$1/4$ cup water

$1/3$ cup raw, unsalted cashews

$1/3$ cup soft silken tofu

$1/4$ cup nutritional yeast flakes

1 tablespoon light miso

1 teaspoon onion granules

1 teaspoon freshly squeezed lemon juice

1 tablespoon chopped fresh parsley

1 Preheat oven to 400°F.

2 Put the potatoes in a medium bowl. Add the olive oil, salt, and pepper; stir to coat. Mist a baking sheet with nonstick cooking oil spray. Arrange the potatoes on the baking sheet in a single layer and roast for 25 minutes or until golden-

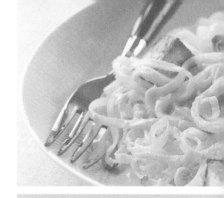

brown on the outside and soft on the inside. Remove from heat and transfer to a large mixing bowl. Stir in beans and set aside.

3 In a blender, combine the water, cashews, tofu, nutritional yeast flakes, miso, onion granules, and lemon juice and process until completely smooth. Transfer to a medium saucepan and heat gently over low heat for several minutes or until warm, stirring constantly. Pour over potato/bean mixture, add the parsley, and stir gently to coat. Serve immediately.

variations

- Use red potatoes instead of white, scrub instead of peeling them, and cut them into bite-size chunks. Add 1 tablespoon fresh rosemary (or 1 teaspoon dried) with the olive oil, salt, and pepper before roasting.

- Sauté or steam a chopped bunch of kale, dandelion greens, or other greens, and add it to the potato/bean mixture.

per serving: 0mg cholesterol • 386 calories • 7g fat • 58g carbohydrate • 25g protein

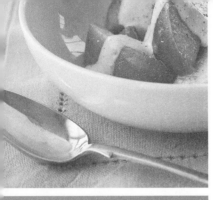

mediterranean tofu
with fresh basil and pine nuts

Israeli couscous is delightfully round and chewy and much larger than regular couscous. Here, it's topped with a flavorful medley of Mediterranean staples.

2 cups water or vegetable broth

1 cup Israeli couscous

1 (6.5-ounce) jar chopped sun-dried tomatoes in olive oil (about $^1/_2$ cup) (see Notes)

1 onion, chopped

2 garlic cloves, minced

1 pound soft, firm, or extra-firm tofu, rinsed, patted dry, and cut into $^1/_2$-inch cubes

$^1/_2$ cup (packed) chopped fresh basil

$^1/_4$ cup sliced kalamata olives

2 tablespoons pine nuts

1 Put the water or vegetable broth in a medium saucepan and bring to a boil. Stir in the couscous, cover, reduce the heat to low, and simmer until the liquid is absorbed, 8 to 10 minutes. Remove from the heat and set aside. (See Notes.)

2 Strain the sun-dried tomatoes, reserving both the tomatoes and the oil.

3 Put 1 tablespoon of the reserved oil in a large, nonstick skillet and heat over medium-high heat. Add the onion and garlic and cook, stirring, until softened, about 7 minutes. Add the tofu and cook, stirring, for 5 minutes. Add the basil, olives, and reserved tomatoes and cook, stirring, for 2 minutes, adding a tablespoon of water, vegetable broth, or reserved oil if the mixture gets dry.

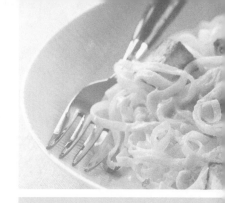

4 Transfer the couscous to a large serving platter or individual dishes. Top with the tofu and vegetable mixture, and sprinkle with pine nuts. Serve immediately. (The remaining oil from the tomatoes can be refrigerated in its jar for future use.)

note Make sure that your oil-packed sun-dried tomatoes do not contain vinegar. Fortunately, most brands do not. However, it is important to check the label because vinegar will ruin the recipe.

note Like other pasta, Israeli couscous starts to stick together after being cooked if it sits in the pot for too long. To prevent this from happening, remove the cover and fluff it up with a fork. Ideally, prepare the vegetables and tofu while the Israeli couscous is cooking so they are both done about the same time.

per serving: 0mg cholesterol • 279 calories • 10g fat • 38g carbohydrate • 13g protein

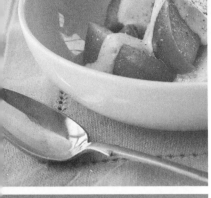

ilyse's crispy cutlets
with creamy dijon sauce

My sister Ilyse whips up these breaded and baked tofu cutlets for impromptu gatherings and it's no wonder why—everyone loves them, and most of the ingredients are typical kitchen standards.

¹/₃ cup tamari or soy sauce

1 tablespoon apricot fruit spread

1 tablespoon water

1 teaspoon freshly squeezed lemon juice

1 teaspoon vegetarian Worcestershire sauce

¹/₄ teaspoon garlic granules

¹/₄ teaspoon onion granules

¹/₄ teaspoon ground ginger

1¹/₃ cups bread crumbs

1 tablespoon nutritional yeast flakes (optional)

1 pound firm or extra-firm tofu, rinsed and patted dry

Creamy Dijon Sauce (recipe follows), for serving

1 Preheat oven to 400°F. Mist a baking sheet with nonstick cooking oil spray; set aside.

2 In a medium bowl, whisk together the tamari, apricot fruit spread, water, lemon juice, Worcestershire sauce, garlic granules, onion granules, and ginger and set aside.

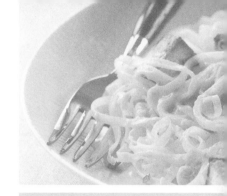

3 Combine the bread crumbs and nutritional yeast flakes (if using) in a shallow baking dish and stir with a wire whisk; set aside.

4 Slice the tofu widthwise into 10 rectangles, each about $1/3$ inch thick. Dip each piece in the marinade and gently dredge in the bread crumbs. Arrange the cutlets on the baking sheet and bake for 20 minutes or until the tops are brown and crispy. Flip the cutlets and bake for 5 minutes or until the tops are brown and crispy.

5 Remove the tofu from the oven, transfer to a serving dish, and serve with a dollop of Creamy Dijon Sauce.

per serving: 0mg cholesterol • 270 calories • 8g fat • 34g carbohydrate • 17g protein

creamy dijon sauce

makes about 1$1/3$ cups

1 cup eggless mayonnaise

2–3 tablespoons Dijon mustard

2 tablespoons relish

Put all the ingredients in a small bowl and mix.

per tablespoon: 0mg cholesterol, 27 calories, 2g fat, 1g carbohydrate, 1g protein

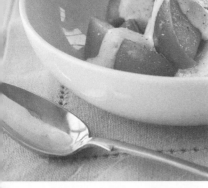

tofu burritos

Keep a container of firm or extra-firm tofu in the freezer just in case you spontaneously decide to whip up this easy dinner, sure to become a favorite. Top with guacamole and serve with brown rice for a satisfying and flavorful Mexican meal.

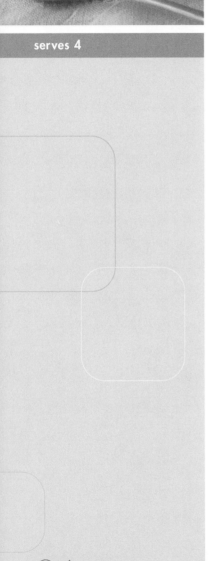

2 tablespoons chili powder

1 teaspoon ground cumin

1 teaspoon paprika

1 teaspoon dried oregano

1 teaspoon salt

1 teaspoon sugar

1 pound firm or extra-firm frozen tofu, defrosted and pressed (see page xv)

1 tablespoon olive oil

1 onion, chopped

1 green bell pepper, chopped

2 garlic cloves

1 tomato, chopped

1 cup fresh or frozen (defrosted) corn

1 tablespoon nutritional yeast flakes (optional)

4 flour tortillas

Sliced avocado, black olives, and/or jalapeño peppers (optional)

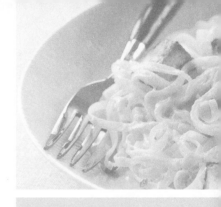

1 In a medium bowl, place the chili powder, cumin, paprika, oregano, salt, and sugar and stir to combine. Crumble the tofu into bite-size chunks and add them to the spice mixture. Stir well until the tofu is completely coated with the spice. Set aside.

2 Heat the olive oil in a large nonstick skillet over medium-high heat. Add the onion, green bell pepper, and garlic and cook, stirring, until softened, 7 to 10 minutes. Add the seasoned tofu and cook, stirring, for 1 minute. Add the tomato and corn and cook, stirring, for 1 minute. Remove from the heat and stir in the nutritional yeast flakes, if using.

3 Wrap the stack of tortilla shells in a clean, damp dishtowel and microwave on high for 30 seconds or until warm and soft. Lay the tortillas on a flat surface and evenly divide the filling onto the middle of each, making rectangular mounds. Top with slices of avocado, olives, and/or jalapeño peppers, if using. Grasp the two ends that are closest to the filling, and fold them over the filling. Fold the bottom end over the filling (and over the two sides), and continue to roll all the way up. Place the burritos seam-side down on plates and serve immediately.

note For a fun and festive burrito party, present the burrito filling in a bowl next to a stack of warm tortilla shells. Arrange little bowls of extras such as guacamole or sliced avocado, chopped onions, shredded lettuce, chopped tomato, dairy-free sour cream, and sliced jalapeño peppers. Invite your guests to choose their fillings and "roll their own!"

per serving: 0mg cholesterol • 313 calories • 13g fat • 38g carbohydrate • 16g protein

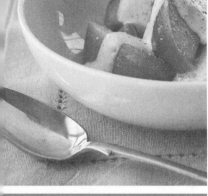

pan-fried tofu filets
with crimini mushroom sauce

Sometimes, even the most basic of ingredients can be brought together for a memorable and satisfying entrée. Here, tofu is pan-fried with salt, pepper, garlic powder, and a splash of white wine, and blanketed with a rich, brown mushroom sauce that you and your family will find irresistible.

1 pound extra-firm tofu, rinsed and pressed

2 tablespoons olive oil

Salt and freshly ground black pepper, to taste

Garlic powder, to taste

3 tablespoons white wine or sherry

6 ounces crimini mushrooms (baby bellas) or white mushrooms, sliced (about 2 cups)

1 tablespoon whole wheat flour

1 cup vegetable broth

1 Slice the tofu widthwise into thin rectangles about $1/4$ inch thick.

2 Heat the olive oil in a large, nonstick skillet over medium-high heat. Add the tofu slices and sprinkle with pinches of salt, pepper, and garlic powder. Cook until the undersides of the tofu are golden, 3 to 5 minutes. Carefully flip the tofu and sprinkle with more salt, pepper, and garlic powder. Drizzle with 1 tablespoon of the white wine and cook for 3 to 4 minutes. When both sides of the tofu are golden brown, transfer the tofu to a serving dish and cover to keep warm. Leave the skillet on the heat and do not wash it out.

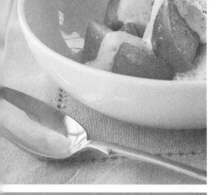

vegetable flecked arborio rice

Most of the ingredients used in this deliciously creamy rice dish are pantry standards, making it a particularly convenient dinner item.

1 tablespoon olive oil

1 red onion, coarsely chopped

3 garlic cloves, minced

1 red bell pepper, chopped

1 teaspoon dried marjoram

1 teaspoon dried basil

$^1/_2$ teaspoon dried thyme

$^1/_4$ teaspoon freshly ground black pepper

1 (16-ounce) bag frozen mixed vegetables, defrosted

1 (14.5-ounce) can diced tomatoes

$3^1/_2$ cups vegetable broth

1 cup Arborio rice

$^1/_2$ cup silken tofu

2 tablespoons dry white wine

3 tablespoons dairy-free Parmesan cheese

Salt, to taste

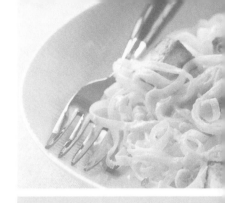

1   Heat the oil in a large, heavy-bottomed pot over medium-high heat. Add the onion and garlic and cook, stirring, for 3 minutes. Add the red bell pepper, marjoram, basil, thyme, and pepper and cook, stirring, until the red bell pepper begins to soften, about 3 minutes. Add the mixed vegetables, diced tomatoes, 3 cups of the vegetable broth, and the rice. Stir and bring to a boil. Cover, reduce the heat, and simmer for 15 to 20 minutes or until the rice is tender.

2   Combine the silken tofu, white wine, and remaining $1/2$ cup vegetable broth in a blender and process until smooth. Stir into the cooked rice mixture along with the Parmesan cheese and salt. Cover and cook for 5 minutes. Remove from the heat and let sit, covered, for 10 minutes before serving.

per serving: 0mg cholesterol • 307 calories • 6g fat • 52g carbohydrate • 10g protein

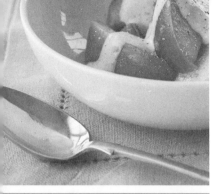

barbecued tofu
with oven-roasted potatoes

Potatoes, onions, and peppers bring garden-variety freshness to this downright succulent dish flavored with your favorite barbecue sauce. I prefer smoky sauces, but if you gravitate towards the sweeter varieties, you will be equally pleased with the results.

3 medium baking potatoes, peeled and cut into bite-size chunks

$1/4$ teaspoon salt

$1/8$ teaspoon freshly ground black pepper

2 tablespoons olive oil

1 large onion, cut into large wedges

1 green bell pepper, cut into 1-inch squares

2 garlic cloves, minced

1 pound frozen extra-firm tofu, defrosted, pressed, and crumbled into bite-size pieces (see page xv)

1 jar barbecue sauce (about 15 ounces)

1 Preheat oven to 400°F. Mist a baking sheet with nonstick cooking oil spray and set aside.

2 Put the potatoes in a large bowl with the salt, pepper, and 1 tablespoon of the olive oil. Stir to coat and spread the potatoes in a single layer on the prepared baking sheet. Bake for 30 minutes or until the tops start to turn golden brown and the insides are soft. Remove from the heat, cover to keep warm, and set aside.

100

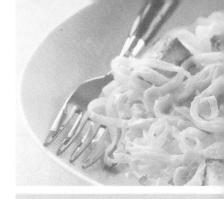

3   Meanwhile, heat the remaining tablespoon of olive oil in a large skillet over medium-high heat. Add the onion, green bell pepper, and garlic and cook, stirring, until the onion and pepper are softened, about 8 minutes. Add the tofu and cook, stirring, for 5 minutes more. Add the barbecue sauce and bring to a boil. Cover, reduce the heat, and simmer over low heat for 30 minutes, stirring occasionally. (Add a few tablespoons of water if it starts to stick while cooking.)

4   Put the potatoes on a large serving platter or on individual dishes. Top with the barbecue tofu and serve.

per serving: 0mg cholesterol • 216 calories • 9g fat • 26g carbohydrate • 7g protein

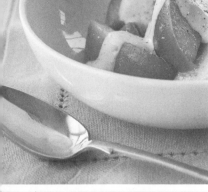

baked stuffed eggplant

Tiny cubes of tofu marinated in balsamic vinaigrette add a tender touch to stuffed eggplant.

$^1/_2$ pound firm or extra-firm tofu, rinsed, pressed, and cut into $^1/_8$-inch cubes (see page xiv)

$4^1/_2$ tablespoons olive oil

1 tablespoon balsamic vinegar

1 garlic clove, minced

$^1/_4$ teaspoon dried oregano

$^1/_8$ teaspoon salt

5 Italian eggplants (smaller than regular eggplants)

1 onion, chopped

2 garlic cloves, minced

1 green bell pepper, chopped

3 plum tomatoes, seeded and chopped

1 tablespoon red or white wine (optional)

1 teaspoon dried oregano

$^1/_4$ teaspoon salt

Freshly ground black pepper, to taste

1 cup plain bread crumbs

$^1/_2$ cup chopped fresh parsley

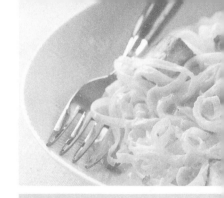

1. Put the tofu cubes into a jar or storage container and set aside. In a small bowl, combine $2^1/_2$ tablespoons of the olive oil, the vinegar, 1 minced garlic clove, the oregano, and $^1/_8$ teaspoon salt, stir with a wire whisk, and pour over the tofu. Cover and refrigerate until later in the recipe, shaking gently after about 10 minutes to evenly distribute the marinade. (This step can be done the night before for enhanced flavor.)

2. Preheat oven to 350°F. Mist a baking sheet with nonstick cooking oil spray.

3. Slice the eggplants in half lengthwise. Using a sharp knife or spoon, scoop out the pulp within $^1/_2$ inch of the skin. Chop the pulp and set aside. Place the skins (face-up) on the baking sheet and drizzle with 1 tablespoon of the remaining olive oil. Bake for 20 to 25 minutes or until the shells are soft. Remove from the oven and let cool.

4. Heat the remaining 1 tablespoon of olive oil in a large nonstick skillet over medium-high heat. Add the onion and 2 minced garlic cloves and cook, stirring, for 3 minutes. Add the bell pepper and reserved eggplant pulp and cook, stirring, for 5 minutes. Add the tomatoes, red wine (if using), oregano, $^1/_4$ teaspoon salt, and pepper and cook, stirring, for 5 minutes more. Remove from the heat and stir in the bread crumbs, parsley, and marinated tofu.

5. Spoon the mixture into the empty eggplant shells and bake for 30 minutes. Remove from the heat and serve.

per serving (2 halves): 0mg cholesterol • 330 calories • 16g fat • 40g carbohydrate • 10g protein

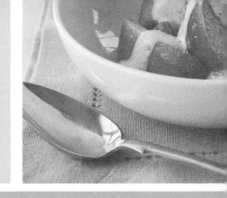

4 savory stews
and soups

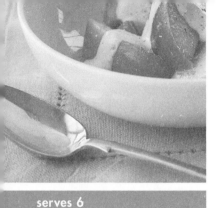

kale and chickpea chardonnay

I've always been drawn to the trio of kale, chickpeas, and potatoes. Here, they come together in a creamy white wine sauce for a rich and satisfying stew.

$^1/_2$ cup soft silken tofu

2 tablespoons Chardonnay or other white wine

$1^1/_2$ tablespoons tamari or soy sauce

1 teaspoon dried thyme

$^1/_2$ teaspoon toasted sesame oil

$^1/_4$ teaspoon salt

$^1/_8$ teaspoon freshly ground black pepper

1 tablespoon olive oil

1 red onion, chopped

2 garlic cloves, minced

2 medium potatoes, peeled and chopped

1 bunch kale, chopped (about 4 cups)

2 cups vegetable broth

1 (15.5-ounce) can chickpeas, rinsed and drained

1 In a blender, combine the tofu, Chardonnay, tamari, thyme, sesame oil, salt, and pepper. Process until smooth and set aside.

tofu 1-2-3

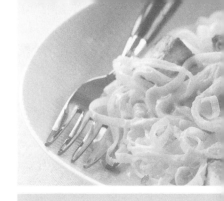

2 Heat the olive oil in a large heavy-bottomed pot over medium-high heat. Add the
   onion and garlic and cook, stirring, until the onion begins to soften, about 5 minutes. Add the potatoes and cook, stirring, for 5 minutes more. Add the kale and
   vegetable broth and bring to a boil. Cover, reduce the heat, and simmer, stirring
   occasionally, until the potatoes and kale are tender, 15 to 20 minutes. Stir in the
   chickpeas, cover, and simmer for 5 minutes.

3 Stir the tofu sauce into the kale mixture and simmer, uncovered, for 5 minutes.
   Remove from the heat, adjust the seasonings to taste, and serve in bowls or
   deep dishes.

per serving: 0mg cholesterol • 394 calories • 9g fat • 61g carbohydrate • 18g protein

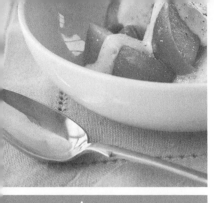

sweet potato stew
with zucchini and peppers

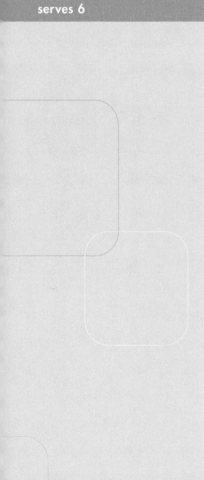

Traditional African "tagine" or stew contains deep-colored vegetables such as sweet potatoes in a rich ginger-peanut stock. Here, firm tofu replaces the chickpeas typically found in this flavorful dish.

1 tablespoon olive oil

1 onion, chopped

2 garlic cloves, minced

1 green bell pepper, chopped

1 red bell pepper, chopped

1 zucchini, chopped

1 sweet potato, peeled and chopped

$1^{1}/_{2}$ teaspoons fresh, minced ginger

$^{1}/_{2}$ teaspoon salt

$^{1}/_{8}$ teaspoon cayenne pepper

$1^{1}/_{2}$ cups vegetable broth

1 (8-ounce) can tomato sauce

1 pound firm or extra-firm tofu, rinsed and cut into $^{1}/_{2}$-inch cubes

2 tablespoons natural creamy peanut butter

1 Heat the olive oil in a large, heavy-bottomed pot over medium-high heat. Add the onion and garlic and cook, stirring, for 3 minutes. Add the bell peppers, zucchini,

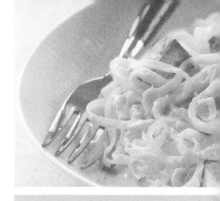

sweet potato, ginger, salt, and cayenne pepper, and cook, stirring, for 7 minutes more. Add the broth and tomato sauce and bring to a boil. Gently stir in the tofu, cover, reduce the heat, and simmer until the sweet potato is tender, about 30 minutes.

2 Using a ladle, transfer about $1/2$ cup of the liquid from the stew into a medium bowl and stir or whisk in the peanut butter. Transfer the peanut butter mixture back into the stew and stir well to combine. Simmer for 5 minutes, remove from the heat, and serve.

per serving: 0mg cholesterol • 193 calories • 9g fat • 19g carbohydrate • 10g protein

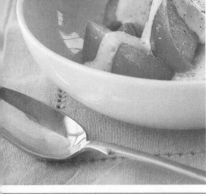

harvest stew

Tofu joins squash and corn in this autumn-inspired stew. Although it makes a wonderful stew on its own, try serving it over brown rice for a hearty meal.

1 tablespoon olive oil

1 onion, coarsely chopped

2 garlic cloves, minced

1 butternut squash, peeled, seeds removed, and cut into 1-inch cubes

1 teaspoon dried oregano

$^1/_2$ teaspoon paprika

$^1/_4$ teaspoon cayenne pepper

1 teaspoon salt

1 pound firm or extra-firm tofu, rinsed, pressed, and cut into $^1/_2$-inch cubes
  (see page xiv)

1 (16-ounce) package frozen corn, defrosted

1 (14.5-ounce) can diced tomatoes

2 cups vegetable broth

3 tablespoons chopped fresh parsley

1 Heat the oil in a large, heavy-bottomed pot over medium-high heat. Add the onion and garlic and cook, stirring, for 5 minutes. Add the butternut squash, oregano, paprika, cayenne pepper, and salt, and cook, stirring, for 5 minutes.

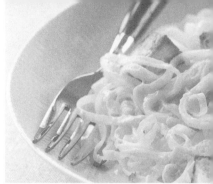

2 Add the tofu, corn, tomatoes, and vegetable broth and stir well to combine. Bring to a boil, cover, reduce the heat, and simmer for 30 minutes. Remove from the heat, stir in the parsley, let sit for 5 to 10 minutes, and serve.

per serving: 0mg cholesterol • 260 calories • 8g fat • 40g carbohydrate • 12g protein

savory stews and soups

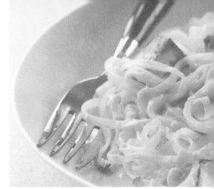

3 Add the mushrooms and 1 tablespoon of the white wine to the skillet and cook, stirring, until soft, 5 to 7 minutes. Sprinkle the mushrooms with the whole wheat flour and stir to coat for 1 minute. Gradually add the vegetable broth, stirring constantly to prevent lumps, and cook until the sauce is thickened, 2 to 3 minutes. Stir in the remaining tablespoon of white wine. Pour the mushroom sauce over the tofu filets and serve immediately.

per serving: 0mg cholesterol • 213 calories • 13g fat • 12g carbohydrate • 11g protein

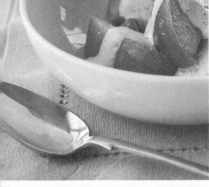

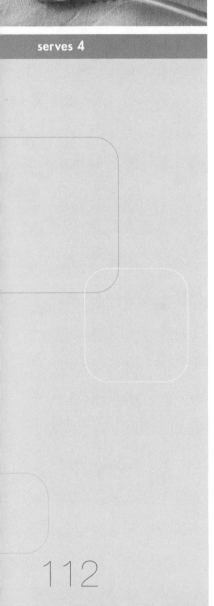

wagemann's falls tofu

In beautiful Pine Bush, New York, my good friends Diane and Dennis Wagemann built their dream home just a few feet from the glorious 30-foot waterfall that Dennis constructed. Diane is an extraordinarily creative cook and this is her recipe pairing vibrant, dark purple prunes with bright orange root vegetables for a meal as tantalizing to the eye as is Wagemann's Falls. Chop your vegetables and prunes as small as the tofu pieces for awesome texture.

1 tablespoon olive oil

1 small onion, chopped

$^1/_2$ sweet potato, peeled and chopped (about 1 cup)

2 carrots, chopped (about 1 cup)

3 garlic cloves, minced

1 teaspoon ground cumin

1 teaspoon paprika

1 teaspoon ground ginger

1 cup vegetable broth or water

1 cup chopped cauliflower florets

$^3/_4$ cup chopped, pitted prunes

$^1/_2$ pound firm or extra-firm tofu, rinsed, pressed, and cut into $^1/_2$-inch dice
   (see page xiv)

2 plum tomatoes, chopped

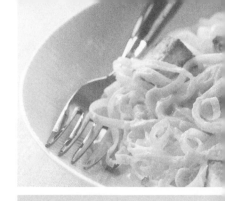

1. Heat the olive oil in a heavy-bottomed pot or saucepan over medium-high heat. Add the onion and cook, stirring, until the onion is softened, about 7 minutes. Add the sweet potato, carrots, garlic, cumin, paprika, and ginger, and cook, stirring, for 2 minutes more.

2. Add the vegetable broth, cauliflower, prunes, tofu, and tomatoes, and bring to a boil. Cover, reduce the heat, and simmer until all of the vegetables are tender, about 30 minutes. It is natural for the tofu cubes to break apart a little bit during cooking. Season to taste and serve.

per serving: 0mg cholesterol • 244 calories • 7g fat • 39g carbohydrate • 8g protein

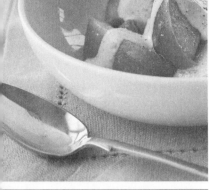

garden vegetable chili
with kale and black beans

serves 6

The secret to great tofu chili is using defrosted frozen tofu, and coating it with spices before sautéing. This recipe gets rave reviews each and every time, so enjoy!

2 tablespoons chili powder

1 teaspoon ground cumin

1 teaspoon paprika

1 teaspoon dried oregano

1 teaspoon salt

1 teaspoon sugar

1 pound firm or extra-firm tofu, frozen, defrosted, and pressed (see page xv)

1 tablespoon olive oil

1 onion, chopped

1 carrot, chopped

2 garlic cloves, minced

1 red bell pepper, chopped

1 (28-ounce) can crushed tomatoes

1 (15-ounce) can black beans, rinsed and drained

1 cup chopped fresh kale or 1 (10-ounce) package frozen chopped kale, defrosted and drained

$^1/_2$ cup sliced black olives (optional)

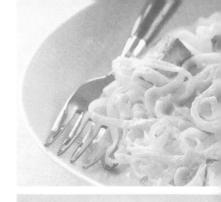

1. In a medium bowl, mix together the chili powder, cumin, paprika, oregano, salt, and sugar and set aside. Crumble the tofu into the bowl of spices and stir until the tofu is thoroughly coated with the spices. Set aside.

2. Heat the oil in a large heavy-bottomed pot over medium-high heat. Add the onion, carrot, and garlic and cook, stirring, for 5 minutes. Add the red bell pepper and cook, stirring, for 5 minutes. Add the reserved tofu and cook, stirring, for 5 minutes. Add the tomatoes, black beans, kale, and olives, if using. Bring to a boil, reduce the heat, and simmer until the kale is tender, 2 to 7 minutes—the cooking time will take longer if you use fresh rather than frozen kale. Season to taste and serve.

per serving: 0mg cholesterol • 375 calories • 8g fat • 57g carbohydrate • 23g protein

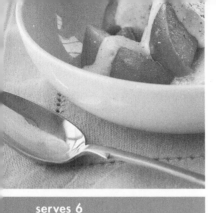

mushroom barley stew

This is best served on a cold, wet day—inside the house, of course!

2 tablespoons olive oil

1 onion, finely chopped

1 garlic clove, minced

1 pound firm or extra-firm tofu, rinsed, pressed, and cut into $3/4$-inch cubes
   (see page xiv)

24 ounces assorted mushrooms, cleaned and cut into bite-size slices (about 8 cups)

2 teaspoons dried marjoram

1 teaspoon dried thyme

1 cup pearled barley

3 cups vegetable broth

$1/4$ cup white wine

1   Heat the oil in a large, heavy-bottomed pot over medium-high heat. Add the onion and garlic and cook, stirring, for 3 minutes. Add the tofu and cook, stirring, for 5 minutes. Add the mushrooms, marjoram, and thyme, and cook, stirring, for 5 minutes.

2   Add the barley and stir to coat. Add the broth and wine and bring to a boil. Cover, reduce the heat, and simmer until barley absorbs the liquid and is tender, about 1 hour.

per serving: 0mg cholesterol • 337 calories • 11g fat • 47g carbohydrate • 15g protein

tofu 1-2-3

southwestern corn chowder

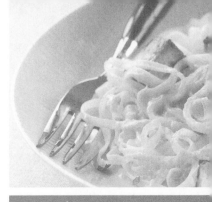

Leeks, red bell peppers, and corn take top billing in this fantastic soup.

1 tablespoon olive oil

2 leeks, chopped

2 garlic cloves, minced

2 red bell peppers, chopped

2 cups vegetable broth

1 (28-ounce) can whole peeled tomatoes

$^1/_3$ cup soft silken tofu, crumbled

2 cups frozen corn

1 tablespoon chopped fresh parsley or 1 teaspoon dried

1 to 2 teaspoons hot sauce

$^3/_4$ teaspoon salt

1 Heat the oil in a large, heavy-bottomed pot over medium-high heat. Add the leeks and garlic and cook, stirring, for 3 minutes. Add the red bell peppers and cook, stirring, for 3 minutes. Add the vegetable broth and tomatoes, breaking apart the tomatoes with a wooden spoon. Bring to a boil, cover, reduce the heat, and simmer for 20 minutes.

2 Remove from the heat, add the tofu, and puree the soup using a hand-held immersion blender. (Alternatively, puree the soup in batches using a traditional blender, then transfer back into the pot.) Stir in the corn, parsley, hot sauce, and salt. Heat gently for 5 minutes or until the corn is hot.

per serving: 0mg cholesterol • 172 calories • 5g fat • 29g carbohydrate • 6g protein

savory stews and soups

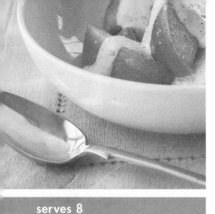

corn chowder

Chock-full of potatoes and vegetables, here's a mellow-flavored chowder that will warm you inside and out.

1 tablespoon olive oil

1 onion, chopped

2 celery stalks, chopped

1 red bell pepper, chopped

2 medium potatoes, peeled and cut into $1/2$-inch cubes

4 cups vegetable broth

$1/2$ cup soft silken tofu

2 teaspoons dry white wine

1 teaspoon dried basil

1 teaspoon salt

Freshly ground black pepper, to taste

Dulse flakes (optional, see Note)

2 cups corn, fresh or frozen (defrosted)

1 Heat the oil in a large, heavy-bottomed pot over medium-high heat. Add the onion, celery, and red bell pepper and cook, stirring, until soft, about 5 minutes. Stir in the potatoes and cook, stirring, for 1 minute. Add the vegetable broth and bring to a boil. Reduce the heat and simmer until the potatoes are soft, about 7 minutes. Remove from the heat.

tofu 1-2-3

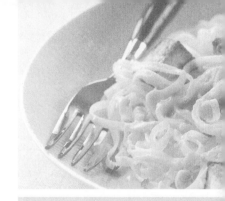

2 Remove 1 cup of the soup liquid and transfer it to the container of a blender. Let cool for 3 to 5 minutes and add the tofu, white wine, basil, salt, pepper, and dulse flakes, if using. Blend until smooth, then pour back into the soup pot along with the corn. Simmer for 5 minutes and serve.

note Dulse is a highly nutritious and richly flavorful sea vegetable. Dulse flakes add a distinctive "ocean taste" when used as a seasoning. Look for prepackaged dulse flakes and other sea vegetables in well-stocked natural food stores.

per serving: 0mg cholesterol • 165 calories • 4g fat • 26g carbohydrate • 6g protein

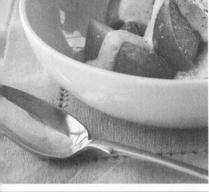

diane's christmas eve soup

My vegan friend and colleague Diane Wagemann developed this cholesterol-free recipe to replace the chicken soup her family traditionally consumed on Christmas Eve. They love her for it because it's delicious and cholesterol-free down to the last drop.

1 tablespoon olive oil

1 onion, coarsely chopped

3 carrots, coarsely chopped

3 celery stalks, coarsely chopped

1 medium potato, peeled and coarsely chopped

$3^1/_2$ cups vegetable broth

$^1/_2$ cup soft silken tofu, crumbled

2 tablespoons dry white wine

1 teaspoon poultry seasoning

2 tablespoons non-hydrogenated soy margarine

1 Heat the oil in a large heavy-bottomed pot over medium-high heat. Add the onion, carrots, celery, and potato and cook, stirring, until the vegetables are softened, about 10 minutes. Add 3 cups of the vegetable broth and bring to a boil. Cover, reduce the heat, and simmer until the vegetables are tender, about 15 minutes.

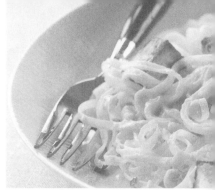

2 Put the silken tofu in a blender along with the wine, poultry seasoning, and remaining ¹/₂ cup of vegetable broth. Blend until smooth. Stir the blended mixture into the soup along with the margarine. Simmer for 2 minutes or until the soup is hot and the margarine has melted. Serve immediately.

per serving: 0mg cholesterol • 198 calories • 9g fat • 23g carbohydrate • 5g protein

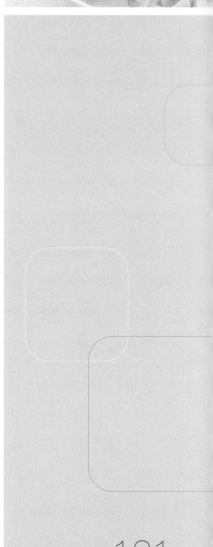

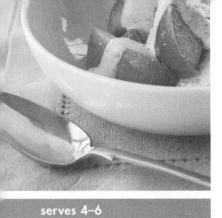

cream of mushroom

Mushrooms need little embellishment when it comes to providing soothing, savory taste. Here, sherry, scallions, and tamari do the trick.

1 tablespoon olive oil

4 scallions, chopped (both green and white parts)

10 ounces mushrooms, sliced (about $3^1/_2$ cups)

$3^1/_2$ cups vegetable broth

1 tablespoon sherry or white wine

$^1/_4$ cup soft silken tofu, crumbled

$^1/_2$ teaspoon tamari or soy sauce

$^1/_8$ teaspoon salt

Pinch ground nutmeg

1　Heat the olive oil in a large, heavy-bottomed pot over medium-high heat. Add the scallions and cook, stirring, for 3 minutes. Add the mushrooms and cook, stirring, for 3 minutes. Add the vegetable broth and sherry and bring to a boil. Cover, reduce the heat, and simmer for 15 minutes.

2　Add the tofu, tamari, salt, and nutmeg. Puree the soup using a hand-held blender. (Alternatively, puree the soup in batches using a traditional blender, then transfer back into the pot.) Season to taste and serve.

per serving: 0mg cholesterol • 168 calories • 6g fat • 22g carbohydrate • 6g protein

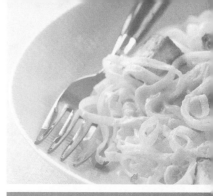

cream of asparagus

For simple sophistication, look no further than this lovely asparagus soup.

1 tablespoon olive oil

1 onion, chopped

3 celery stalks, chopped

1 garlic clove, minced

1 pound asparagus (tough ends removed and discarded), chopped (about 4 cups)

4 cups vegetable broth

$^1/_3$ cup soft silken tofu, crumbled

Salt and freshly ground black pepper, to taste

1 Heat the oil in a large heavy-bottomed pot over medium-high heat. Add the onion, celery, and garlic and cook, stirring, for 3 minutes. Add the asparagus and cook, stirring, for 5 minutes more.

2 Add the vegetable broth and bring to a boil. Cover, reduce the heat, and simmer until the vegetables are tender, about 20 minutes. Remove from the heat, add the tofu, and puree the soup using a hand-held blender. (Alternatively, puree the soup in batches using a traditional blender, then transfer back into the pot.) Season with salt and pepper to taste and serve hot or chilled.

per serving: 0mg cholesterol • 155 calories • 5g fat • 21g carbohydrate • 6g protein

savory stews and soups

123

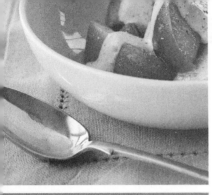

cream of tomato soup

Grilled cheese's best friend gets a makeover with silken tofu and red wine.

1 tablespoon olive oil

1 onion, chopped

1 garlic clove, minced

1 (28-ounce) can whole, peeled tomatoes

2 cups vegetable broth

1/4 cup soft silken tofu

1 to 3 teaspoons red wine

1/2 teaspoon salt

1/2 teaspoon dried basil

Freshly ground black pepper, to taste

1/2 cup chopped escarole, kale, or spinach (optional)

1 Heat the oil in a large, heavy-bottomed pot over medium-high heat. Add the onion and garlic and cook, stirring, until the onion is softened, about 5 minutes. Add the tomatoes and break apart with a wooden spoon. Add the vegetable broth and bring to a boil. Cover, reduce the heat, and cook for 20 minutes.

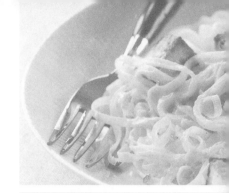

2 Add the tofu, red wine, salt, basil, and pepper and puree the soup using a hand-held blender. (Alternatively, puree the soup in batches using a traditional blender, then transfer back into the pot.) If using the escarole, add it now and simmer until tender, 8 to 10 minutes. Otherwise, season to taste and serve.

per serving: 0mg cholesterol • 135 calories • 5g fat • 19g carbohydrate • 4g protein

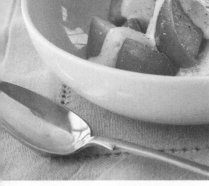

cream of artichoke

Artichoke lovers will take notice of this soft and creamy soup, light enough to enjoy through summer.

1 tablespoon olive oil

1 onion, chopped

2 garlic cloves, minced

2 celery stalks, chopped

2 (9-ounce) packages frozen artichoke hearts, defrosted (see Note)

$1/2$ teaspoon dried marjoram

3 cups vegetable broth

$1/4$ cup soft silken tofu

2 teaspoons freshly squeezed lemon juice

1 teaspoon dry white wine

$1/4$–$1/2$ teaspoon salt

Freshly ground black pepper, to taste

1 Heat the oil in a large, heavy-bottomed pot over medium-high heat. Add the onion and garlic and cook, stirring, until the onion is softened, about 5 minutes. Add the celery and cook, stirring, for 2 minutes. Add the artichoke hearts and marjoram and cook, stirring, for 2 minutes. Add the vegetable broth and bring to a boil. Cover, reduce the heat, and simmer for 20 minutes.

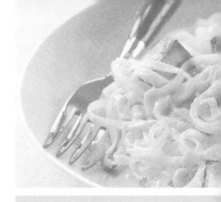

2   Add the tofu, lemon juice, wine, salt, and pepper and puree the soup using a hand-held blender. (Alternatively, puree the soup in batches using a traditional blender, then transfer back into the pot.) Season to taste and serve.

note   Frozen artichoke hearts are available in most large grocery stores but can be hard to find amidst all the other more popular frozen vegetables. Call ahead before shopping to make sure that your local supermarket has them in stock. Canned artichoke hearts are too bland and soft for use in this recipe.

per serving: 0mg cholesterol • 192 calories • 5g fat • 29g carbohydrate • 8g protein

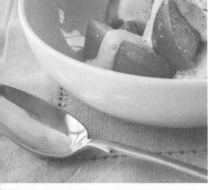

dream of cannellini with kale

I used to call this "Cream of Cannellini with Kale" until a friend tasted it, fell in love with the recipe, and strongly suggested that I rename it "Dream of . . ." Cannellini beans and kale pair fabulously with toasted sesame oil and lemon juice in this exquisitely flavored soup.

1 tablespoon coconut oil or olive oil

4 scallions, chopped (both green and white parts)

1 garlic clove, minced

$3^1/_2$ cups vegetable broth

1 (15.5-ounce) can cannellini beans, rinsed and drained

$^1/_4$ cup soft silken tofu, crumbled

1 cup sliced kale, cut into very thin 1-inch ribbons

1–$1^1/_2$ tablespoons freshly squeezed lemon juice

$^1/_8$ teaspoon toasted sesame oil

$^1/_4$ teaspoon paprika

$^1/_8$ teaspoon salt

Freshly ground black pepper, to taste

1. Heat the oil in a large, heavy-bottomed pot over medium-high heat. Add the scallions and garlic and cook, stirring, for 3 minutes. Add the vegetable broth and half of the beans and bring to a boil. Cover, reduce the heat, and simmer for 15 minutes.

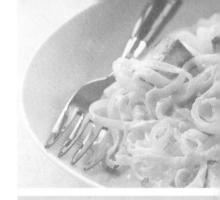

2 Add the tofu and puree the soup using a hand-held blender. (Alternatively, puree the soup in batches using a traditional blender, and transfer the soup back into the pot.) Stir in the remaining beans, kale, lemon juice, sesame oil, paprika, salt, and pepper. Simmer until the kale is tender, 10 to 15 minutes. Season to taste and serve.

per serving: 0mg cholesterol • 383 calories • 5g fat • 63g carbohydrate • 22g protein

savory stews and soups

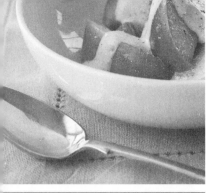

curried october pumpkin

Pumpkin's gorgeous hue celebrates the colors of fall in this creamy, curry-spiked soup.

1 tablespoon olive oil

1 onion, finely chopped

4 cups vegetable broth

$^1/_2$–1 teaspoon curry powder

$^1/_4$ teaspoon salt

1 (15-ounce) can pumpkin puree

$^1/_4$ cup soft silken tofu, crumbled

1 tablespoon soy margarine

1   Heat the oil in a large, heavy-bottomed pot over medium-high heat. Add the onion and cook, stirring, until soft and caramelized, about 15 minutes. Add the vegetable broth, curry powder, and salt and stir well. Bring to a boil, reduce the heat, cover, and simmer, stirring occasionally, for 5 minutes.

2   Remove 1 cup of the soup and puree it in a blender with the pumpkin puree and tofu. Pour the pureed mixture back into the soup. Simmer for 5 minutes, stir in the soy margarine, season to taste, and serve.

per serving: 0mg cholesterol • 166 calories • 5g fat • 25g carbohydrate • 5g protein

tofu 1-2-3

carrot-ginger soup

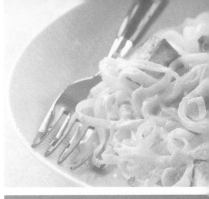

Coconut oil and fresh ginger make this cold-weather soup especially warm in flavor.

1 tablespoon coconut oil or olive oil

1 red onion, chopped

4 large carrots, chopped (about $2^{1}/_{2}$ cups)

1 red bell pepper, chopped

2 teaspoons minced fresh ginger

4 cups vegetable broth

$^{1}/_{2}$ cup soft silken tofu, crumbled

1 tablespoon smooth almond butter

$^{1}/_{2}$ teaspoon salt

1 Heat the oil in a large, heavy-bottomed pot over medium-high heat. Add the onion and carrots and cook, stirring, until the onion is softened, about 5 minutes. Add the red bell pepper and ginger and cook, stirring, for 3 minutes. Add the vegetable broth and bring to a boil. Cover, reduce the heat, and simmer until the carrots are soft, about 20 minutes.

2 Add the tofu, almond butter, and salt and puree the soup using a hand-held blender. (Alternatively, puree the soup in batches using a traditional blender, and transfer the soup back into the pot.) Season to taste and serve.

per serving: 0mg cholesterol • 189 calories • 7g fat • 25g carbohydrate • 6g protein

savory stews and soups

131

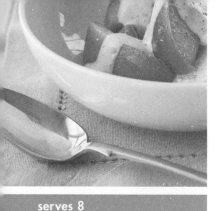

cauliflower leek soup

Perfect for a mild summer night, this soup is smooth, creamy, and easy on the lips.

1 tablespoon coconut oil or olive oil

1 head cauliflower, cored and chopped

3 leeks, trimmed, washed well, and chopped

2 garlic cloves, minced

8 cups vegetable broth

1 cup soft silken tofu

Salt and freshly ground black pepper, to taste

Chopped fresh chives (optional)

1 Heat the oil in a large heavy-bottomed pot over medium-high heat. Add the cauliflower, leeks, and garlic and cook, stirring, for 8 to 10 minutes. Add the broth and bring to a boil. Cover, reduce the heat, and simmer for 45 minutes.

2 Remove from the heat and add the tofu. Using a hand-held blender, blend the soup until completely smooth. (Alternatively, blend the soup in batches using a traditional blender, and transfer the soup back into the pot.) Season to taste with salt and pepper and serve hot or chilled. Garnish with chives, if desired.

per serving: 0mg cholesterol • 213 calories • 6g fat • 30g carbohydrate • 8g protein

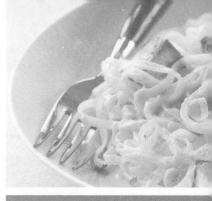

ivy's thai noodle express

Students and busy people take notice: single-serving instant Thai noodle soups can be embellished for super-easy, nutrition-packed meals. This recipe is also a great use for leftover tofu, since it doesn't really matter how much you use; the amount can be anywhere from a few chunks to half a pound.

serves 2

2 cups water

1 (1.6-ounce) package instant Thai rice noodle soup or vegetarian ramen noodles (any flavor)

Up to $1/2$ pound soft, firm, or extra-firm tofu, rinsed and cubed

$1/4$ cup frozen peas

$1/4$ cup frozen corn

Put the water in a medium pot and bring to a boil. Add the entire contents of the instant Thai noodle soup packet (noodles, spice pack, and oil pack if included). Return to a boil, reduce the heat to a simmer, and stir in the tofu, peas, and corn. Cook, stirring occasionally, until the noodles reach the desired consistency, 5 to 10 minutes. (They will continue to soften and absorb the broth even after being removed from the heat.) Remove from the heat and let cool for 5 minutes before serving.

per serving: 0mg cholesterol • 187 calories • 4g fat • 31g carbohydrate • 8g protein

savory stews and soups

133

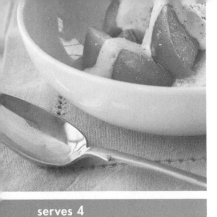

udon noodle soup

The only way to describe this soup is "totally yummy!" Look for udon noodles in natural food stores, Asian grocery stores, and in the Asian or natural foods sections of large grocery stores.

1 (8-ounce) package udon noodles

1 tablespoon peanut oil or olive oil

1 red bell pepper, cut into thin, 2-inch strips

1 carrot, thinly sliced on the diagonal

3 scallions, thinly sliced (both green and white parts)

3 cups vegetable broth

1½ teaspoons tamari or soy sauce

1½ teaspoons grated fresh ginger

⅛ teaspoon freshly ground black pepper

1½ cups thinly sliced shiitake mushrooms (stems removed)

1 pound soft, firm, or extra-firm tofu, rinsed and cut into ½-inch cubes

1 Cook the udon noodles according to the package directions. Rinse, drain, and transfer to large, individual serving bowls.

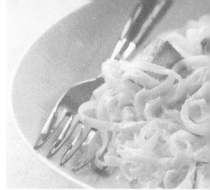

2 Heat the oil in a large heavy-bottomed pot over medium-high heat. Add the red bell pepper, carrot, and scallions and cook, stirring, for 5 minutes. Add the broth, tamari, ginger, and pepper. Bring to a boil, stir in the mushrooms and tofu, reduce the heat, and simmer for 5 minutes. Ladle the soup over the noodles and serve immediately.

per serving: 0mg cholesterol • 375 calories • 10g fat • 55g carbohydrate • 17g protein

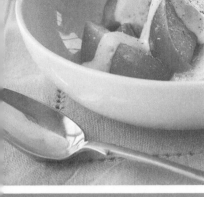

miso soup

You'll forgo prepackaged instant miso soup once you see how fast and easy it is to make this nourishing soup from scratch.

4 cups water

$^1/_2$ pound soft tofu, rinsed and cut into $^1/_2$-inch cubes

$^1/_2$ cup sliced kale, cut into 1-inch ribbons

$^1/_4$ cup dark miso

3 scallions, chopped (both green and white parts)

$^1/_4$ teaspoon toasted sesame oil

$^1/_4$ teaspoon tamari or soy sauce

Put the water in a medium pot and bring to a boil. Add the tofu and kale, reduce the heat, and simmer for 5 minutes. Transfer $^1/_3$ cup of the cooking liquid to a small bowl. Add the miso into the $^1/_3$ cup cooking liquid and stir until completely dissolved. Stir the miso mixture back into the soup and simmer for 1 minute over very low heat until the soup is smooth and becomes "cloudy" from the miso. Stir in the scallions, sesame oil, and tamari. Remove from the heat, season to taste, and serve.

per serving: 0mg cholesterol • 88 calories • 4g fat • 7g carbohydrate • 7g protein

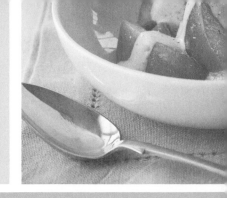

sumptuous salads
and sandwiches

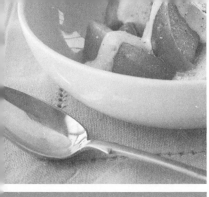

thai salad

Crunchy and flavorful, this bright purple and orange salad makes excellent use of prepackaged baked tofu. Serve the salad on a bed of greens or wrapped in warm flour tortillas.

$1/2$ small purple cabbage, coarsely chopped

1 large carrot, coarsely shredded

5 scallions, sliced (both green and white parts)

$1/3$ cup chopped fresh cilantro

1 (8-ounce) package Thai-style baked tofu, cut into $1/2$-inch dice (see Notes)

$1/3$ cup pure maple syrup

2 tablespoons tamari or soy sauce

1 tablespoon toasted sesame oil

1 garlic clove, minced

$1/2$ teaspoon minced fresh ginger

$1/4$ teaspoon cayenne pepper

1 tablespoon toasted sesame seeds (optional, see Notes)

1 In a large bowl, combine the cabbage, carrot, scallions, cilantro, and tofu. Toss gently and set aside.

2 In a medium bowl, whisk together the maple syrup, tamari, sesame oil, garlic, ginger, and cayenne pepper and whisk together. Pour over the vegetables and

tofu 1-2-3

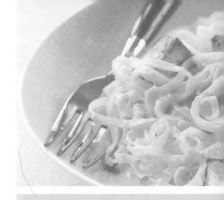

stir gently to coat. Sprinkle with toasted sesame seeds, if using. Serve chilled or at room temperature.

note If you've yet to try prepackaged, flavored baked tofu, you're in for a treat. Readily available in the refrigerated section of natural food stores, baked tofu comes in irresistible flavors such as barbecue, Italian, and Thai as used here. Baked tofu is already cooked and tastes phenomenal even when eaten straight from the package.

note To toast sesame seeds, place them in a dry pan on medium heat. Stir constantly until the seeds become aromatic and start to turn golden brown, about 2 to 3 minutes.

per serving: 0mg cholesterol • 203 calories • 7g fat • 29g carbohydrate • 7g protein

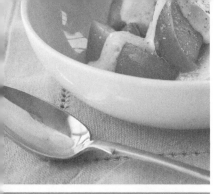

broccoli salad

Crunchy, sweet, and tangy, this awesome use of broccoli is great as a side dish, tucked into pita bread, or as filler for whole wheat wraps.

3 cups broccoli florets

1 cup chopped red onion

1 cup dark raisins

$^1/_2$ cup sunflower seeds

$^1/_3$ cup firm silken tofu

2 tablespoons olive oil

2 tablespoons rice vinegar

2 tablespoons pure maple syrup

$^1/_2$ teaspoon salt

1. Fill half of a medium pot with water and bring to a boil. Add the broccoli and boil for just 1 minute. Rinse the broccoli with cold, running water to stop it from cooking further and transfer to a large mixing bowl. Stir in the onion, raisins, and sunflower seeds.

2. In a blender, combine the tofu, olive oil, vinegar, maple syrup, and salt and process until smooth. Pour over the broccoli mixture and stir well to coat. Refrigerate for at least 30 minutes before serving.

per serving: 0mg cholesterol • 207 calories • 8g fat • 31g carbohydrate • 5g protein

tofu 1-2-3

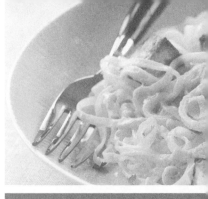

chickenless salad

Defrosted frozen tofu lends chewy texture to this easy yet tasty lunch staple. Try it in a pita pocket with lettuce and tomato, and enjoy every bite to your heart's content knowing that it doesn't contain cholesterol, and has only 12 grams of fat per serving. (The same amount of white-meat chicken salad would contain about 85 milligrams of cholesterol and 20 grams of fat.)

1 pound firm or extra-firm tofu, frozen, defrosted, and pressed (see page xv)

$^1/_3$ cup eggless mayonnaise

1 celery stalk, minced

1 scallion, minced (both green and white parts)

1 teaspoon poultry seasoning

$^1/_4$ teaspoon salt

$^1/_8$ teaspoon freshly ground black pepper

In a medium bowl, crumble the defrosted tofu into small, bite-size chunks. Add the eggless mayonnaise, celery, scallion, poultry seasoning, salt, and pepper and stir well to combine. Serve immediately or chill for at least 1 hour for optimal flavor.

per serving: 0mg cholesterol • 173 calories • 12g fat • 5g carbohydrate • 12g protein

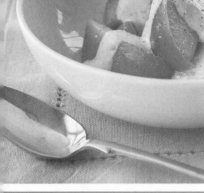

coconut rice salad

A blend of wild rice, brown rice, vegetables, and coconut flakes meld together with a zippy dressing to knock your socks off.

2 cups water

$^3/_4$ cup brown rice

$^1/_4$ cup wild rice

$^1/_2$ cup frozen peas, defrosted

1 small red bell pepper, chopped

2 scallions, sliced (both green and white parts)

$^1/_3$ cup unsweetened dried coconut flakes

1 (12-ounce) package extra-firm silken tofu (1$^1/_2$ cups)

3 tablespoons olive oil

2 tablespoons apple cider vinegar

2 tablespoons pure maple syrup

1 tablespoon freshly squeezed lime juice

$^1/_2$ teaspoon toasted sesame oil

$^1/_2$ teaspoon tamari or soy sauce

2 garlic cloves, minced

1 teaspoon minced fresh ginger or $^1/_4$ teaspoon dried

1–2 teaspoons curry powder

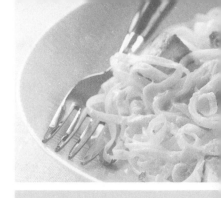

1. Bring the water to a boil in a medium pot. Stir in the brown rice and wild rice. Return to a boil, cover, reduce the heat, and simmer until the rice is tender, about 40 minutes.

2. Meanwhile, in a large bowl, combine the peas, red bell pepper, scallions, and coconut flakes and set aside.

3. To make the dressing, in a blender, combine the tofu, olive oil, vinegar, maple syrup, lime juice, sesame oil, tamari, garlic, ginger, and curry powder and process until smooth.

4. Add the cooked rice and dressing to the vegetables and toss to coat. Serve warm, chilled, or at room temperature.

per serving: 0mg cholesterol • 200 calories • 8g fat • 26g carbohydrate • 6g protein

sumptuous salads and sandwiches

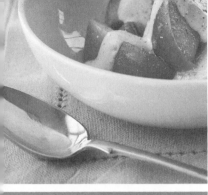

eggless salad

Grated tofu gives this deli-style salad a somewhat fluffy consistency. It's delicious in wraps, pita pockets, and on whole wheat toast with lettuce and tomato.

1 pound firm or extra-firm tofu, rinsed and patted dry

1 celery stalk, minced

2 tablespoons minced red bell pepper

2–3 tablespoons eggless mayonnaise

2 tablespoons relish

1 tablespoon nutritional yeast flakes (optional)

$1/4$ teaspoon ground mustard

$1/4$ teaspoon salt

$1/4$ teaspoon freshly ground black pepper

$1/8$ teaspoon turmeric

1 Grate the tofu (like cheese) into a medium bowl. Gently stir in the celery and red bell pepper.

2 In a small bowl, combine the eggless mayonnaise, relish, nutritional yeast flakes (if using), mustard, salt, pepper, and turmeric and stir well. Fold into the tofu mixture and stir gently. Serve immediately or transfer to a storage container and chill for at least 1 hour for optimal flavor.

per serving: 0mg cholesterol • 125 calories • 7g fat • 7g carbohydrate • 11g protein

tofu 1-2-3

waldorf salad

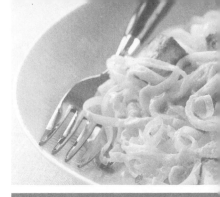

Apples, raisins, dates, and celery are dressed in a delicately sweet lemon cream sauce for a heavenly fruit salad perfect any time of day. Use Fuji apples for optimal texture and flavor, and consider making this the night before so flavors can "marry."

6 red apples, cored and cut into bite-size pieces

Juice of 2 lemons

3 celery stalks, chopped

$1/3$ cup golden raisins

6 dates, pitted and chopped

$1/4$ cup almonds, chopped

1 (12-ounce) package firm silken tofu ($1^{1}/_2$ cups)

3 tablespoons pure maple syrup

2 teaspoons vanilla extract

1 tablespoon grated lemon zest

$1/4$ teaspoon ground cinnamon

$1/4$ teaspoon ground nutmeg

1 Put the apples in a large bowl and stir in the juice of 1 lemon. Add the celery, raisins, dates, and almonds. Stir and set aside.

2 In a blender, combine the tofu, maple syrup, vanilla, lemon zest, cinnamon, nutmeg, and remaining juice of 1 lemon and process until smooth. Pour over the apple mixture and stir well to coat. Chill for at least 1 hour before serving.

per serving: 0mg cholesterol • 155 calories • 3g fat • 31g carbohydrate • 4g protein

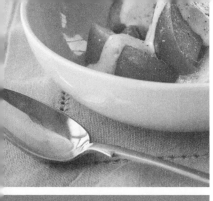

ambrosia

You could categorize this gussied-up fruit salad as a breakfast or lunch, even a dessert. One thing for sure, though, is that fruit, pecans, and coconut flakes are a rather tempting combination.

1 orange, peeled, membrane removed, and cut into $1/2$-inch dice

1 banana, cut into $1/2$-inch slices

1 cup diced ($1/2$-inch dice) fresh pineapple

1 cup halved red or green seedless grapes

$1/2$ cup coarsely chopped pecans

$1/2$ cup unsweetened dried coconut flakes

$3/4$ cup firm or extra-firm silken tofu

2 tablespoons pure maple syrup

$1/2$ teaspoon vanilla extract

Pinch salt

Pinch ground nutmeg

1   Put the orange, banana, pineapple, and grapes in a medium bowl. Stir and set aside.

2   Put the pecans and coconut flakes in a dry skillet over medium heat and toast them, stirring constantly, until they become aromatic and the coconut flakes start to turn golden, about 3 minutes. Stir into the fruit and set aside.

tofu 1-2-3

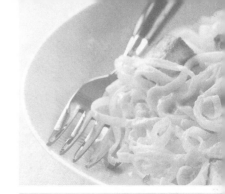

3   In a food processor, combine the tofu, maple syrup, vanilla, salt, and nutmeg and blend until completely smooth. Pour over the fruit mixture and stir to combine. Serve immediately or transfer to a storage container and refrigerate until ready to serve.

per serving: 0mg cholesterol • 142 calories • 6g fat • 20g carbohydrate • 3g protein

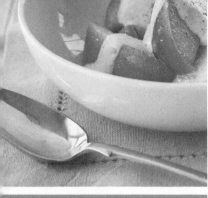

potato "egg" salad

Tiny pieces of soft tofu imitate bits of cooked egg in this picnic favorite.

4 large potatoes, peeled and cut into large chunks

1 cup eggless mayonnaise

4 scallions, sliced (both green and white parts)

1 tablespoon chopped fresh parsley

$1/2$ teaspoon salt

$1/8$ teaspoon freshly ground black pepper

$1/2$ pound soft tofu, rinsed, patted dry, and cut into tiny $1/8$-inch cubes

1 Cook the potatoes in a pot of boiling water until tender, about 15 minutes; do not overcook. Drain, cool, and cut into bite-size chunks. Put the potatoes in a large bowl.

2 Stir the eggless mayonnaise into the potatoes. Add the scallions, parsley, salt, and pepper and stir. Gently fold in the tiny cubes of tofu. Adjust the seasonings to taste and refrigerate for at least 2 hours before serving.

per serving: 0mg cholesterol • 118 calories • 7g fat • 10g carbohydrate • 3g protein

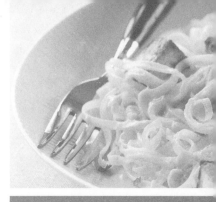

california coleslaw

serves 6

The addition of avocado makes this new take on traditional coleslaw especially creamy and delicious. Serve as a side dish or wrapped in a soft flour tortilla with a dab of spicy mustard.

1 small purple cabbage or $1/2$ medium green cabbage, shredded

3 medium carrots, shredded

$3/4$ cup firm silken tofu

$1/2$ ripe avocado

3 tablespoons pure maple syrup

3 tablespoons apple cider vinegar

$1/4$ teaspoon vegetarian Worcestershire sauce

1 scallion, chopped (both green and white parts)

$3/4$ teaspoon salt

$1/4$ teaspoon ground mustard

$1/8$ teaspoon freshly ground black pepper

1 Put the cabbage and carrots in a large bowl and set aside.

2 In a blender, combine the tofu, avocado, maple syrup, vinegar, Worcestershire sauce, scallion, salt, mustard, and pepper and process until smooth. Pour over the vegetables and stir well. Chill for at least 2 hours before serving.

per serving: 0mg cholesterol • 115 calories • 3g fat • 19g carbohydrate • 4g protein

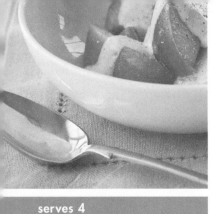

sunny carrot tostadas

If you've yet to try the delicious mixture of tahini, nutritional yeast flakes, and miso, then you are in for a wonderful surprise. Here, these three ingredients bring rich flavor to a carrot spread that goes perfectly on warm corn tortillas. I encourage my guests to fold these in half and eat them like soft tacos, although the more timid at heart tend to opt for knife and fork. Feel free to add a healthy heap of sprouts to each tostada as the sheer height of the dish adds to its beauty.

$1/4$ pound soft tofu (about $1/2$ cup)

$1/3$ cup tahini (sesame paste)

2 garlic cloves, minced

2 tablespoons nutritional yeast flakes

1 tablespoon balsamic vinegar

1 tablespoon tamari or soy sauce

2 teaspoons light or dark miso

2 large carrots, shredded (about 2 cups)

3 scallions, chopped (both green and white parts)

4 corn tortillas

1 small bunch alfalfa or other sprouts

1   Put the tofu in a medium bowl and mash with a fork or potato masher. Mix in the tahini. Add the garlic, nutritional yeast flakes, vinegar, tamari, and miso and stir well. Add the carrots and scallions and mix/mash with the back of a spoon until

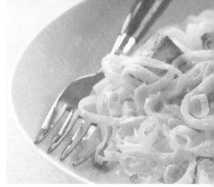

the mixture forms a thick paste. (The recipe can be prepared up to this step from several hours to one day in advance and stored, covered, in the refrigerator.)

2 Mist a skillet with nonstick cooking oil spray and heat over medium-high heat. Cook the tortillas for about 1 minute on each side. Lay each tortilla on a plate and spread with the carrot mixture. Top each with a handful of sprouts and serve.

per serving: 0mg cholesterol • 258 calories • 13g fat • 26g carbohydrate • 13g protein

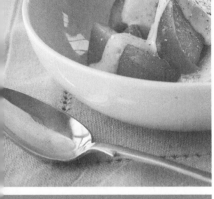

tofu-avocado pita

Nutritional yeast flakes give tofu a cheesy flavor in this overstuffed pita with roasted red peppers, avocado, and fresh sprouts.

$1/3$ cup nutritional yeast flakes

1 pound firm or extra-firm tofu, rinsed and pressed (see page xiv)

3 tablespoons olive oil

3 tablespoons eggless mayonnaise

6 pita breads, sliced open across the top

6 slices of roasted pepper

1 avocado, cut into thin slices

1 cup alfalfa sprouts

1 Put the nutritional yeast flakes in a large, shallow baking dish. Cut the tofu lengthwise into 6 equal slices and place in the nutritional yeast flakes. Gently shake the baking dish back and forth to coat the tofu. Flip the tofu over to coat completely.

2 Heat the olive oil in a large nonstick skillet over medium-high heat. Cook the tofu until golden brown on each side, about 7 minutes per side. Remove from the heat and set aside.

3 Spread the eggless mayonnaise inside the pita breads and fill each one with a piece of tofu. Stuff each with roasted red pepper, avocado slices, and sprouts. Serve immediately.

per serving: 0mg cholesterol • 387 calories • 17g fat • 43g carbohydrate • 19g protein

tofu 1-2-3

sloppy joes

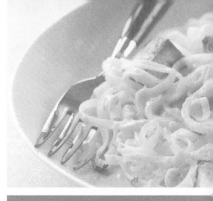

Defrosted, frozen tofu is a nutritious base for the ultimate, overflowing sandwich.

$^3/_4$ cup ketchup

2 tablespoons tamari or soy sauce

2 tablespoons yellow mustard

1 tablespoon pure maple syrup

2 teaspoons cider vinegar

1 tablespoon olive oil

$^1/_2$ onion, finely chopped

1 celery stalk, finely chopped

1 pound firm or extra-firm tofu, frozen, defrosted, and pressed (see page xv)

4 whole grain buns

1   In a small bowl, combine the ketchup, tamari, mustard, maple syrup, and vinegar. Mix well and set aside.

2   Heat the olive oil in a nonstick skillet over medium-high heat. Add the onion and celery and cook, stirring, for 5 minutes. Crumble the tofu into the pan and cook, stirring, for 2 minutes. Add the ketchup mixture and stir to coat. Cook, stirring frequently, until the bottom of the pan is deglazed and the mixture is heated through, about 2 minutes.

3   Divide the Sloppy Joe filling between the 4 buns and serve immediately.

per serving: 0mg cholesterol • 399 calories • 12g fat • 58g carbohydrate • 19g protein

sumptuous salads and sandwiches

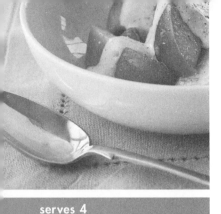

teriyaki wrap

Eastern flavor meets Western convenience in this scrumptious meal to go. For a special indulgence, serve with fried potato wedges.

1 tablespoon peanut oil, olive oil, or vegetable oil

1 onion, chopped

2 garlic cloves, minced

1 cup chopped broccoli florets

3 ounces mushrooms, sliced (about 1 cup)

1 medium zucchini, sliced

1 pound firm or extra-firm tofu, frozen, defrosted, and pressed (see page xv)

3 tablespoons tamari or soy sauce

2 tablespoons toasted sesame oil

2 tablespoons pure maple syrup

1 tablespoon unsalted sesame seeds

1 teaspoon chopped fresh ginger or $1/4$ teaspoon ground

4 warm flour tortillas

Chinese mustard or other spicy mustard (optional)

1   Heat the peanut oil in a wok or large, nonstick skillet over medium-high heat. Add the onion and garlic and cook, stirring, for 3 minutes. Add the broccoli, mushrooms, and zucchini and cook, stirring, for 5 minutes. Crumble the tofu into bite size pieces, stir it into the mixture, and cook, stirring, for 5 minutes more.

tofu 1-2-3

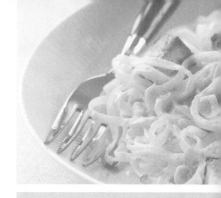

2 Meanwhile, in a small bowl, mix together the tamari, sesame oil, maple syrup, sesame seeds, and ginger. Add to the tofu mixture and stir to coat. Cook, stirring, for 3 minutes and remove from the heat.

3 Take ¼ of the filling and form it into a rectangular mound in the center of a tortilla. Top with Chinese mustard, if using. Grab the two sides of the tortilla that are closest to the filling, and fold them over the filling. Fold the bottom half all the way over the filling, then roll up the rest of the way. Repeat with the remaining 3 tortillas and serve immediately.

per serving: 0mg cholesterol • 365 calories • 19g fat • 34g carbohydrate • 16g protein

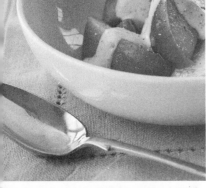

curried tofu chapatis

Pan-fried tofu seasoned with Indian spices is sensational when wrapped in chapatis with sautéed cauliflower and fresh cilantro. Feel free to substitute flour tortillas for the chapatis if you can't find this soft, flat Indian bread locally.

2^1/$_2$ teaspoons curry powder

^{3}/$_4$ teaspoon salt

^{3}/$_4$ teaspoon freshly ground black pepper

^{3}/$_4$ teaspoon garlic granules

^{1}/$_2$ teaspoon ground ginger

^{1}/$_2$ teaspoon ground cumin

1 pound extra-firm tofu, rinsed and patted dry

3 tablespoons olive oil

2 cups chopped cauliflower florets

^{1}/$_2$ cup chopped, fresh cilantro

4 chapatis

1 In a small bowl, combine the curry powder, salt, pepper, garlic granules, ginger, and cumin.

2 Cut the tofu widthwise into ^{1}/$_4$-inch-thick slices. (You will have about 12 rectangles.) Set aside.

3 Heat 2 tablespoons of the oil in a large nonstick skillet over medium-high heat. When the oil is hot, lay the sliced tofu in the pan and sprinkle with half of the spice

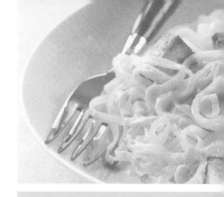

mixture. Cook for 4 minutes, then flip the tofu, and sprinkle with the remaining spice mixture. Cook for 2 minutes, flip once more, and cook for 1 minute. Transfer the tofu to a plate and cover to keep warm.

4   Add the remaining tablespoon of oil to the unwashed pan. Add the cauliflower and cook, stirring, until softened and coated with the spice remnants, about 4 minutes. Remove the pan from the heat and stir in the cilantro.

5   Lay the chapatis on a flat surface. Evenly divide the tofu between the centers of each chapati, and top with cauliflower. Roll up and serve.

per serving: 0mg cholesterol • 321 calories • 18g fat • 27g carbohydrate • 15g protein

variation

Quick Curried Tofu Sub

• Prepare the tofu as directed, but omit the cauliflower, cilantro, and chapatis. Serve the sautéed tofu on rolls with lettuce and eggless mayonnaise.

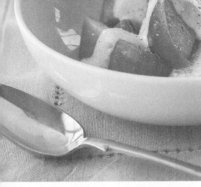

serves **4**

tofu reuben

You're going to love the healthy makeover of this timeless sandwich.

1 pound firm or extra-firm tofu, rinsed and patted dry

2 tablespoons vegetable oil

3 tablespoons tamari or soy sauce

4 slices of dairy-free cheese (your choice)

$^1/_3$ cup eggless mayonnaise

2 tablespoons ketchup

2 teaspoons dried oregano

8 slices rye bread, toasted

1 cup sauerkraut, drained well

1 Slice the tofu lengthwise into 6 equal rectangles. Heat the oil in a nonstick skillet over medium-high heat. Lay each piece of tofu in the pan, and cook until golden brown on the bottom, 7 to 10 minutes. Carefully flip the tofu, sprinkle with the tamari, and cook until the bottom is golden brown, about 5 minutes. Flip one more time and cook for 1 minute.

2 Remove the entire pan from the heat and top each piece of tofu with a slice of cheese. Cover the pan and let the cheese melt for about 3 minutes. Remove 2 of the cheese-topped tofu pieces from the pan and cut them in half. Set all of the tofu aside.

tofu 1-2-3

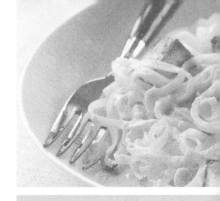

3 In a small bowl, mix together the eggless mayonnaise, ketchup, and oregano. Spread onto one side of each of the pieces of toast.

4 Top 4 slices of the rye toast with one and a half pieces of "cheesy" tofu and ¼ cup of drained sauerkraut. Cover with remaining rye toast, slice in half, and serve immediately.

per serving: 0mg cholesterol • 400 calories • 18g fat • 43g carbohydrate • 18g protein

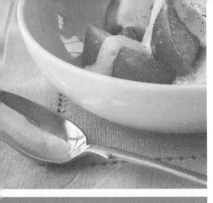

tofu parmesan grinder

When it comes to the urge to sink your teeth into a mouthwatering taste sensation, look no further than this ultimate, Italian-inspired favorite.

$^{1}/_{3}$ cup unbleached all-purpose flour

6 tablespoons water

1 tablespoon flax seeds

$1^{1}/_{2}$ cups plain bread crumbs

2 tablespoons Italian seasoning

4 tablespoons dairy-free Parmesan cheese

1 pound firm or extra-firm tofu, rinsed and pressed (see page xiv)

$^{1}/_{4}$ cup vegetable oil

4 medium rolls

1 (16-ounce) jar spaghetti sauce

1 cup jarred roasted red peppers, sliced

1   Preheat oven to 350°F.

2   Put the flour in a shallow dish and set aside. Put the water and flax seeds in a blender and process until emulsified. Transfer to a shallow dish and set aside. In a medium bowl, mix together the bread crumbs, Italian seasoning, and 2 table-spoons of the Parmesan cheese and set aside.

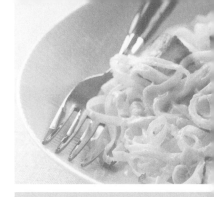

3 Cut the tofu lengthwise into 8 rectangles. Heat a thin layer of oil in a nonstick skillet over medium-high heat. Dip the tofu pieces into the flour, then into the flax mixture, then gently dredge them in the bread crumbs, coating well. Fry the tofu until brown and crispy, about 3 minutes per side. Remove from the pan and drain on a wire rack.

4 Partially cut each roll in half lengthwise and open them up like books to make room for the filling. Coat the insides of the rolls with spaghetti sauce. Lay 2 pieces of tofu inside each roll and top with the sliced roasted peppers. Sprinkle the remaining 2 tablespoons of dairy-free Parmesan cheese over the peppers. Arrange the open grinders on a cookie sheet. Place in the oven and bake for 8 to 10 minutes or until the bread turns light brown.

5 Remove the grinders from the oven. Close them, slice in half, and let cool for 5 minutes before serving.

per serving: 0mg cholesterol • 481 calories • 21g fat • 60g carbohydrate • 17g protein

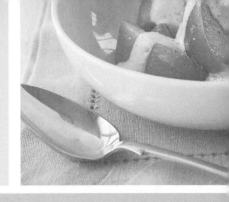

6 smoothies and other bubbly blender concoctions

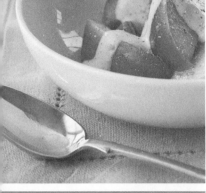

tropical sunrise

This is best served in the early morning after a rousing frolic in the sea.

1 cup mango nectar

$^1/_2$ cup frozen strawberries

$^1/_2$ cup fresh pineapple

2 tablespoons silken tofu

1 tablespoon pure maple syrup

Combine all of the ingredients in a blender and process until smooth.

per serving: 0mg cholesterol • 103 calories • 1g fat • 23g carbohydrate • 1g protein

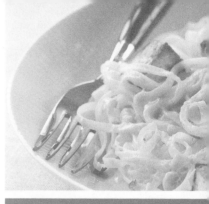

almond jubilation

Drink the flavors of chocolate, coconut, and almond to reconnect with the flavor of that classic childhood candy bar.

$^2/_3$ cup coconut milk

$^1/_3$ cup almonds (see Note)

$^2/_3$ cup apple juice

3 tablespoons silken tofu

2 tablespoons pure maple syrup

2 teaspoons cocoa powder

1 teaspoon vanilla extract

$^2/_3$ cup ice

Combine the coconut milk and almonds in a blender and process until smooth. Add the remaining ingredients except the ice, and process until smooth. Add the ice and process until blended. Serve immediately.

 It is preferable but not necessary to use almonds with their skins removed. To remove the skins, drop the almonds into boiling water for 20 seconds. Drain them and plunge them into a bowl of very cold water. Squeeze the ends of the almonds and they will pop out of their skin.

per serving: 0mg cholesterol • 233 calories • 16g fat • 20g carbohydrate • 3g protein

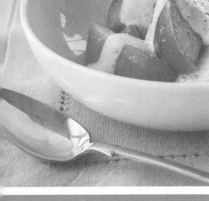

blueberry thrill

Blueberries can be blended with nearly any sweet juice for an equally delicious beverage.

$1^1/_2$ cups fresh or frozen blueberries

1 cup blueberry nectar (see Note)

$^1/_4$ cup silken tofu

$^1/_4$ cup apple juice

Combine all of the ingredients in a blender and process until smooth.

 Blueberry nectar is available in most natural food stores and in the natural foods section of large grocery stores.

per serving: 0mg cholesterol • 151 calories • 1g fat • 33g carbohydrate • 2g protein

tofu 1-2-3

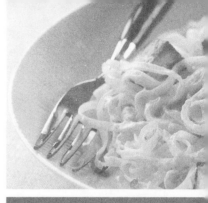

piña colada

Tofu takes on the flavors of whatever it's prepared with, so how does the ultimate beach drink taste with tofu? The same!

$^2/_3$ cup ice

$^1/_2$ cup fresh pineapple

$^1/_2$ cup coconut milk

$^1/_3$ cup pineapple juice

$^1/_4$ cup silken tofu

2 tablespoons pure maple syrup

Combine all of the ingredients in a blender and process until smooth.

 The fresh pineapple and the pineapple juice can be substituted with canned pineapple in its own juice.

per serving: 0mg cholesterol • 242 calories • 15g fat • 25g carbohydrate • 3g protein

smoothies and other bubbly blender concoctions

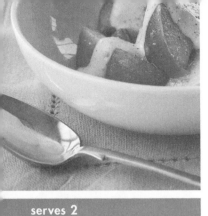

black forest

Cherries and chocolate, these are the flavors of love!

1 frozen banana

$^1/_2$ cup black cherry juice

$^1/_2$ cup frozen or fresh (pitted) cherries

$^1/_4$ cup silken tofu

2 tablespoons pure maple syrup

1 tablespoon cocoa powder

Combine all of the ingredients in a blender and process until smooth.

per serving: 0mg cholesterol • 168 calories • 2g fat • 37g carbohydrate • 3g protein

raspberry smoothie

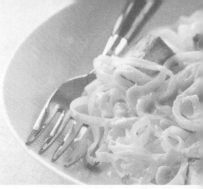

Pucker up and say "I love you!" with this pink-hued raspberry blend.

1 frozen banana

$^1/_2$ cup pineapple juice

$^1/_2$ cup orange juice

$^1/_3$ cup frozen raspberries

$^1/_4$ cup silken tofu

Combine all of the ingredients in a blender and process until smooth.

per serving: 0mg cholesterol • 123 calories • 1g fat • 26g carbohydrate • 2g protein

smoothies and other bubbly blender concoctions

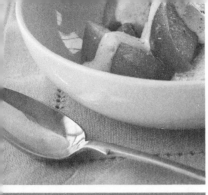

mango tenderness

This is soft and smooth and easy on the lips.

Flesh of 1 ripe mango

1 ripe banana

1 cup mango nectar, apricot nectar, or apple juice

$1/4$ cup silken tofu

Combine all of the ingredients in a blender and process until smooth.

per serving: 0mg cholesterol • 146 calories • 1g fat • 33g carbohydrate • 2g protein

avocado cooler

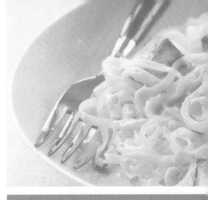

Avocado's mild flavor doesn't make a significant impact on smoothie flavor, but boy does it add ultra-smoothness!

serves 3

1$^{1}/_{3}$ cups orange juice

$^{1}/_{2}$ ripe Haas avocado

$^{1}/_{2}$ cup ice

$^{1}/_{3}$ cup fresh pineapple chunks

$^{1}/_{4}$ cup silken tofu

3 frozen strawberries

2 tablespoons pure maple syrup

Combine all of the ingredients in a blender and process until smooth.

per serving: 0mg cholesterol • 340 calories • 5g fat • 77g carbohydrate • 4g protein

smoothies and other bubbly blender concoctions

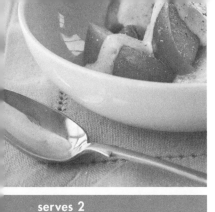

strawberry fields

This basic strawberry smoothie can be made with nearly any kind of sweet juice.

1 cup apple juice

1 cup frozen strawberries

$1/4$ cup silken tofu

1 tablespoon pure maple syrup

Combine all of the ingredients in a blender and process until smooth.

per serving: 0mg cholesterol • 124 calories • 1g fat • 26g carbohydrate • 2g protein

almond peach sunset

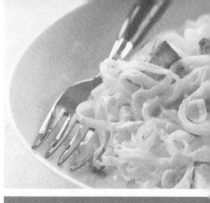

Almonds blended with peach nectar make a subtly sophisticated base for this frozen peach creation.

serves 2

$^1/_4$ cup almonds

1 cup peach nectar

1 banana

$^1/_3$ cup frozen peaches

$^1/_4$ cup silken tofu

Combine the almonds and $^1/_3$ cup of the peach nectar in a blender and process until smooth. Add the banana, frozen peaches, tofu, and remaining peach nectar, and process until smooth.

per serving: 0mg cholesterol • 201 calories • 5g fat • 37g carbohydrate • 4g protein

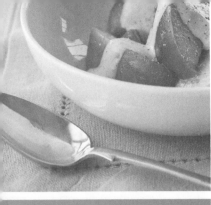

orange jubilee

Creamy, vanilla-spiked orange juice aims to please.

1$^1/_2$ cups orange juice

$^1/_4$ cup silken tofu

2 tablespoons pure maple syrup

1 teaspoon vanilla extract

Combine all of the ingredients in a blender and process until smooth.

variation

- Pour a few tablespoons of cherry juice in the bottom of a tall glass and fill with Orange Jubilee.

per serving: 0mg cholesterol • 157 calories • 1g fat • 33g carbohydrate • 3g protein

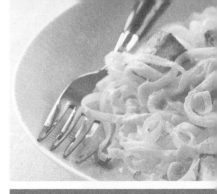

chocolate chill

Think of it as the polar opposite of hot chocolate.

1$^1/_2$ cups rice milk

$^1/_3$ cup silken tofu

3 tablespoons cocoa powder

3 tablespoons pure maple syrup

$^2/_3$ cup ice

Combine all of the ingredients except the ice in a blender and process until smooth. Add the ice and process until smooth.

per serving: 0mg cholesterol • 208 calories • 4g fat • 42g carbohydrate • 4g protein

smoothies and other bubbly blender concoctions

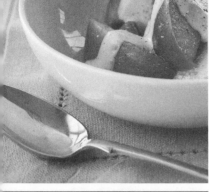

cherry citrus frost

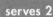
Frozen cherries and orange juice concentrate deliver maximum, heat-busting satisfaction.

$^1/_2$ cup frozen cherries

$^1/_3$ cup silken tofu

$^1/_3$ cup water

$^1/_3$ cup frozen orange juice concentrate

1 tablespoon pure maple syrup

1 teaspoon vanilla extract

Combine all of the ingredients in a blender and process until smooth.

per serving: 0mg cholesterol • 173 calories • 1g fat • 36g carbohydrate • 4g protein

kiwi blackberry delight

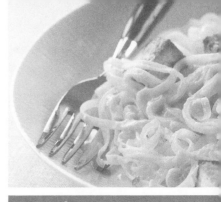

Blackberries and kiwis pair fabulously for great taste and vivid color.

    2 whole kiwis, peeled

    $2/_3$ cup apple juice

    $2/_3$ cup ice

    $1/_3$ cup fresh blackberries

    $1/_4$ cup silken tofu

    1 tablespoon pure maple syrup

Combine all of the ingredients in a blender and process until smooth.

per serving: 0mg cholesterol • 142 calories • 1g fat • 31g carbohydrate • 3g protein

177

smoothies and other bubbly blender concoctions

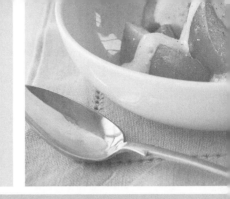

7 happy endings

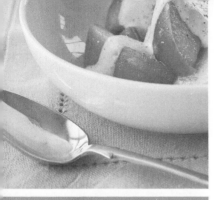

lemon dream pie
with blueberry glaze

Perfect in spring or summer, this creamy yellow pie with a striking blueberry topping is refreshing in taste, not to mention gorgeous in sight.

1 unbaked flaky pie crust

1 pound soft tofu, rinsed and patted dry

²/₃ cup sugar

4 teaspoons freshly squeezed lemon juice

2 teaspoons lemon extract

2 teaspoons freshly grated lemon zest

1 teaspoon vanilla extract

Blueberry Glaze (recipe follows)

1 Preheat oven to 350°F. Prebake the pie crust for 7 minutes. Remove from the oven and set aside.

2 In a blender or food processor, combine the tofu, sugar, lemon juice, lemon extract, lemon zest, and vanilla and blend until completely smooth, at least 2 minutes. Pour the mixture into the pie crust and smooth the top of the filling with the back of a spoon.

3 Bake for 45 minutes. Cool, refrigerate for at least 2 hours, and top with Blueberry Glaze. Can be served immediately or chilled for a firmer topping that is the same temperature as the (chilled) cake.

per serving: 0mg cholesterol • 205 calories • 8g fat • 27g carbohydrate • 5g protein

tofu 1-2-3

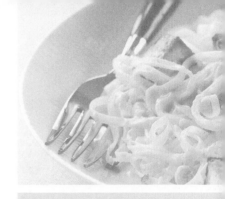

blueberry glaze

makes about 1 1/2 cups

1/2 cup apple juice

1 tablespoon arrowroot or cornstarch

1 1/2 cups fresh or frozen blueberries (don't strain away their juice, if any)

Stir together the juice and arrowroot in a small bowl and set aside. Put the blueberries in a medium pot and heat over high heat for several minutes until the juices are released and it starts to simmer. Add the arrowroot mixture and stir constantly until it thickens, about 2 minutes. Remove from the heat and let cool 5 minutes before using.

 Blueberry Glaze is also good over Delectable Cream Cheese Pie (page 188) and Almond Cream Pie (page 185). When topping either one of those pies, feel free to substitute strawberries or cherries for the blueberries. It will be necessary, though, to chop the fruit into blueberry-size pieces before simmering it, and to add a few tablespoons of pure maple syrup to taste if using strawberries.

per serving: 0mg cholesterol • 29 calories • .1g fat • 7g carbohydrate • .2g protein

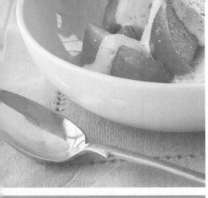

pumpkin pie

A serving of pumpkin pie usually contains about 19 grams of fat and 133 milligrams of cholesterol. But here, where tofu replaces the eggs, cream, and milk, you get less than half the fat and absolutely none of the cholesterol. Now that's what I call the ultimate finish to a perfect Thanksgiving feast!

> 1 (12-ounce) package extra-firm silken tofu (1$^1/_2$ cups)
>
> 1 (15-ounce) can pumpkin puree
>
> $^3/_4$ cup sugar
>
> 1$^1/_2$ teaspoons ground cinnamon
>
> 1$^1/_2$ teaspoons vanilla extract
>
> $^3/_4$ teaspoon ground ginger
>
> $^3/_4$ teaspoon salt
>
> $^1/_2$ teaspoon ground nutmeg
>
> 1 unbaked flaky pie crust

1 Preheat oven to 350°F.

2 In a food processor, combine the tofu, pumpkin puree, sugar, cinnamon, vanilla, ginger, salt, and nutmeg and blend until completely smooth, about 2 minutes, stopping once or twice to scrape down the sides of the bowl. Pour into the pie crust. Bake for 1 hour, cool, and refrigerate for at least 3 hours or overnight before serving.

per serving: 0mg cholesterol • 217 calories • 8g fat • 33g carbohydrate • 5g protein

tofu 1-2-3

chocolate cream pie

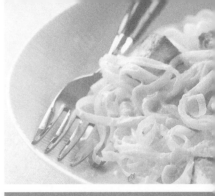

Simply stated, everyone who tastes this pie loves this pie.

serves 8

1 recipe Chocolate Mousse (page 204, made with extra-firm silken tofu)

1 graham cracker crust

Prepare the Chocolate Mousse; instead of transferring the mixture into a storage container, pour it into the pie crust. Cover with plastic wrap and refrigerate for several hours or overnight until firm.

per serving: 0mg cholesterol • 323 calories • 15g fat • 42g carbohydrate • 5g protein

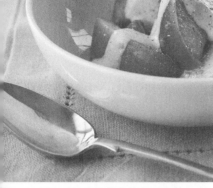

peanut butter cup pie

A creamy, dreamy way to serve tofu to chocolate-and-peanut-butter lovers.

1 (12-ounce) package extra-firm silken tofu (1$^1/_2$ cups)

$^1/_2$ cup natural smooth peanut butter

$^1/_3$ cup pure maple syrup

2 teaspoons vanilla extract

1 cup dairy-free chocolate chips, melted (see Note)

1 graham cracker crust

Put silken tofu in a food processor and blend until smooth, about 1 minute. Add the peanut butter, maple syrup, and vanilla and blend until smooth. Add the melted chocolate chips and blend until smooth. Pour into the graham cracker crust. Refrigerate for at least 3 hours or overnight before serving.

 Melt chocolate chips in a double-boiler, stirring constantly to prevent burning, or in the microwave oven, on the defrost setting for approximately 3 minutes, stopping to stir at least once.

per serving: 0mg cholesterol • 334 calories • 18g fat • 36g carbohydrate • 7g protein

almond cream pie

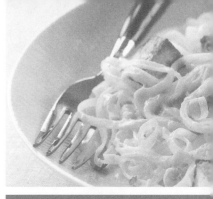

Creamy, luscious almond butter lends outstanding flavor to this smooth, delectable pie. Serve with Blueberry or Strawberry Glaze for the ultimate touch.

1 unbaked flaky pie crust

1 pound soft tofu

$1/2$ cup almond butter (unsalted)

$1/2$ cup pure maple syrup

1 teaspoon almond extract or almond liqueur

$1/8$ teaspoon ground cinnamon

Pinch salt

Blueberry or Strawberry Glaze (page 181), for serving (optional)

1 Preheat oven to 350°F. Prebake the pie crust for 7 minutes. Remove from the oven and set aside. Do not turn off the oven.

2 Put the tofu in a food processor and blend until completely smooth and creamy, about 2 minutes; all of the graininess from the tofu should be gone. Add the almond butter, maple syrup, almond extract, cinnamon, and salt and blend until smooth, about 2 minutes more, stopping at least once to scrape down the sides.

3 Pour into the pie crust and bake for 45 minutes. Cool and refrigerate for at least 2 hours or overnight. Top with Blueberry or Strawberry Glaze or serve plain.

per serving: 0mg cholesterol • 295 calories • 18g fat • 27g carbohydrate • 8g protein

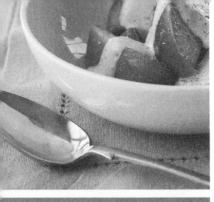

mochaccino pie

Here, instant grain coffee is blended with melted chocolate chips and other tasty ingredients to make a decidedly adult-flavored cream pie. Instant grain coffee is naturally caffeine-free—it's usually based on barley, chickory, and/or rye—and can be found in natural food stores and in the natural foods aisle of large grocery stores.

1 pound soft tofu

$1/3$ cup pure maple syrup

$2^1/_2$ tablespoons instant grain coffee powder (not reconstituted)

2 tablespoons cashew butter

1 teaspoon coffee liqueur

Pinch of ground cinnamon

$1/_2$ cup dairy-free chocolate chips, melted (see Note)

1 graham cracker crust

1   Put the tofu in a food processor and blend until completely smooth, about 2 minutes, stopping at least once to scrape down the sides of the bowl. (The tofu should be smooth and creamy with no graininess.) Add the maple syrup, coffee powder, cashew butter, coffee liqueur, and cinnamon and blend until smooth, about 2 minutes more.

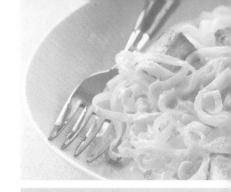

2 Add the melted chocolate chips and pulse one or two short times; the melted chocolate will be swirled into the tofu mixture, not blended together. Carefully pour the swirled filling into the pie crust, minimizing disruption of the majority of the swirl. Refrigerate for at least 3 hours or until firm to the touch before serving.

 Melt chocolate chips in a double-boiler, stirring constantly to prevent burning, or in the microwave oven, on the defrost setting for approximately 3 minutes, stopping to stir at least once.

per serving: 0mg cholesterol • 312 calories • 15g fat • 38g carbohydrate • 6g protein

happy endings

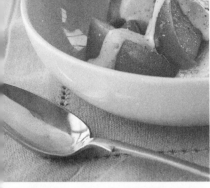

delectable cream cheese pie

Heaven on Earth is a glorious dairy-free cheesecake served au naturel or topped with delectable fruit glaze.

1 unbaked flaky pie crust

1 pound soft tofu

1 (8-ounce) container dairy-free cream cheese

$1/2$ cup sugar

1 tablespoon vanilla extract

Blueberry, Strawberry, or Cherry Glaze (page 181), for serving (optional)

1   Preheat oven to 350°F. Prebake the pie crust for 7 minutes. Remove from the oven and set aside. Do not turn off the oven.

2   Put the tofu in a food processor and blend until completely smooth and creamy, about 2 minutes; all of the graininess from the tofu should be gone. Add the cream cheese, sugar, and vanilla and blend until smooth, about 2 minutes more, stopping at least once to scrape down the sides. Pour into the pie crust and bake for 40 minutes. Refrigerate for 3 hours or overnight until the top is firm. Top with Blueberry, Strawberry, or Cherry Glaze or serve plain.

per serving: 0mg cholesterol • 303 calories • 10g fat • 35g carbohydrate • 6g protein

reed's fruit-swirled cheesecake

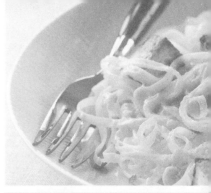

When you really want to impress friends or family, make cheesecake with a beautiful swirl. (Shhh, don't tell anyone how easy it is—nor that it contains tofu!)

1 unbaked flaky pie crust

1 recipe Delectable Cream Cheese Pie (filling only, page 188)

$^{1}/_{2}$ cup fruit spread (blueberry, strawberry, raspberry, or cherry)

1 teaspoon freshly squeezed lemon juice

1 Preheat oven to 350°F. Prebake the pie crust for 7 minutes. Remove from the oven and set aside. Do not turn off the oven.

2 Pour half of the prepared Delectable Cream Cheese Pie filling into the pie crust. Mix the fruit spread with the lemon juice in a small bowl. Spoon half of the spread over the filling and use a knife to swirl it into the pie. Pour the remaining cheese-cake filling on top. Wipe the knife clean and use it to swirl the remaining spread on top of the pie in a decorative pattern.

3 Bake for 40 minutes. Let cool and refrigerate for 4 hours or overnight until the top is very firm before serving.

per serving: 0mg cholesterol • 352 calories • 15g fat • 48g carbohydrate • 7g protein

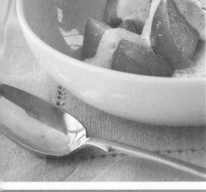

fudge brownies

I love making Fudge Brownies for my kids and my niece and nephews because they smile when I pull them out of the oven, and they tell me that I really know how to make brownies.

1 cup unbleached all-purpose flour

$^1/_2$ cup cocoa powder

$^1/_3$ cup sugar

$^1/_2$ teaspoon salt

1 cup pure maple syrup

$^1/_2$ cup soft silken tofu

$^1/_3$ cup vegetable oil

2 teaspoons vanilla extract

1 cup dairy-free chocolate chips, melted (see Note)

1 Preheat oven to 350°F. Mist an 8 × 8-inch baking dish with nonstick cooking oil spray. Set aside.

2 In a large mixing bowl, combine the flour, cocoa powder, sugar, and salt and stir with a wire whisk. In a blender, combine the maple syrup, tofu, vegetable oil, and vanilla and process until smooth. Add the melted chocolate chips and process until smooth. Pour the liquid ingredients into the dry ingredients and mix well.

190

tofu 1-2-3

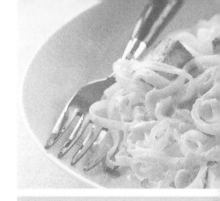

3 Transfer the batter into the prepared baking dish and bake for 25 to 30 minutes or until a toothpick comes out dry. Cool for at least 30 minutes before cutting into squares.

 Melt chocolate chips in a double-boiler, stirring constantly to prevent burning, or in the microwave oven, on the defrost setting for approximately 3 minutes, stopping to stir at least once.

per square: 0mg cholesterol • 198 calories • 8g fat • 31g carbohydrate • 2g protein

happy endings

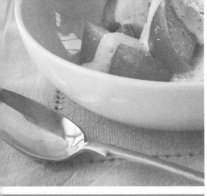

chocolate chip cookie bars

Can't decide between brownies and chocolate chip cookies? Get the best of both worlds with the all-time favorite soft-baked chocolate chip cookies baked in a pan and cut into squares like brownies. Or, for a giant cookie that can be sliced like a pie, forgo the specified rectangular pan in favor of a round springform pan. Just bake, cool, and decorate as desired!

4 cups unbleached all-purpose flour

1 cup sugar

2 teaspoons baking powder

$1/4$ teaspoon salt

1 cup vegetable oil

$3/4$ cup pure maple syrup

$1/3$ cup soft silken tofu

1 teaspoon vanilla extract

1 cup dairy-free chocolate chips

1 Preheat oven to 350°F. Mist an 8 × 11-inch baking pan with nonstick cooking oil spray.

2 In a large bowl, combine the flour, sugar, baking powder, and salt and stir with a wire whisk. In a blender, combine the oil, maple syrup, tofu, and vanilla and process until smooth. Pour the liquid ingredients into the dry ingredients and mix well with a spoon. Stir in the chocolate chips.

tofu 1-2-3

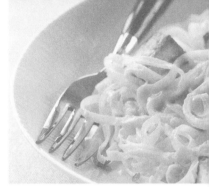

3 Transfer the mixture into the prepared baking pan, using the back of a spoon to spread the mixture and press it down until the top is smooth. Bake for 15 minutes, cool, and refrigerate for at least 1 hour before cutting into squares.

per bar: 0mg cholesterol • 250 calories • 11g fat • 35g carbohydrate • 2g protein

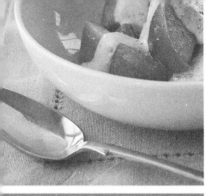

oatmeal cookies

Chewy and delicious, add raisins for an extra-flavor boost.

2 cups unbleached all-purpose flour

1$^1/_2$ teaspoons baking soda

$^1/_2$ teaspoon salt

$^1/_2$ teaspoon ground cinnamon

2 cups rolled oats

$^3/_4$ cup sugar

$^3/_4$ cup vegetable oil

$^3/_4$ cup pure maple syrup

$^1/_3$ cup rice milk

$^1/_4$ cup silken tofu

1 teaspoon vanilla extract

$^1/_2$ cup dark raisins (optional)

1 Preheat oven to 350°F. Line a cookie sheet with parchment paper or mist with nonstick cooking oil spray.

2 In a large mixing bowl, combine the flour, baking soda, salt, and cinnamon and stir with a wire whisk. Add the rolled oats and sugar and stir with a wire whisk. In a blender, combine the oil, maple syrup, rice milk, tofu, and vanilla and process until smooth. Pour the liquid ingredients into the dry ingredients and stir until combined. Stir in the raisins if using.

tofu 1-2-3

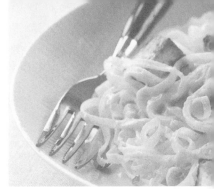

3 Drop the batter by the rounded teaspoon onto the prepared cookie sheet. Bake each batch for 15 minutes or until golden brown. Transfer to a wire cooling rack for 5 minutes and serve.

per cookie: 0mg cholesterol • 133 calories • 5g fat • 19g carbohydrate • 2g protein

happy endings

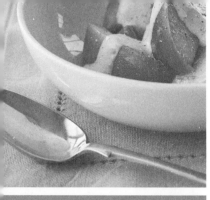

all-occasion white cake

The magic in this all-purpose white cake lies not only in its simplicity, but also in the fact that it's completely free of eggs and dairy.

$2^1/_2$ cups unbleached all-purpose flour

$1^1/_2$ teaspoons baking powder

1 teaspoon baking soda

$^1/_4$ teaspoon salt

$1^1/_2$ cups rice milk

1 cup pure maple syrup

$^1/_3$ cup soft silken tofu

$^1/_4$ cup vegetable oil

2 teaspoons vanilla extract

Chocolate Frosting (page 205)

1 Preheat oven to 350°F. Mist two 9-inch round cake pans or an 8 × 11-inch baking pan with nonstick cooking oil spray. Dust with flour and set aside.

2 In a large bowl, combine the flour, baking powder, baking soda, and salt and stir with a wire whisk. In a blender, combine the rice milk, maple syrup, tofu, oil, and vanilla and process until smooth. Pour the liquid ingredients into the dry ingredients and stir until blended.

196

tofu 1-2-3

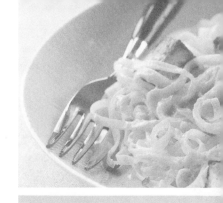

3   Transfer the batter to the pan(s) and bake for 25 minutes or until a toothpick inserted into the center of the cake comes out dry.

4   Remove from the oven. If using round layer pans, let cool 15 to 20 minutes, then carefully release the cakes from the pans. It can be tricky to remove the cake from larger pans, so if using a rectangular pan, you may prefer to frost and serve right from the pan. Cool completely and frost with Chocolate Frosting.

per serving: 0mg cholesterol • 224 calories • 5g fat • 40g carbohydrate • 3g protein

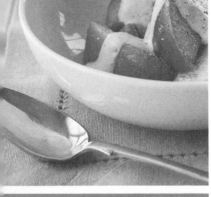

serves 12

ultra-chocolate cake

Cocoa powder and melted chocolate chips make an unforgettable duo when it comes to creating this rich, deep chocolate cake.

2$^1/_2$ cups unbleached all-purpose flour

$^1/_2$ cup cocoa powder

1 tablespoon baking powder

1 tablespoon baking soda

1 teaspoon salt

1 cup sugar

1 cup soft silken tofu

1 cup soy milk

$^1/_2$ cup vegetable oil

$^1/_2$ cup pure maple syrup

2 teaspoons vanilla extract

$^1/_4$ teaspoon almond extract

$^1/_2$ cup chocolate chips, melted (see Note)

Chocolate Frosting (page 205)

1 Preheat oven to 350°F. Mist two 9-inch round cake pans or an 8 × 11-inch baking pan with nonstick cooking oil spray. Dust with flour and set aside.

tofu 1-2-3

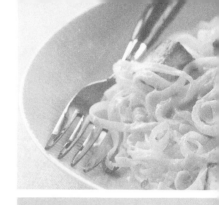

2　Into a large bowl, sift together the flour, cocoa powder, baking powder, baking soda, and salt. Add the sugar and stir with a wire whisk. In a blender, combine the tofu, soy milk, oil, maple syrup, vanilla, and almond extract, and process until smooth. Add the melted chocolate chips and process until smooth. Pour the liquid ingredients into the dry ingredients and stir until combined.

3　Transfer the batter into the prepared cake pan(s) and bake for 20 to 25 minutes or until a toothpick inserted into the center of the cake comes out dry.

4　Remove from the oven. If using round layer pans, let cool 15 to 20 minutes, then carefully release the cakes from the pans. It can be tricky to remove the cake from larger pans, so if using a rectangular pan, you may prefer to frost and serve right from the pan. Cool completely and frost with Chocolate Frosting.

 Melt chocolate chips in a double-boiler, stirring constantly to prevent burning, or in the microwave oven, on the defrost setting for approximately 3 minutes, stopping to stir at least once.

per serving: 0mg cholesterol　•　322 calories　•　10g fat　•　59g carbohydrate　•　4g protein

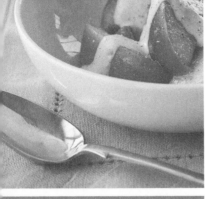

carrot spice snack cake

Sweet enough for a birthday treat but nutritious enough for a post-workout snack, this cake packs carrots, walnuts, raisins, and of course tofu into moist squares that taste delicious with or without frosting.

2 cups unbleached all-purpose flour

2 teaspoons ground cinnamon

1 teaspoon ground nutmeg

1 teaspoon baking powder

$^1/_2$ teaspoon salt

1 cup sugar

$^2/_3$ cup soft silken tofu

$^1/_2$ cup pure maple syrup

$^1/_2$ cup vegetable oil

3 cups shredded carrots (about 4 large carrots)

$^1/_2$ cup chopped walnuts

$^1/_2$ cup golden raisins

Cashew-Coconut Frosting (page 207) or Coconut Frosting (page 206) (optional)

1 Preheat oven to 350°F. Mist a 9 × 13-inch baking pan with nonstick cooking oil spray. Set aside.

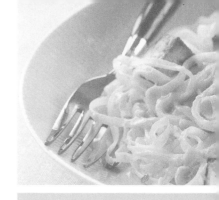

2   Into a large bowl, sift together the flour, cinnamon, nutmeg, baking powder, and salt. Add the sugar and stir with a wire whisk. In a blender, combine the tofu, maple syrup, and oil and process until smooth. Pour the liquid ingredients into the dry ingredients and stir until combined.

3   Add the carrots, walnuts, and raisins and stir well. The mixture will be thick and sticky.

4   Transfer the mixture to the prepared baking pan. Bake for 45 minutes or until a toothpick inserted into the center of the cake comes out clean. Remove from the oven, cool, cut into squares, and serve as is. This can also be frosted with Cashew-Coconut Frosting or Coconut Frosting.

per square: 0mg cholesterol • 148 calories • 5g fat • 24g carbohydrate • 1g protein

happy endings

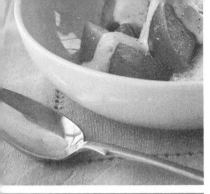

chocolate chip peanut butter cupcakes

Large, fluffy, and delicious, these delightful baked goodies make great birthday party fare.

2 cups unbleached all-purpose flour

1 tablespoon baking powder

$1/2$ teaspoon salt

1 cup pure maple syrup

$2/3$ cup soft silken tofu

$1/2$ cup natural smooth peanut butter

3 tablespoons dairy-free milk (soy-, rice-, almond-, or oat-based)

1 teaspoon vanilla extract

$1/2$ cup dairy-free chocolate chips

Chocolate Frosting (page 205) or Peanut Butter Frosting (page 207)

1   Preheat oven to 350°F. Mist 12 muffin cups with nonstick cooking oil spray and set aside.

2   Into a large bowl, sift together the flour, baking powder, and salt and set aside. In a blender, combine the maple syrup, tofu, peanut butter, dairy-free milk, and vanilla and process until smooth. Pour the liquid ingredients into the dry ingredients and stir until blended. Stir in the chocolate chips.

tofu 1-2-3

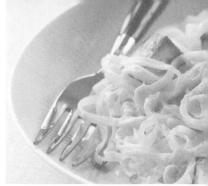

3 Transfer the batter into the prepared muffin cups and bake for 20 minutes or until a toothpick inserted into the center of a muffin comes out dry. Remove from the oven, cool for 10 minutes, and release the cupcakes. Frost with Chocolate Frosting or Peanut Butter Frosting when completely cool.

per cupcake: 0mg cholesterol • 257 calories • 8g fat • 41g carbohydrate • 6g protein

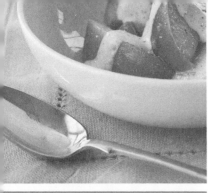

chocolate mousse

For kids, it's simply pudding, but for adults, it's exquisite mousse—especially when spiked with almond liqueur.

1 (12-ounce) package firm or extra-firm silken tofu (1½ cups)

1 cup dairy-free chocolate chips, melted (see Note)

⅓ cup pure maple syrup

2 teaspoons vanilla extract

1 tablespoon almond liqueur or ¼ teaspoon almond extract (optional)

1 Put the tofu in a food processor and blend until completely smooth, about 2 minutes. Add the melted chocolate chips, maple syrup, vanilla, and almond liqueur or extract, if using. Blend until smooth.

2 Transfer to six serving bowls or glasses, cover the top of each with plastic wrap, and refrigerate for at least 2 hours before serving.

 Melt chocolate chips in a double-boiler, stirring constantly to prevent burning, or in the microwave oven, on the defrost setting for approximately 3 minutes, stopping to stir at least once.

per serving: 0mg cholesterol • 234 calories • 10g fat • 30g carbohydrate • 5g protein

chocolate frosting

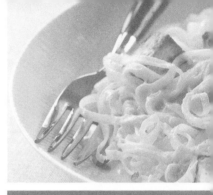

A rich and creamy frosting that adds the perfect touch to birthday cakes. Frosts one 8-inch or 9-inch round layer cake, one 9 × 13-inch sheet cake, or 24 to 36 cupcakes.

1 (12-ounce) package extra-firm silken tofu (1¹/₂ cups)

3 tablespoons pure maple syrup

2 teaspoons pure vanilla extract

1¹/₂ cups dairy-free chocolate chips, melted (see Note)

1 Put the tofu in a food processor and blend until completely smooth, about 2 minutes. Add the maple syrup and vanilla and blend until smooth. Add the melted chocolate chips and blend until smooth.

2 Transfer to a storage container with a lid and refrigerate for at least 4 hours or overnight before using.

note Melt chocolate chips in a double-boiler, stirring constantly to prevent burning, or in the microwave oven, on the defrost setting for approximately 3 minutes, stopping to stir at least once.

per tablespoon: 0mg cholesterol • 41 calories • 2g fat • 5g carbohydrate • 1g protein

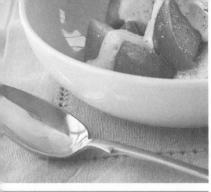

coconut frosting

This frosting is very thick and rich, ideal for small areas such as the tops of cupcakes.

¹/₂ pound soft tofu

¹/₂ cup agave nectar or pure maple syrup

1 teaspoons coconut extract

³/₄ cup dried unsweetened coconut flakes

Put the tofu in a food processor and blend until completely smooth, about 2 minutes, stopping at least once to scrape down the sides of the bowl. (It should be free of all graininess.) Add the agave nectar and coconut extract and blend until smooth. Add the coconut flakes and pulse several times until it is mixed in. The mixture will be smooth except for the coconut flakes. Use immediately or refrigerate in a storage container for up to one day before use.

per tablespoon: 0mg cholesterol • 55 calories • 1g fat • 10g carbohydrate • 1g protein

tofu 1-2-3

cashew frosting

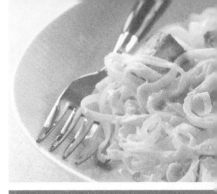

Best used on cakes that are medium to light in both color and flavor. One batch is sufficient for 12 cupcakes or the top of a regular-size sheet cake, so double the recipe to frost a layer cake.

$1/2$ pound soft tofu, rinsed and patted dry

$1/3$ cup smooth cashew butter

$1/3$ cup sugar

$1/2$ teaspoon vanilla extract

Pinch salt

Put the tofu in a food processor and blend until completely smooth, for at least 2 minutes, stopping to scrape down the sides of the bowl at least once. (It should be free of all graininess.) Add the cashew butter, sugar, vanilla, and salt and blend until smooth. Use immediately or refrigerate in a storage container for up to one day before use.

variations

Cashew-Coconut Frosting

- Leave the completed frosting in the food processor and add $1/3$ cup coconut flakes. Pulse several times to mix (do not blend). Use as desired.

Peanut Butter Frosting

- Replace the cashew butter with $1/2$ cup smooth peanut butter and omit the vanilla extract.

per tablespoon: 0mg cholesterol • 57 calories • 3g fat • 5g carbohydrate • 2g protein

happy endings

index

index

tofu 1-2-3